Science of Diving
Concepts and Applications

Science of Diving
Concepts and Applications

Bruce Wienke

Applied and Computational Physics Division
Los Alamos National Laboratory
Los Alamos, N.M. 87545

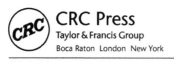

CRC Press
Taylor & Francis Group
Boca Raton London New York

CRC Press is an imprint of the
Taylor & Francis Group, an **informa** business
A SCIENCE PUBLISHERS BOOK

Cover illustrations reproduced by kind courtesy of Suunto, Luminox, Advanced Diver Magazine, and NAUI Technical Diving.

CRC Press
Taylor & Francis Group
6000 Broken Sound Parkway NW, Suite 300
Boca Raton, FL 33487-2742

First issued in paperback 2020

© 2015 by Taylor & Francis Group, LLC
CRC Press is an imprint of Taylor & Francis Group, an Informa business

No claim to original U.S. Government works

ISBN-13: 978-1-4987-2513-2 (hbk)
ISBN-13: 978-0-367-73827-3 (pbk)

Visit the Taylor & Francis Web site at
http://www.taylorandfrancis.com

and the CRC Press Web site at
http://www.crcpress.com

FOREWORD

As land dwelling, air breathing creatures, we have evolved perceptions, behaviors, practices, and procedures for living in an air atmosphere. Venturing into the underwater world, many things change. A number of important physical changes affect this underwater world, and are important to us as technical and commercial divers. This monograph discussed these changes and suggested application problems that hopefully quantified underlying physical principles affecting underwater life and activities.

Technical diving used to be the pervue of just commercial and military divers. Today, highly motivated and well trained recreational divers are pushing diving to new depths, on mixed gases, with sophisticated electronic sensors and dive computers, using modern rebreathers, wearing special exposure suits, in the oceans, lakes, and at high altitude. This new breed of diver receives training from any one of a number of new technical agencies, like Technical Diving International (TDI), International Association of Nitrox and Technical Divers (IANTD), and Association of Nitrox Diving Instructors (ANDI), as well as the established recreational agencies, NAUI, PADI, YMCA, SSI, and NASDS. For the technical diver and working commercial diver, this monograph is intentionally both a training tool and extended reference.

Technical diving encompasses a wide spectrum of related disciplines, from geosciences to biosciences, atmospherics sciences to hydrodynamics, medical sciences to engineering sciences, and mathematical physics to statistical analysis. The scope is immense, and so any monograph need be selective, and probably not in depth as possible. And diving physics can be a tedious exercise for readers. Obviously, physiology is an even more complicated mix of physics, chemistry, and biology. Like comments apply to decompression theory, a combination of biophysics, physiology, and biochemistry in a much cloudier picture within perfused and metabolic tissue and blood. Biological systems are so complex, beyond even the fastest and biggest supercomputers for modeling analysis. The marine and geosciences are also beyond comprehensive treatment. Often, tedium relates to a proliferation of equations and deduced results without practical application.

So, selectivity with mathematical application was a direction taken here in narrative. Mathematical equations were kept at definitional level to facilitate description. The hope was to better encapsulate a large body of underlying physical principle in hopefully readable form. Sample problems, with solutions, were included to enhance quantitative description and understanding. Topics were fundamental and chosen in their relevance to technical diving. Bibliographies offer full blown treatments of all principles detailed for diving. For highlight, Figures included some mathematical definitions for completeness, with intended purpose of extending discourse. Problems employed quantitative relationships detailed in the text, using data and information from Tables and Figures.

Thanks again to all of you who have added impetus to this monograph. Hope it has met all of your particular needs. Please contact me with any comments, questions, or concerns.

Safe and fun diving always.

Tim O'Leary
Director, NAUI Technical Diving Operations
Tampa, FL

PREFACE

The physics, biology, engineering, physiology, medicine, and chemistry of diving center on pressure, and pressure changes. The average individual is subjected to atmospheric pressure swings of 3% at sea level, as much as 20% a mile in elevation, more at higher altitudes, and all usually over time spans of hours to days. Divers and their equipment can experience compressions and decompressions orders of magnitude greater, and within considerably shorter time scales. While the effects of pressure change are readily quantified in physics, chemistry, and engineering applications, the physiology, medicine, and biology of pressure changes in living systems are much more complicated. Caution is needed in transposing biological principles from one pressure range to another. Incomplete knowledge and biochemical complexities often prevent extensions of even simple causal relationships in biological science. Causal relationships between observables are the pervue of physics and that difficult process in living systems is biophysics.

This complex science translated to technical diving is discussed in a Five Part series, with each topic self contained and strategically developed in relationship to diving. Topics span many disciplines and focus on a number of technical arenas. Targeted audience is the commercial diver, instructor, hyperbaric technician, underwater researcher, and technical diver looking for greater detail, and especially the doctor, physiologist, physicist, chemist, mathematician, engineer, or biologist by training. Topics include energy and matter interactions, thermodynamics, pressure and density, mechanics, gas kinetics, free and dissolved phase transfer, nucleation and cavitation, bubbles and surfactants, oxygen dose, gas mixtures, buoyancy, gauges and tanks, compressors and regulators, maladies and drugs, statistics, profile and diving model comparisons, risk and probability, data banks and fitting, distributions, waves, transport, currents, geology, oceanography, geophysics, global warming and cooling, solar energy and radiation. References are included. Appendix A reviews basic physical laws and associated concepts and Appendix B details and discusses diveware and dive planning software. A suite of application exercises is provided for example at strategic points in the text. This monograph extends, updates, and rewrites an earlier work published in 2001. Additional material focusing on diving data, statistical correlations, underwater tests, and risk is presented and additional applications (numerical exercises) are included. For the experienced diver, this is a workbook. For the neophyte diver, it is likely primer and workbook.

Bruce Wienke
Applied and Computational Physics Division
Los Alamos National Laboratory
Los Alamos, N.M. 87545

ACKNOWLEDGMENTS

Many thanks go to my colleagues here at Los Alamos National Laboratory, to collaborators in the industrial, military, and academic sectors, and to investigators and teachers over the years who ask interesting diving questions. Affiliations with the American Physical Society, American Nuclear Society, American Academy of Underwater Sciences, Undersea and Hyperbaric Medical Society, South Pacific Underwater Medicine Society, and Society of Industrial and Applied Mathematics are also gratefully acknowledged. Thanks to the diver training agencies for their constant support, but especially the technical training agencies, NAUI, TDI, IANTD, and ANDI, and Divers Alert Network (DAN). Warm thanks to Marco Cressi and Pippo Marenco of CressiSub, Giuseppe Giovanelli of Mares, Jim Clymer of Huish Scuba, Kees Hofwegen of GAP Software, Brent Goetzel of ConneXon, Yuval Malka of UTC, Ari Nikkol, Toni Leskila, and Alastair Ansell of Suunto, Sergio Angelini of Scubapro, Doug Toth and Dean Garafola of Atomic Aquatics, Chris Parrett and Peter Baker of Abysmal Diving, Tim O'Leary, Jan Neal, Peter Oliver, Jim Bram, and Jed Livingstone of NAUI Technical Diving, Charlie Lehner and Ed Lanphier (late) of the University of Wisconsin, Dick Vann of Duke University, David Yount (late) of the University of Hawaii, Tom Kunkle and Jim Morel of Los Alamos National Laboratory (LANL), Lee Somers of the University of Michigan, Peter Readey of Steam Machines, Gene Melton of HydroSpace Engineering, Bret Gilliam of SDI/TDI, Tom Mount of IANTD, Curt Bowen of Advanced Diver Magazine, Drew Richardson of PADI, Peter Bennett of the UHMS, Alessandro Marroni of DAN Europe, Ed Betts of ANDI, the Finnish and Irish Diving Federations, Lonnie Sharp of the USN, Alf Brubakk of the University of Trondheim, George Irvine and Jarrod Jablonski of the Woodville Karst Plain Project (WKPP), Mike Powell and Mike Gernhardt of NASA, Murat Egi of Istanbul University, Mike Lang of the Smithsonian Institut, Wayne Gerth of the Naval Experimental Diving Unit (NEDU), the LANL NEST Team, and USN Special Warfare Command. And I must thank my diving, skiing, tennis, and windsurfing cronies, Dave Padilla, Mike Sorem, Jerry Byrd, Mike Stout, Joe Quintana, Tom Seed, Craig Mechem, Gordon Jio, Hugh Casey, Tim O'Leary, Gary Lewis, Andy White, and the Staff of ATOMIC USA.

Bruce Wienke
Los Alamos National Laboratory
Los Alamos, N.M. 87545
6/1/14

CONTENTS

CONVENTIONS AND UNITS

Standard (SI) and English units are employed. By convention, by usage, or for ease, some nonstandard units are employed. Pressure and depth are both measured in feet of sea water (*fsw*) and meters of sea water (*msw*), with 1 *atm* = 33 *fsw* = 10 *msw* to good approximation. Specific densities, η (dimensionless), in pressure relationships are normalized to sea water density. Table 1 summarizes some useful unit equivalences.

Table 1. Equivalence And Unit Conversion Table.

Time
$$1 \; megahertz = 10^6 \; hertz = 10^6 \; sec^{-1}$$

Length
$$1 \; m = 3.28 \; ft = 1.09 \; yd = 39.37 \; in$$
$$1 \; \mu m = 10^4 \; angstrom = 10^3 \; nm = 10^{-6} \; m$$
$$1 \; km = .62 \; mile$$
$$1 \; fathom = 6 \; ft$$
$$1 \; nautical \; mile = 6,080 \; ft = 1.15 \; mile = 1.85 \; km$$
$$1 \; light \; year = 9.46 \times 10^{12} \; km = 6.31 \times 10^4 \; AU$$

Speed
$$1 \; km/hr = 27.77 \; cm/sec$$
$$1 \; mi/hr = 1.47 \; ft/sec$$
$$1 \; knot = 1.15 \; mi/hr = 51.48 \; cm/sec$$

Volume
$$1 \; cm^3 = .06 \; in^3$$
$$1 \; m^3 = 35.32 \; ft^3 = 1.31 \; yd^3$$
$$1 \; l = 10^3 \; cm^3 = .04 \; ft^3 = .91 \; qt$$

Mass and Density
$$1 \; g = .04 \; oz$$
$$1 \; kg = 32.27 \; oz = 2.20 \; lb$$
$$1 \; g/cm^3 = .57 \; oz/in^3$$
$$1 \; kg/m^3 = .06 \; lb/ft^3$$

Table 1 contd....

Table 1 contd.

Force and Pressure

$1\ newton = 10^5\ dyne = .22\ lb$

$1\ g/cm^2 = .23\ oz/in^2$

$1\ kg/m^2 = .20\ lb/ft^2$

$1\ atm = 33\ fsw = 760\ mmHg = 1.03\ kg/cm^2 = 14.69\ lbs/in^2$

Energy and Power

$1\ cal = 4.19\ joule = 3.96 \times 10^{-3}\ btu = 3.09\ ft\ lb$

$1\ joule = 10^7\ ergs = .74ft\ lb$

$1\ keV = 10^3\ eV = 1.60 \times 10^{-16}\ joule$

$1\ amu = 931.1\ MeV$

$1\ watt = 3.41\ btu/hr = 1.34 \times 10^{-3}\ hp$

Electricity and Magnetism

$1\ coul = 2.99 \times 10^9\ esu$

$1\ amp = 1\ coul/sec = 1\ volt/ohm$

$1\ volt = 1\ newton\ m/coul = 1\ joule/coul$

$1\ gauss = 10^{-4}\ weber/m^2 = 10^{-4}\ newton/amp\ m$

$1\ f = 1\ coul/volt$

Standard mathematical and physical conventions are followed. Bold face quantities are vectors, while roman face quantities are scalars. Bold face vectors with hat denote unit vectors in the indicated direction, for instance, $\hat{r}$, $\hat{\theta}$, and $\hat{\phi}$, are units vectors in the r, θ, and ϕ directions. Fundamental constants are tabulated below in Table 2. Full discussion of constants and impacts can be found in the References, particularly the physics and chemistry entries.

Metrology is the science of measurement, and broadly construed, encompasses the bulk of experimental science. In the more restricted sense, metrology refers to the maintenance and dissemination of a consistent set of units, support for enforcement of equity in trade by weights and measure laws, and process control for manufacturing.

A measurement is a series of manipulations of physical objects or systems according to experimental protocols producing a number. The objects or systems involved are test objects, measuring devices, or computational operations. The objects and devices exist in and are influenced by some environment. The number relates to the some unique feature of the object, such as the magnitude, or the intensity, or the weight, or time duration. The number is acquired to form the basis of decisions effecting some human feature or goal depending on the test object.

In order to attain the goal of useful decision, metrology requires that the number obtained is functionally identical whenever and wherever the measurement process is performed. Such a universally reproducible measurement is called a *proper measurement* and leads to describing *proper quantities*. The equivalences in Table 1 relate *proper quantities* and the fundamental constants in Table 2 permit codification of these quantities into physical laws.

Table 2. Fundamental Constants.

$$g_0 = 9.80 \; m/sec^2 \quad (Sea \; Level \; Acceleration \; Of \; Gravity)$$
$$G_0 = 6.67 \times 10^{-11} \; newton \; m^2/kg^2 \quad (Gravitational \; Constant)$$
$$M_0 = 5.98 \times 10^{24} \; kg \quad (Earth \; Mass)$$
$$\Gamma_0 = 1.98 \; cal/min \; cm^2 \quad (Solar \; Constant)$$
$$c = 2.998 \times 10^8 \; m/sec \quad (Speed \; Of \; Light)$$
$$h = 6.625 \times 10^{-34} \; joule \; sec \quad (Planck \; Constant)$$
$$R = 8.317 \; joule/gmole \; ^oK \quad (Universal \; Gas \; Constant)$$
$$k = 1.38 \times 10^{-23} \; joule/gmole \; ^oK \quad (Boltzmann \; Constant)$$
$$N_0 = 6.025 \times 10^{23} \; atoms/gmole \quad (Avogadro \; Number)$$
$$m_0 = 9.108 \times 10^{-31} \; kg \quad (Electron \; Mass)$$
$$e_0 = 1.609 \times 10^{-19} \; coulomb \quad (Electron \; Charge)$$
$$r_0 = .528 \; angstrom \quad (First \; Bohr \; Orbit)$$
$$\varepsilon_0 = (4\pi)^{-1} \times 1.11 \times 10^{-10} \; f/m \quad (Vacuum \; Permittivity)$$
$$\mu_0 = 4\pi \times 10^{-7} \; h/m \quad (Vacuum \; Permeability)$$
$$\kappa_0 = (4\pi\varepsilon_0)^{-1} = 8.91 \times 10^9 \; m/f \quad (Coulomb \; Constant)$$
$$\alpha_0 = \mu_0/4\pi = 1 \times 10^{-7} \; h/m \quad (Ampere \; Constant)$$
$$\sigma_0 = 5.67 \times 10^{-8} \; watt/m^2 \; ^oK^4 \quad (Stefan-Boltzmann \; Constant)$$

Keyed Exercises

• *How many nautical miles to a kilometer?*

$$1 \; nautical \; mile = 1.85 \; km, \quad 1 \; km = \frac{1}{1.85} \; nautical \; mile = .54 \; nautical \; mile$$

• *How many electrostatic units (esu) to a coulomb?*

$$1 \; coul = 2.99 \times 10^9 \; esu, \quad 1 \; esu = \frac{1}{2.99 \times 10^9} \; coul = 3.34 \times 10^{-10} \; coul$$

• *How many light years to a mile?*

$$1 \; light \; yr = 5.88 \times 10^{12} \; mile, \quad 1 \; mile = \frac{1}{5.88 \times 10^{12}} \; light \; yr = 1.70 \times 10^{-13} \; light \; yr$$

• *Convert depth, $d = 38 \; fsw$, to depth, ffw, in fresh water?*

$$38 \; fsw \times \frac{1 \; ffw}{.975 \; fsw} = 38.9 \; ffw$$

• *Convert ascent rate, $r = 60 \; fsw/min$, to msw/sec?*

$$r = 60 \; fsw/min \times \frac{msw}{3.28 \; fsw} \times \frac{min}{60 \; sec} = .305 \; msw/sec$$

- *Convert volume, $V = 6.2\ m^3$, to ft^3?*

$$V = 6.2\ m^3 \times \frac{353.2\ ft^3}{m^3} = 2189\ ft^3$$

- *Convert pressure, $P = 5.3\ kg/m^2$, to lb/in^2?*

$$P = 5.3\ kg/m^2 \times \frac{.20\ lb/ft^2}{1\ kg/m^2} \times \frac{1\ ft^2}{144\ in^2} = .0074\ lb/in^2$$

- *Convert acceleration, $g = 32\ ft/sec^2$, to m/sec^2?*

$$g = 32\ ft/sec^2 \times \frac{1\ m}{3.28\ ft} = 9.8\ m/sec^2$$

- *What is the specific density, η, of mercury (Hg) with respect to seawater?*

$$\rho_{Hg} = 13.55\ g/cm^3, \quad \rho_{seawater} = 1.026\ gm/cm^3$$

$$\eta = \frac{\rho_{Hg}}{\rho_{seawater}} = \frac{13.55}{1.026} = 13.21$$

DIVING HISTORY

Man has probably practised breath hold diving in some form across all stages of development, first becoming adept at swimming and then recovering food from lakes and oceans. Now, breath hold diving and snorkeling are popular sports. Breath hold and inverted bell diving reach back over many centuries, like fifty or so. Written records of Cretan sponge divers (3000 *BC*) and Chinese pearl divers (2000 *BC*) exist today. Detailed military accounts link to Xerxes who employed combat divers to recover treasure from sunken ships (519 *BC*), as chronicled by the Greek historian, Herodotus. Alexander the Great (356 *BC*) also deployed breathold divers in the siege for Tyre. Depths rarely exceeded 60 *fsw* in these exploits. According to Pliny (77 *AD*), reed breathing tubes were employed by Roman Legions, hiding or waiting in ambush. Aristotle (384 *BC*), pupil of Plato, and tutor of Alexander, writes of diving bells used to recover treasure. These inverted receptacles, utilizing trapped compressed air as breathing mixture, gained renown in Europe in the 1600s. Ancient Assyrians and Persians also carried air in goatskins underwater. Some Korean and Japanese breathold divers (armaghs) still gather pearls and sponges with lung power, but most of the fishing, pearling, and sponging divers of the world today have gone over to SCUBA. Terroists in Southeast Asia avoided capture by lying beneath swamp surfaces and breathing through hollow reeds. SEALs adopted similar assault tactics in the Mekong Delta in Vietnam.

Halley patented a large diving bell in 1690, refurbished with surface air for periods beyond an hour. In 1770, Le Havre developed a manual air compressor. Surface supplied air and demand regulators were employed in hard hat diving by the 1800s, with the first demand regulator, patented by Rouquayrol in 1866, supplied by hand bellows. The first case of nitrogen narcosis was reported by Junod in 1835. Full diving suits, in which air escapes through a one way exhaust valve, were invented by Siebe in 1840, and a few are still around. Quietly, the revolutionary *aqua lung* of Cousteau, a refinement of the Rouquayrol surface supplied demand regulator, ushered the modern era of SCUBA in wartime Europe in 1943. Diving would never be the same afterward. In the US Navy, elite SRs, NCDUs, and UDTs (SEALs now) honed their skills above and below the surface, extending the meaning of combat utility. Freed from surface umbilical, open and closed circuit units enhanced the mobility and range of tactical operations for sure, but the impact on nonmilitary diving was orders of magnitude greater. Coupled to high pressure compressed air in tanks, SCUBA offered the means to explore the underwater world for fun and profit.

Commercial availability of the demand regulator in 1947 initiated sport diving and a fledgling equipment industry. Serious diver training and certifying agencies, such as the National Association of Underwater Instructors, YMCA, and Professional Association of Diving Instructors, strong and vital today, organized in the late 1950s and 1960s. In the mid 1950s, the Royal Navy released their bulk diffusion decompression tables, while a little later, in 1958, the US Navy compiled their modified Haldane tables with six perfusion limited compartments. Both would acquire biblical status over the next 25 years, or so. In the mid to late 1950s, Fredrickson in the USA and Alinari in Italy designed and released the first analog decompression meters, or decometers, emulating tissue gas uptake and elimination with pressure gauges, porous plugs, and distensible gas bags. The first digital computers, designed by DCIEM in Canada, appeared in the mid 1950s. Employed by the Canadian Navy, they were based on a four compartment analog model of Kidd and Stubbs. Following introduction of a twelve compartment Haldanian device, linked to Doppler technology, by Barshinger and Huggins in 1983, decompression computers reached a point in addressing repetitive exposures and staging regimens for the first of maturation and acceptance. Flexible, more reliable to use, and able to emulate almost any mathematical model, digital computers rapidly replaced pneumatic devices in the 1980s. Their timely functionality and widespread use heralded the present era of high tech diving, with requirements for comprehensive decompression models across a full spectrum of activity. Computer usage statistics, gathered in the 1990s, suggest an enviable track record of diver safety, with an underlying decompression sickness (DCS) incidence below 0.05% roughly.

Diver mobility concerns ultimately fostered development of the modern SCUBA unit, and the quest to go deeper led to exotic gas breathing mixtures. High pressure cylinders and compressors similarly expedited deeper diving and prolonged exposure time. The world record dives of Keller to 1,000 *fsw* in 1960 not only popularized multiple gas mixtures, but also witnessed the first real use of computers to generate decompression schedules. Saturation diving and underwater habitats followed soon after, spurred by a world thirst for oil. Both multiple gas mixtures and saturation diving became a way of life for some commercial divers by the 1970s, particularly after the oil embargo. Oil concerns still drive the commercial diving industry today.

Cochrane in England invented the high pressure caisson in 1830. Shortly afterward, the first use of a caisson in 1841 in France by Triger also precipitated the first case of decompression sickness, aptly termed the bends because of the position assumed by victims to alleviate the pain. Some fifty years later, in 1889, the first medical lock was employed by Moir to treat bends during construction of the Hudson River Tunnel. Since that time many divers and caisson workers have been treated in hyperbaric chambers. Indeed, the operational requirements of diving over the years have provided the incentives to study hyperbaric physiology and its relationship to decompression sickness, and impetus for describing fundamental biophysics. Similarly, limitations of nitrogen mixtures at depth, because of narcotic reactivity, prompted recent study and application of helium, nitrogen, hydrogen, and oxygen breathing mixtures at depth, especially in the commercial sector.

Increases in pressure with increasing depth underwater impose many of the limitations in diving, applying equally well to the design of equipment used in this environment. Early divers relied on their breathholding ability, while later divers used diving bells. Surface supplied air and SCUBA are rather recent innovations. With increasing depth and exposure time, divers encountered a number of physiological and medical problems constraining activity, with decompression sickness perhaps the most restrictive. By the 1800s, bubbles were noted in animals subject to pressure reduction. In the 1900s, they were postulated as the cause of decompression sickness in caisson workers and divers. Within that postulate, and driven by a need to both optimize diver safety and time underwater, decompression modeling has consolidated early rudimentary schedules into present more sophisticated tables and meters. As knowledge and understanding of decompression sickness increase, so should the validity, reliability, and range of applicability of models.

A consensus of opinions, and for a variety of reasons, suggests that modern diving began in the early 1960s. Technological achievements, laboratory programs, military priorities, safety concerns, commercial diving requirements, and international business spurred diving activity and scope of operation. Diving bells, hot water heating, mixed gases, saturation, deep diving, expanded wet testing, computers, and efficient decompression algorithms signaled the modern diving era. Equipment advances in open and closed circuit breathing devices, wet and dry suits, gear weight, mask and fin design, high pressure compressors, flotation and buoyancy control vests, communications links, gauges and meters, lights, underwater tools (cutting, welding, drilling, explosives), surface supplied air, and photographic systems paced technological advances. Training and certification requirements for divers, in military, commercial, sport, and scientific sectors, took definition with growing concern for underwater safety and well being.

In the conquest and exploration of the oceans, saturation diving gained prominence in the 1960s, thereby permitting exploitation of the continental shelf impossible within exposure times permitted by conventional regimens. Spurred by both industrial and military interests in the ability of men to work underwater for long periods of time, notable *habitat* experiments, such as Sealab, Conshelf, Man In Sea, Gulf Task, and Tektite established the feasibility of living and working underwater for extended periods. These efforts followed proof of principle validation, by Bond and coworkers (USN) in 1958, of saturation diving. Saturation exposure programs and tests have been conducted from 35 *fsw* down to 2,000 *fsw*.

The development and use of underwater support platforms, such as habitats, bell diving systems, lockout and free flooded submersibles, and diver propulsion units also accelerated in the 1960s and 1970s, for reasons of science and economics. Support platforms extended both diver usefulness and bottom time, by permitting him to live underwater, reducing descent and ascent time, expanding mobility, and lessing physical activity. Today, operating from underwater platforms themselves, remotely operated vehicles (ROVs) scan the ocean depths at 6,000 *fsw* for minerals and oil.

Around 1972, strategies for diving in excess of 1,000 *fsw* received serious scrutiny, driven by a commercial quest for oil and petroleum products, and the needs of the commercial diving industry to service that quest. Questions concerning pharmacological additives, absolute pressure limits, thermal exchange, therapy, compression-decompression procedures, effective combinations of mixed breathing gases, and equipment functionality addressed many fundamental issues, unknown or only partially understood. By the early 1980s, it became clear that open sea water work in the 1,000 to 2,000 *fsw* range was entirely practical, and many of the problems, at least from an operational point of view, could be solved. So, the need for continued deep diving remains, with demands that cannot be answered with remote, or 1 *atm*, diver systems. Heliox and trimix have become standards for deep excursion breathing gases, with heliox the choice for shallower exposures, and trimix a choice for deeper exposures in the field.

Yet, despite tremendous advances in deep diving technology, most of the ocean floor is outside human reach. Breathing mixtures that are compressible are limiting. Breathing mixtures that are not compressible offer interesting alternatives. In the 1960s, serious attention was given to liquid breathing mixtures, physiological saline solutions. Acting as inert respiratory gas diluents, oxygenated fluids have been used as breathing mixtures, thereby eliminating decompression requirements. Some synthetic fluids, such as fluorocarbon (*FX*80), exhibit enormous oxygen dissolution properties.

AUTHOR SKETCH

Bruce Wienke is Director of the Computational Testbed for Industry (CTI), a DOE User Facility providing cooperative opportunities for American Industry in high performance supercomputing, software development, and training, and is a Program Manager in the Nuclear Weapons Technology/Simulation And Computing Office at the Los Alamos National Laboratory (LANL), with interests in computational physics, neutron and photon transport, mathematical and numerical methods, particle and nuclear physics, high performance and parallel computing, hydrodynamics, plasma physics, cavitation, decompression testing, deep diving and models, gas diffusion, and phase mechanics. He contributes to professional symposia, educational publications, technical journals and topical workshops, having authored 11 monographs *(Diving Physics with Bubble Mechanics and Decompression Theory in Depth, Hyperbaric Physics and Phase Mechanics, The Technical Diver, Reduced Gradient Bubble Model in Depth, Technical Diving in Depth, Decompression Theory, Physics, Physiology and Decompression Theory for the Technical and Commercial Diver, High Altitude Diving, Basic Diving Physics and Application, Diving Above Sea Level, Basic Decompression Theory and Application)* and some 300+ peer reviewed journal articles. He functions on the LANL Nuclear Emergency Strategy Team (NEST), in exercises involving Special Operations (SEAL, Delta, PJ, Recon, Ranger), above and below water and leads the C & C Dive Team. He heads Southwest Enterprises, a consulting company for research and applications in overlapping areas of applied science and simulation, functions as an Expert Witness in litigation, and works with DHS Rescue and Recovery Teams.

He has taught physics (all levels from basic to quantum mechanics), mathematics (algebra, geometry, calculus, advanced calculus, numerical methods), and computer science (programming, high performance systems, parallel algorithms) at Marquette, Northwestern, University of New Mexico, LANL, and College of Santa Fe in both undergraduate and graduate programs. Wienke has served as Thesis Advisor for MS and PhD students. He helped formulate the instructional programs in weapons phenomenology at LANL. A number of his books serve as college texts in decompression theory and diving physics in both commercial diving schools and training agency programs.

Extracurricular activities combine work and recreation in many cases. Wienke is a Workshop Director/Instructor Trainer with the National Association of Underwater Instructors (NAUI), serves on the Board of Directors (Vice Chairman for Technical Diving, Technical and Decompression Review Board Member), and is a Master

Instructor with the Professional Association of Diving Instructors (PADI) serving in various capacities. Wintertime he hobbies racing, skiing, coaching, and teaching as a Racing Coach and Instructor, certified United States Ski Coaches Association (USSCA) and Professional Ski Instructors of America (PSIA). Wienke races in the United States Ski Association (USSA) Masters Series Competition, holding a 8 NASTAR racing handicap while winning NASTAR National Championships in his age class in 2002, 2007, 2009, 2011, and 2012 and Rocky Mountain Masters combined and individual DH, SG, SC, GS, SL championships in 2010 and 2012. Other interests include tennis, windsurfing, and mountain biking. He quarterbacked the 63 Northern Michigan Wildcats to an NCAA II Championship (Hickory Bowl) garnering All American honors.

Wienke received a BS in physics and mathematics from Northern Michigan University, MS in nuclear physics from Marquette University, and PhD in particle physics from Northwestern University. He belongs to the American Physical Society (APS), American Nuclear Society (ANS), Society of Industrial and Applied Mathematics (SIAM), South Pacific Underwater Medical Society (SPUMS), Undersea and Hyperbaric Medical Society (UHMS), and American Academy of Underwater Sciences (AAUS). He is a Fellow of the American Physical Society, and a Technical Committee Member of the American Nuclear Society. He serves as an Associate/ Review Editor for a number of professional journals, such as Journal of Computational Physics, Physical Review, Nuclear Science and Engineering, Computers in Biology and Medicine, to name a few.

His teaching background, job tasks, and research interests also overlap in useful ways. As a former dive shop owner in Santa Fe, he also serves as a Consultant for decompression algorithms in the diving industry. He has worked with Divers Alert Network (DAN) on applications of high performance computing and communications to diving, and is a Regional Data Coordinator for Project Dive Exploration. Scubapro, Suunto, Mares, Dacor, Liquivision, HydroSpace, CressiSub, ConneXon, Abysmal Diving, GAP, Steam Machines, and Atomic Aquatics engage him (or have) as Consultant for meter algorithms, and Industry Representative in dive product legalities. He is the developer of the Reduced Gradient Bubble Model (RGBM), a dual phase approach to staging diver ascents over an extended range of diving applications (altitude, nonstop, decompression, multiday, repetitive, multilevel, mixed gas, and saturation). A number of dive computers (Mares, Dacor, Suunto, Liquivision, CressiSub, ConneXon, HydroSpace, Atomic Aquatics, UTC, and others coming online) incorporate the modified and full iterative RGBM into staging regimens, for technical and recreational diving. GAP, RGBM Simulator, and ABYSS, commercial software products, feature some of the RGBM dynamical diving algorithms developed by him for Internet users and technical divers. He is also Associate Editor for the International Journal Of Aquatic Research And Education, and is a former Contributing Editor of *Sources*, the NAUI Training Publication. NAUI Technical Training has adopted the RGBM for technical and recreational training, having released RGBM trimix, helitrox, nitrox, and air tables. Wienke is a Contributing Editor of *Advanced Diver Magazine*.

Part 1

EARTH ATMOSPHERE, TERRASPHERE, AND HYDROSPHERE

Cosmology

Modern science began with the discovery that the Earth is not the center of the Universe. *Antianthropocentrism* has been incorporated into scientific mentality, and none would suggest that the Earth, nor the Solar System, nor the Milky Way, nor our local group of galaxies occupies any specially favored position in the cosmos. Rather, our perceptions run counter. Modern cosmology hypothesizes that all positions in the Universe are equivalent, when smeared out over 10^8 to 10^9 light years. It also appears that the Universe is spherically symmetric, essentially isotropic in composition about every point. Such is the *Cosmological Principle*.

Current philosophy on the structure on the Universe commences from two observable assumptions, primarily postulated in the present century:

- in the large, the Universe is homogeneous and isotropic (apart from fluctuations on galactic scales);
- the Universe is expanding uniformly in all directions, with noted increasing speed at the outermost boundaries (red shift);

so that it possible to assign Hubble's law to the mean recessional velocity, ζ, in terms of separation in megaparsecs (*mpsec*),

$$\zeta = \Upsilon r$$

with Υ Hubble's constant,

$$\Upsilon \approx 50 \ km/sec \ mpsec$$

and r the separation in *mpsec* (1 *mpsec* $= 3.26 \times 10^6$ *light yr* $= 3.086 \times 10^{21}$ *km*). The first assumption means that the Universe looks the same when viewed from any galaxy. The second assumption implies that well separated bits of matter are on the average moving apart. Further, it is thought the Universe was *detonated* at the *beginning* from a very hot, localized, dense state, affectionately called the *big bang*.

The big bang sent the galactic components outward with increasing radial velocities, observed presently as red shifts in their electromagnetic spectra.

Evidence for homogeneity on larger scales is seen in the high degree of isotropy of the microwave and X-ray background radiation. The microwave background is thought to be a remnant from an early, hot, dense phase of an expanding Universe, while the X-ray background is consistent with hot galaxies, galactic clusters, quasars, and very hot extracluster formations uniformly distributed out to 50 *mpsec* at the 1% accuracy level.

The origin of planets and stars is taken as a problem for astrophysics and geophysics, while the provenance of galaxies and clusters is left to cosmology. The division is historical and not necessarily rational. Opinion on the significance of clumping of matter (gravitation) tend to fall into two camps. One asserts that present clumping is a remnant of an initially chaotic Universe and that we can compute present conditions independent of initial conditions at big bang time. The other holds that the homogeneity is unstable, and that at big bang time the Universe was more isotropic than it is now.

Fundamental to cosmology are the concepts of gravitation and radiation, perhaps just different sides of the same coin according to modern field theories in particle physics and astrophysics. Even on the geophysical scale, gravitation and radiation are paramount in the shape and evolution of planets and asteroids, and on much shorter time scales than cosmology wants to admit. So, on smaller time scales and over shorter distances, the observable features of the Earth, Sun, and Moon system are manifest. Then the interactions of the Earth, Sun, and Moon form basis for geophysical processes. Fundamental to those processes are planetary attraction and solar energy production. Consider the former first, the fundamental attraction between objects with mass.

Gravitation

Newton first recognized that the motions of the planets, as well as many other terrestrial phenomena, such as falling apples and feathers, rest on a single precise statement relating the separation of two bodies, their masses, and an attractive force between them, ultimately called the law of universal attraction. A simple descriptor is *gravitation*. The law of universal attraction states that every particle in the Universe attracts every other particle with a force, **F**, directly proportional to the product of their two masses, M and m, and inversely proportional to the square of their separation, r. More specifically, the law takes the form,

$$\mathbf{F} = -G_0 \frac{Mm}{r^2} \hat{\mathbf{r}},$$

with G_0 the gravitational constant. Many regard the law of universal attraction as the most important single event in the history of science. Published in the Principia in 1686 along with the laws of motion, both provided the basis for all developments in classical mechanics.

The gravitational force exerted by the Earth on any object is local *gravity*, obviously a function of the mass and position of the object. For geophysical applications, is convenient to write the gravitational law in the form,

$$\mathbf{F} = m\mathbf{g},$$

for m the mass of the object, $\mathbf{g}$ the local gravitational acceleration,

$$\mathbf{g} = -G_0 \frac{M_0}{r^2} \hat{\mathbf{r}},$$

and M_0 the mass of the Earth. The gravitational acceleration, $\mathbf{g}$, is directed vertically downward, toward the center of the Earth. Denoting the surface radius of the Earth, R, and the elevation, h, so that, any position on, or above, the surface, r, can be written,

$$r = R + h,$$

the magnitude of the gravitational acceleration, g, varies as,

$$g = G_0 \frac{M_0}{R^2(1 + h/R)^2} = \frac{g_0}{(1 + h/R)^2},$$

for g_0 the sea level acceleration of gravity,

$$g_0 = G_0 \frac{M_0}{R^2}.$$

The Earth is not perfectly spherical, exhibiting radial asymmetry across the polar and Equatorial regions, with the surface radius, R, possessing polar and Equatorial bounds,

$$3941.3 \text{ } miles \leq R \leq 3954.6 \text{ } miles,$$

that is, R slightly larger at the Equator than at the Poles. This variation in radius causes a 0.2% difference in polar and Equatorial gravitational acceleration, certainly very small. There are also small local variations in g_0 associated with mountains, deserts, and the in homogeneous density distribution of the crust. At low elevations, h, that is, $h/R \ll 1$, gravitational acceleration can be approximated by,

$$g \approx g_0(1 - 2h/R),$$

in obviously linear scaling. At 250 *miles* above the Earth, gravity is still 80% of sea level value.

The force acting on a static mass object on the surface of the Earth, or above, which is measured in a fixed laboratory is not exactly that given in the preceding paragraph, because the reference frame in which the measurement is made is an accelerating (rotating) reference frame, with centripetal acceleration, $\mathbf{a}$, given by,

$$\mathbf{a} = \omega^2 \mathbf{r},$$

for ω the angular frequency of Earth rotation, and $\mathbf{r}$ the position vector from the center of the Earth to the static object. Net gravity, $\mathbf{g}$, is then written,

$$\mathbf{g} = \frac{g_0}{(1 + h/R)^2} + \mathbf{a} = -G_0 \frac{M_0}{R^2(1 + h/R)^2} \hat{\mathbf{r}} + \omega \times (\omega \times \mathbf{r}),$$

$$\mathbf{r} = \mathbf{R} + \mathbf{h} = (R+h)\hat{\mathbf{r}},$$

Gravitational attraction and centrifugal acceleration have opposite signs, with net effect that centrifugal forces reduce gravitational attraction. Assuming that $\mathbf{g}_0$ and $\omega \times \mathbf{r}$ are roughly in the same direction, gives the simple expression for the magnitude of effective gravity,

$$g = g_0 - \omega^2(R+h)\sin\theta,$$

at latitude, θ. The effect is, however, relatively small. Net gravity at the Equator is only 0.5% less than at the Poles, roughly 983 cm/sec^2 at the Poles and 978 cm/sec^2 at the Equator.

For a body of mass, m, to be raised in elevation, h, from the surface of the Earth, work must be done against gravity. To define the work, the geopotential, Φ, is useful,

$$\Phi = G_0 \frac{M_0 m h}{R(R+h)} - \omega^2 \sin\theta \left[R + \frac{h}{2}\right] h,$$

with corresponding force, $\mathbf{F}$, as before,

$$\mathbf{F} = -\nabla\Phi.$$

The energy, Φ_0, required to enable a body to escape from the gravitational field, can be found from the geopotential difference at the surface, $h = 0$, and very far away, $h = \infty$, neglecting the small centrifugal contribution,

$$\Phi_0 = G_0 \frac{m M_0}{R} = m g_0 R.$$

Equating kinetic energy to required geopotential energy, we find that the escape velocity, v_0, is given by,

$$v_0 = (2g_0 R)^{1/2}.$$

Escape velocity on the Earth is about 11 km/sec, while the lunar value is much less, that is, some 2.5 km/sec. At the Equator, the tangential surface velocity, due to Earth rotation, is nearly 0.47 km/sec, so there are benefits to launching satellites from low latitudes in the direction of rotation, to the east.

Significant manifestations of gravitation are the tides, hydrospheric and atmospheric. The gravitational forces exerted on the Earth are equal and opposite to those exerted by the Earth on the Moon and the Sun. The Earth, Moon, and Sun form a three body system rotating about a common center of mass point, as seen in Figure 1. Because the Sun is so far away, it is possible to neglect the gravitational effect of the Sun on Earth tides, so that we can envision a two body system of the Earth and the Moon. The common center of mass of the Earth-Moon system is about 1/80 the distance between the geometrical centers of both, some 1,000 *miles* below the surface of the Earth. The Earth and Moon rotate about this point once every 27.3 *days*, giving rise to both atmospheric and hydrospheric tides, that is, gravitational and centrifugal bulges at opposite sides of the globe. By virtue of this rotation, all mass within the Earth system experiences equal and parallel centrifugal forces, balanced by opposite equal and parallel gravitational Moon forces.

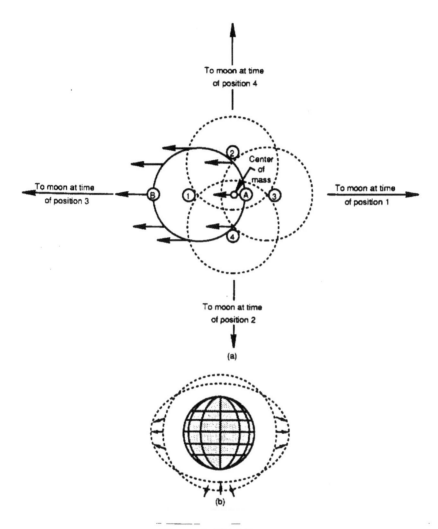

Figure 1. Tidal Forces

The Earth and Moon revolve about their center of mass, some 1,000 miles below the surface of the Earth. The rotation produces equal and opposite centrifugal forces on the Earth, balanced by the gravitational pull of the Sun and Moon. Successive positions of the Earth with respect to the center of mass are shown in (a), with parallel arrows representing centrifugal force when the Earth is in position 1. The resultants of centrifugal and gravitational forces generating tides, and the distortion of the atmospheric shell are depicted in (b).

The magnitude of the tide generating force per unit mass, W, can be estimated by replacing the farside centrifugal force, acting at a distance, D, center of the Earth to the Moon, by the gravitational force, and subtracting the nearside lunar gravitational force, that is,

$$W \approx G_0 M \left[\frac{1}{D^2} - \frac{1}{(D-R)^2} \right] \approx -2 G_0 M \frac{R}{D^3},$$

for M the mass of the Moon, and R the Earth radius, assuming that $D >> R$. Numerically, the tidal force works out to be 10^{-4} *dyne/g*. The results are hydrospheric and atmospheric bulges on opposite sides, with depressions in between. Relative to a point on the rotating Earth, these bulges, or waves, travel around the Earth each day, producing a semidiurnal lunar tide. An analogous semidiurnal solar tide is also present. Amplitudes for both are greatest at lower latitudes, and least at higher ones.

Centrifugal and Coriolis Effects

Many surprises await the study of nature regarding parity, or handedness. Nature is left-handed with regard to the DNA helix, while man himself tends to be right-handed. Clocks, gauges, speedometers, and tachometers operate clockwise, while the orbital motions of the planets and Moon are counterclockwise. The Earth rotates about its axis in counterclockwise motion. While the fundamental reasons are not known, the mechanical implications of such handedness in rotating systems are understood.

Terrestrial measurements are made with respect to the Earth, more particularly with respect to a fixed coordinate system which rotates with constant angular velocity, ω, relative to the Sun. Because it is rotating, the Earth is not an inertial frame, while the Sun can be considered a fixed frame of reference. This rotation imparts centrifugal and Coriolis forces to the equations of motion, ultimately reducing gravitational acceleration and causing deflections in rectilinear particle trajectories. Tides, weather, and ocean currents are manifestations of these rotational forces.

A simple mathematical definition of the time rate of change in a rotating coordinate system serves to quantify both effects. The vectorial time rates of change, d/dt, in two systems, one rotating with respect to the other with angular frequency, ω, are connected symbolically in operator form,

$$\left[\frac{d}{dt} \right]_{fix} = \left[\frac{d}{dt} \right]_{rot} + \omega \times,$$

with subscripts denoting fixed and rotating frames. Velocities are thus connected, using the definition for the radius vector, r, drawn from origin of the rotating system,

$$\mathbf{v}_{fix} = \mathbf{v}_{rot} + \omega \times \mathbf{r},$$

while accelerations take similar form,

$$\mathbf{a}_{fix} = \left[\frac{d\mathbf{v}_{fix}}{dt} \right]_{rot} + \omega \times \mathbf{v}_{fix},$$

which, using the above for $\mathbf{v}_{fix}$, yields,

$$\mathbf{a}_{fix} = \mathbf{a}_{rot} + 2\,\omega \times \mathbf{v}_{rot} + \omega \times (\omega \times \mathbf{r}),$$

To an observer standing in the rotating system, an acceleration, $\mathbf{a}_{rot}$, is observed (measured),

$$\mathbf{a}_{rot} = \mathbf{a}_{fix} - 2\,\omega \times \mathbf{v}_{rot} - \omega \times (\omega \times \mathbf{r}).$$

The nature of each of the terms in $\mathbf{a}_{rot}$ is interesting, leading to centrifugal and Coriolis accelerations. The first term, $\mathbf{a}_{fix}$, is the actual (real) inertial acceleration, like gravity. The last term, $\omega \times (\omega \times \mathbf{r})$, is a vector, normal to ω and pointing outward, the familiar centrifugal acceleration, $\mathbf{a}_{cen}$. The middle term, $\omega \times \mathbf{v}_{rot}$ is the Coriolis acceleration, $\mathbf{a}_{cor}$, perpendicular to both ω and $\mathbf{v}_{rot}$. In the Northern Hemisphere, the Coriolis deflection acts to the right of the particle trajectory, while in the Southern Hemisphere, the deflection acts to the left of the particle trajectory. We summarize by writing,

$$\mathbf{a}_{rot} = \mathbf{a}_{fix} - \mathbf{a}_{cor} - \mathbf{a}_{cen}.$$

When $\omega = 0$, obviously, $\mathbf{a}_{rot} = \mathbf{a}_{fix}$. Defining the latitude, θ, and the angle, ζ, between ω and $\mathbf{v}_{rot}$, the magnitudes of the centrifugal and Coriolis accelerations, a_{cen} and a_{cor}, are easily written,

$$a_{cen} = \omega^2\,r\,\sin\,\theta,$$

$$a_{cor} = \omega\,v_{rot}\,\sin\,\zeta.$$

Order of magnitude estimates of both accelerations can be made at the surface of the Earth. The Earth rotates counterclockwise about its North Pole, with angular frequency, ω,

$$\omega = \frac{2\pi}{24 \times 3600} = 7.29 \times 10^{-5}\;sec^{-1},$$

so that, at the surface at the Equator, $R = 6378\;km$, the centrifugal acceleration is given by,

$$a_{cen} = \omega^2\,R = .034\;m/sec^2,$$

or about a 3% correction to gravity, g_0. While small, this correction is not completely negligible. Centrifugal acceleration is always outward, and at the Equator will be parallel to the radius vector, $\mathbf{R}$. At other latitudes, the radius vector and centrifugal acceleration will not lineup. Hence, except at the Equator, a plumb bob will not point exactly downward to the center of the Earth. No correction is made for this phenomenon, because the vertical is defined as the direction of the plumb bob, rather than the direction of the radius vector. Actually, a better definition of vertical is the normal to a surface of a liquid in equilibrium. The centrifugal acceleration of revolution of the Earth about the Sun is $0.007\;m/sec^2$, another 0.6% correction to g_0, but certainly an even smaller contribution.

The magnitude of the Coriolis acceleration is always less than,

$$2\omega v_{rot} = 1.46 \times 10^{-4}\;sec^{-1}\;v_{rot},$$

which, for velocities, v_{rot}, up to 2,000 mi/hr, is less than .15 m/sec^2, or some 0.015% of gravity. Normally, such corrections are small, but for global trajectories of airplanes and projectiles, the effects are more important. For instance, a projectile fired from the North Pole with a flight time, t, would suffer an apparent angular deflection, θ_{cor}, given by,

$$\theta_{cor} = \omega\, t,$$

because of the rotation of the Earth. For a flight time of 1,000 sec, an angular deflection, θ_{cor}, of some 7×10^{-2} radians would be observed, some 0.4^o longitude, which is not inconsiderable. Coriolis effects are of greater significance in meteorological problems of winds and cyclonic circulation. Wind is simply air in motion, and in the absence of Coriolis forces, the direction of air flow would be along the pressure gradient, from high to low. However, in the Northern Hemisphere, for instance, forces deflect the wind flow to the right of the gradient, producing a counterclockwise cyclonic flow about low pressure systems. In the Southern Hemisphere, cyclonic flows are reversed, clockwise about the lows. Wind flows roughly parallel the isobars, but are not exactly parallel due to viscosity. The actual inclination to the isobars is between 15° and 30°. Another example of the Coriolis effect is seen in a freely falling body. The deflection, x_{cor}, in a body falling from height, z, at latitude, θ, is given by,

$$x_{cor} = \frac{\omega}{3} \left[\frac{(2z)^3}{g} \right]^{1/2} sin\ \theta.$$

From height of 100 ft at the Equator, the deflection, x_{cor}, is .15 in. Determining Coriolis deflections in freely falling bodies is not easy, winds, local disturbances, and the viscosity of air all affect measurements.

Solar Radiation

In spite of its importance to virtually all processes on Earth, the Sun is by no means unique. Among the billions of stars in our Milky Way Galaxy, the Sun is about average mass, but below average size, and the Milky Way Galaxy is, of course, only one of millions of other galaxies. The importance of the Sun results from its closeness to the Earth, about 93 million *miles* away, whereas the next nearest star, Alpha Centauri, is 2.8×10^5 times farther away (4.4 *light years*). Our galactic neighbor, Andromeda Galaxy, is about 1.8×10^6 *light years* away. Radiation from the Sun takes about 8.3 *minutes* to reach the Earth.

The Sun is a gaseous sphere with a diameter of some 88×10^4 *miles*, and an average surface temperature of about 6,000 ^oK. Temperatures increase toward deeper layers, until sufficiently high enough to sustain nuclear reactions, near 10^9 ^oK. The source of solar energy is fusion, more particularly, the synthesis of four hydrogen atoms into one helium atom, and the slight decrease in mass which occurs in the reaction released as energy in the solar interior. This energy is transferred by radiation and convection to the surface, and is then emitted as both electromagnetic waves and charged particles. Each square centimeter of the solar surface emits, on the average, some 6.2 *kilowatts*, or 9×10^4 *cal/min*. This immense power intensity is maintained by the generation of only some 3.8×10^{-6} *cal/min* cm^3 in the solar interior, whereas a corresponding value for burning coal is typically 10^9 times larger. Solar energy is radiated uniformly in all directions, and nearly all of the energy disappears into the vastness of the Universe. Only a minute fraction of the radiative and particulate output of the Sun ever reaches the Earth. Although there is no reason to assume that the Sun emits at a constant rate, measurements so far indicate that such is the case.

The distribution of electromagnetic radiation emitted by the Sun approximates black body radiation near 6,000 ^oK. Similarity between solar and black body radiation provides the basis for estimates of the temperature of the visible surface layer of the Sun. The spectrum, I, as a function of photon frequency, f, is approximated by Wien's law,

$$I(f) = \left[\frac{8\pi \varepsilon f^2}{c^3} \right] exp\ (-\varepsilon/kT),$$

with,

$$\varepsilon = hf = \frac{hc}{\lambda},$$

as before. The distribution peak, $I_{max}(f)$, occurs at wavelength, λ_{max}, that is,

$$\left[\frac{dI}{d\lambda} \right]_{\lambda=\lambda_{max}} = 0,$$

for,

$$\lambda_{max}\ T = 2.898 \times 10^{-3}\ m\ ^oK.$$

At 6,000 ^oK, the corresponding wavelength, λ_{max}, is approximately 0.475 μm.

To the eye armed with only a smoked glass, the Sun seems to have a uniform brightness, or texture. On closer inspection with a telescope, the surface is granular, with bright areas averaging between 185 and 930 *miles* in diameter, and lifetimes of a few minutes, suggesting violent convection. Larger scale structures, called *sunspots*, have also been observed, persisting for longer times. Sunspot activities effect communications on the Earth, probably due to emissions of charged particles and attendant solar flares. Their origin and dynamics are still uncertain, though magnetic fields near the surface must play an important role. Because the solar gas (plasma) consists of charged particles, a magnetic field exerts a force on particles moving in the collective field, and this force may prevent development of convection, and the transport of hot interior matter upward to the photosphere. This may account for the fact that sunspots appear as comparatively darker areas, notably cooler than the surrounding photosphere. Sunspots are more stable than the granulae, possessing a lifetime varying from a few days to a month or more. In the vicinity of sunspots, very bright emissions, called flares, often produce violent emanations into space for thousands of miles.

Solar Constant

Even though solar radiation striking the Earth is attenuated by scattering and absorption in passing through the atmosphere, the intensity of solar radiation at the top of the atmosphere, Γ_0, is constant. According to Beer's law, the monochromatic intensity, γ, for wavelength λ, at any point in the atmosphere, can be written in terms of the intensity at the top of the atmosphere, γ_0, and its exponential attenuation,

$$\gamma = \gamma_0 \, exp \, (-\sigma\mu sec \, \theta),$$

with θ the zenith angle, μ the optical thickness in terms of the integrated density, ρ, over elevation, h,

$$\mu = \int_0^\infty \rho dh,$$

and σ the extinction coefficient, combining the effects of absorption and scattering. Beer's law is a specialized statement of the more general radiative transport equation, treating scattering as a small perturbation on absorption. The total intensity, Γ, is just the integral of the monochromatic intensity over all wavelengths,

$$\Gamma = \int_0^\infty \gamma d\lambda.$$

Assuming that the amount of radiation passing through the top of the atmosphere, Γ_0, of radius, R_0, passes through any other radial shell, R, we find,

$$4\pi R_0^2 \, \Gamma_0 = 4\pi R^2 \, \Gamma,$$

so that,

$$\Gamma_0 = \left[\frac{R}{R_0} \right]^2 \Gamma.$$

Rocket probes sent into the atmosphere to measure Γ have provided good estimates of Γ_0, using the above relationship, Presently, the solar constant is estimated to be,

$$\Gamma_0 = 1.98 \pm .02 \, cal/min \, cm^2,$$

based on both long and short wavelength data.

Most solar radiation never reaches the surface of the Earth, much is reflected and a large percentage is absorbed as energy by the particles that comprise the atmosphere. The net effect is a shift in the wavelength of light reaching the surface. Approximately 65% of the sunlight reaching Earth is infrared, 10% is ultraviolet, and the remaining 25% is visible. The perceived color of the sky and oceans results from scattering of the shortest wavelength component the most, that is, the more energetic blue component.

Seasons

Sunlight reaching the Earth is responsible for life and a chain of energy transfer processes. All energy, save a small fraction of nuclear energy production, comes from the Sun. Electromagnetic radiation causes the temperature structure of atmosphere and hydrosphere. All absorbed energy is turned into heat, chemical, or kinetic energy, or is lost by radiation, convection, or conduction. From year to year, the heat content of the oceans and atmosphere varies little, resulting in nearly constant temperatures. If at constant temperature, the Earth must ultimately be radiating energy to space at the same rate it receives it from the Sun.

As seen in Figure 2, solar radiation hitting the Earth depends on both orientation of the axis of the Earth, as well orbital distance from the Sun. The relative angle of the Earth with respect to the Sun varies as one moves from the Equator. This change in the amount of light falling on the Earth as one moves from the Poles to the Equator is responsible for the seasons. In winter, the Northern Hemisphere is 3 million miles closer to the Sun than in summer, yet winter is colder. The temperature difference does not result from the closeness, but rather from the attitude of the Earth with respect to the Sun, some 23°, reflected by the Tropic of Cancer and Tropic of Capricorn in marking the northernmost and southernmost latitudes for 90° insolation. During the summer, The Northern Hemisphere is tilted toward the Sun, receiving more direct radiation. At the Equator, the attitude of the Earth changes little with respect to the amount of solar radiation, and consequentially the climate and temperature are constant year round. The regular changes in sunlight cause the seasons, but local changes such as clouding and wind patterns, cause the weather. Of course, winds and clouds are also the result of the Sun, so all weather results from solar radiation, over the short and long time span, locally and globally.

All life on the planet depends on the small amount of light received from the Sun. Solar energy is directly responsible for heating and photosynthesis, the basic process by which food for higher organisms is generated. Most of the stored chemical energy on the Earth is a direct consequence of sunlight.

Of the radiant energy absorbed by the Earth and its atmosphere, most is absorbed by the Earth surface. Here it is transformed into internal energy, with resultant larger horizontal and vertical temperature gradients. Thus, the immediate source of energy driving atmospheric processes is the surface internal energy distribution. A variety of processes may bring about subsequent energy transformations, such as evaporation, conduction into the Earth, long wavelength radiation, and upward atmospheric conduction and convection, with each depending on the physical properties of the surface and atmosphere of the Earth. In the atmosphere, oxygen and nitrogen, constituting over 99% of atmospheric gases by volume, strongly absorb radiation with wavelengths shorter than 0.3 μm. The atmosphere is much more transparent for shorter wavelength radiation, than longer wavelength radiation. The result is that solar energy passes through the atmosphere and is absorbed at the surface.

Equinoctial Precession and Nutation

When a top (gyroscope) is rapidly spinning about its axis of symmetry, and is subject to a torque, such as the gravitational torque depicted in Figure 3, the plane containing the top axis and vertical will rotate about the vertical axis. This motion of the top is called precession. If initial conditions are suitably chosen, the precessional angular frequency, ω, will be constant. If not, the axis of the top will bob up, down, and sidewise, producing a trace as seen in Figure 4. Such periodic motion, superimposed on steady precession, is called nutation.

The physical basis for precession is the torque, **L**, exerted on the top by gravity, the magnitude of which is written,

$$L = mgl\sin\theta$$

where m is the mass of the top, and l is the distance from the point of support to the center of mass (Figure 3). The direction of the torque is perpendicular to the plane containing the vertical and top axis. If the plane containing the top axis and the vertical precesses through an angle, $d\phi$, in time, dt, and if, **J**, is the spin angular momentum of the top, the magnitude of the change in angular momentum in time is just $J\sin\theta\, d\phi$. Since torque is the time rate of change of angular momentum, we have,

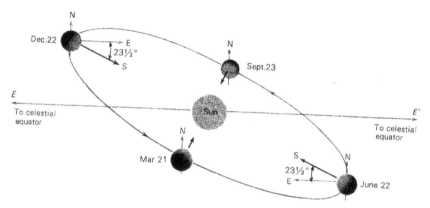

Figure 2. Earth Solar Orbit And Seasons

The plane of the elliptic orbit of the Earth about the Sun is tilted some 23° with respect to axis of rotation of the Sun, producing variation in the angle of sunlight hitting the Northern and Southern Hemispheres, which in turn causes the seasons. Corresponding latitudes in the Northern and Southern Hemispheres (Tropic of Cancer and Tropic of Capricorn) mark the boundaries of the Torrid Zone. Both latitudes are limits for 90° insolation of the Earth's surface (northerly and southerly).

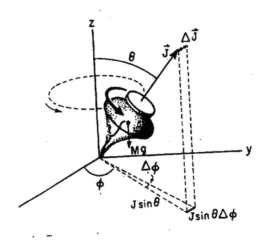

Figure 3. Torque, Angular Momentum, And Precession In A Gravitational Field

When a top (gyroscope) is rapidly spinning about its axis and is subject to a gravitational torque, as shown below, the plane containing the top axis and vertical will rotate about the vertical axis, popularly termed precession.

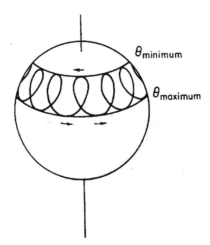

Figure 4. Nutation Of A Spinning Top

Generally, the precessional motion and frequency of a gyroscope in a gravitational field will vary . In periodic fashion, the axis of the spinning top will bob up and down, and sidewise, producing the trace below, called nutation.

$$L = J sin\,\phi \frac{d\phi}{dt} = mgl sin\,\phi$$

Consequently, the precessional angular frequency, ω, takes the form,

$$\omega = \frac{d\phi}{dt} = \frac{mgl}{J}$$

The Earth is very much like the top, with a spin axis precessing about the normal to the ecliptic, astronomically called the Precession of the Equinoxes. Were the Earth completely spherical, none of the other members of the Solar System could exert a gravitational torque on it. But the Earth is slightly flat at the Poles, and bulges to a small extent at the Equator. It is just the net torque on these bulges due to gravitational attraction that sets the Earth's axis precessing in space. The largest part of this precession is caused by pull of the Sun and the Moon on the ellipsoidal Earth. The other planets in the Solar System also exert a gravitational torque on the Earth, but in opposite direction and considerably less in magnitude. The overall gravitational torque is small, so the precession, ω, is extremely slow,

$$\omega = \frac{2\pi}{26000}\,yr^{-1} = 0.00023\,yr^{-1}$$

Total torque is not constant in time, because the torques of the Sun and Moon have slightly different orientations to the ecliptic, varying as the three bodies move around each other. Because of these irregularities, the precessional drift exhibits recurring patterns of nutation, seen in Figure 4.

Having opened on a cosmological scale, a few words about our Solar System might be appropriate in closing.

Solar System

The Sun is a middle size, middle age, field star (loner) in a rather sparse outer arm of the galaxy, about 10,000 *parsec* (3×10^{17} *km*) from the center of the Milky Way Galaxy. Its neighbors consist of mainly nine planets, as mentioned, with properties tabulated in Table 3, in terms of Earth masses (*EM*) and astronomical units (*AU*).

Table 3. Bodies Of The Solar System

Body	Mass	Density	Rotational Period	Satellites	Solar Distance	Orbital Period
	(EM)	(g/cm)	(days)		(AU)	(yrs)
Sun	3.3×10^5	1.4	25.36			
Mercury	0.06	5.4	58.66	0	0.39	0.24
Venus	0.82	5.2	242.98	0	0.72	0.61
Earth	1.00	5.5	1.00	1	1.00	1.00
Mars	0.11	3.9	1.03	2	1.52	1.87
Jupiter	317.84	1.3	0.40	13	5.20	11.86
Saturn	95.15	0.70	0.43	10	9.54	29.47
Uranus	14.60	1.7	0.53	2	19.19	164.81
Neptune	17.21	1.3	0.89	2	30.06	84.06
Pluto	0.18		6.39	0	39.53	248.58

The principal physical interaction between bodies of the Solar System is gravitation, though the Sun casts enormous radiation pressure on all other inhabitants, as a thermonuclear furnace. The orbits of the planets are such that they do not come at all close to each other. For the six largest planets, mean eccentricities are less than 0.05, and their mean inclinations with respect to the invariant plane (plane normal to the total angular momentum vector) are all less than 2%. Even the three smallest planets (Mercury, Mars, Pluto) are not in danger of collision. Pluto is locked in resonance orbit with Neptune. The planetary system appears to be very stable, and should continue so until the Sun undertakes its terminal expansion (death) some 5×10^9 *yrs* hence. The satellite orbits about the planets enjoy similar stability.

In addition to gravitational attraction, the Sun bathes planets with radiative energy, at the Earth some 1.4×10^6 *ergs/cm sec*, as described. Most of this is in visible wavelengths, $0.4 - 0.7$ μm. The Sun also streams matter in a solar wind, an expansion of the solar atmosphere at rate about 10^{13} *g/sec*, mostly protons moving in the $400 - 500$ *km/sec* range. The solar wind density is roughly 5 *particles/cm³*. Associated with the solar wind is a magnetic field of 10^{-4} *gauss* near the Earth. Both the particle energies and magnetic field intensities undergo dramatic fluctuations, linked to sunspot activity. These fluctuations source the interaction of the solar wind with the magnetospheres and atmospheres of the planets. Interactions also vary widely with the magnetic and atmospheric characteristics of the individual planets.

The elemental composition of the Sun is estimated from its spectrum and other means to be (by mass) 74.8% hydrogen, 24% helium and neon, 1% carbon, nitrogen and oxygen, and 0.2% heavier elements. The densities of planets are affected by both composition and compression. They are grouped into four classes:

- iron—Mercury;
- silicate—Venus, Earth, Mars;
- hydrogen—Jupiter, Saturn;
- ice—Uranus, Neptune, Pluto.

Other silicate bodies are the Moon and inner two satellites, Io and Europa, of Jupiter, while ice bodies are the outer two Jovian satellites Ganymede and Callisto, and the big satellite, Titan, orbiting Saturn.

Satellites are all less than 0.04 EM in size, and total 0.13 EM. The asteroids, mostly silicate bodies between Mars and Jupiter, sum to 0.0003 EM. Comets are ice bodies in highly elliptical orbits, with total mass less than 10^{-7} EM, but many believe that a much larger reservoir of comets exist beyond Neptune and Pluto. The last category of small bodies are meteorites, providing data about the evolution of the Solar System, but representing very small total mass.

Radiochronological data suggests the Solar System formed some 4.6×10^9 *yrs* ago. Astronomical observations of star formation hint that the Solar System formed from clouds of gas and dust. Mean densities indicate planetary compositions were determined mainly by the Sun, that is, from solar heat on condensation of dust from the gas. Exceptions are Jupiter and Saturn, large enough to capture gas gravitationally, and Moon, Io, and Europa apparently formed from higher temperature condensates than those corresponding to their present solar positions. The solar wind in the early stages of the evolution of the Solar System is thought to have been nearly 10^7 times stronger than present, thus expelling hydrogen and other gases away from planets.

Keyed Exercises

• *If the age of the Earth is 4.7 billion years, what is the recessional speed of a galaxy on the fringes of the Universe whose light just reached us, assuming transmission at the birth of the Earth?*

$$r = 2.7 \times 10^9 \ light \ yr, \quad \Upsilon = 50 \ km/sec \ mpsec$$

$$\zeta = \Upsilon r = 50 \times 2.7 \times 10^9 \times \frac{1}{3.26 \times 10^6} \ km/sec = 72 \times 10^3 \ km/sec$$

On the average, how fast, ζ, are two galaxies separated a distance, $r = 3.9 \ mparsec$, moving apart from each other?

$$\Upsilon = 50 \ km/sec \ mpsec, \quad \zeta = \Upsilon r$$

$$\zeta = 50 \times 3.9 \ km/sec = 195 \ km/sec$$

What fraction, ξ, of the speed of light, c, is this mean recessional velocity?

$$\xi = \frac{\zeta}{c}, \quad c = 2.998 \times 10^5 \ km/sec$$

$$\xi = \frac{195}{2.998 \times 10^5} = .65 \times 10^{-3}$$

• *What is the magnitude of the gravitational force, F, between a hard hat diver of mass, m = 60 kg, and surface platform of mass, M = 6000 kg, separated a distance, r = 30 m, underwater?*

$$m = 60 \ kg, \quad M = 6000 \ kg, \quad r = 30 \ m$$

$$G_0 = 6.67 \times 10^{-11} \ newton \ m^2/kg^2$$

$$F = G_0 \frac{mM}{r^2} = 6.67 \times 10^{-11} \times \frac{60 \times 6000}{30^2} \ newton = 2.67 \times 10^{-6} \ newton$$

What is the magnitude of the gravitational force, F, between the Earth and the hard hat diver?

$$m = 60 \ kg, \quad g = 9.8 \ m/sec^2$$

$$F = mg = 60 \times 9.8 \ kg \ m/sec^2 = 588 \ newton$$

- *What is the acceleration of gravity, g, at an elevation, h = 1560 mi, above the Earth?*

$$g_0 = 32 \ ft/sec^2, \quad R = 3948 \ mi$$

$$g = \frac{g_0}{(1 + h/R)^2} = \frac{32}{(1 + 1560/3948)^2} \ ft/sec^2 = 16.4 \ ft/sec^2$$

- *A freely falling body has instantaneous (vertical) trajectory, y, given by the relationship,*

$$y = y_i + v_i t - \frac{1}{2} g t^2$$

with t the time, y_i the initial position, v_i the initial velocity, and g the acceleration of gravity. What is the instantaneous velocity, v, and instantaneous acceleration, a?

$$y = y_i + v_i t - \frac{1}{2} g t^2, \quad v = \frac{dy}{dt}, \quad a = \frac{dv}{dt}$$

$$v = \frac{d(y_i + v_i t - 1/2 g t^2)}{dt} = v_i - gt$$

$$a = \frac{d(v_i - gt)}{dt} = -g$$

- *The geopotential, V, of the Earth, in the radial direction is given by, V = $-G_0 Mm/r$, with Earth mass, M, particle mass, m, gravitational constant, G_0, and r the separation of Earth and particle masses? What is magnitude of the force (radially), F, between masses?*

$$F = -\frac{\partial V}{\partial r} = G_0 \frac{\partial(-mM/r)}{\partial r} = G_0 \frac{mM}{r^2}$$

- *Formulate Kepler's laws as a succinct mathematical statement (3rd law), using the period of planetary rotation, T, and the semimajor axis of the elliptic orbit, a?*

$$T^2 \propto a^3$$

$$T^2 = \kappa a^3 \quad (\kappa \; constant)$$

If the period of rotation of the Earth is $T = 365$ days, and the semimajor axis of its orbit is $a = 105 \times 10^6$ miles, what is the proportionality constant, κ?

$$\kappa = \frac{T^2}{a^3} = \frac{365^2}{(105 \times 10^6)^3} = \frac{1.332 \times 10^5}{1.124 \times 10^{18}} = 1.300 \times 10^{-13} \; days^2/miles^3$$

- *At $1,000\,^oK$, what is the corresponding wavelength, λ_{max}, which maximizes the blackbody spectrum of solar electromagnetic radiation?*

$$\lambda_{max}T = 2.898 \times 10^{-3} \; m\,^oK$$

$$\lambda_{max} = \frac{2.898 \times 10^{-3}}{T}\, m = \frac{2.898 \times 10^{-3}}{1000}\, m = 2.898 \mu m$$

- *What is the precessional frequency, ω, for a marine gyroscope, $m = 10$ gm, spinning with angular momentum, $J = 26000$ g cm^2/sec, about a displacement, $l = 3.5$ cm?*

$$\omega = \frac{mgl}{J} = \frac{10 \times 980 \times 3.5}{26000} \; sec^{-1} = 1.32 \; sec^{-1}$$

- *If the radius, R, of the Earth is 3963.3 mi, what is the circumference, C?*

$$R = 3963.3 \; mi, \quad C = 2\pi R = 2 \times 3.14 \times 3963.3 \; mi = 12,451.1 \; mi$$

What would be the arc length, l_{24}, at the Equator of 24 equal time zones?

$$l_{24} = \frac{12451.1}{24} = 518.7 \; mi$$

Atmospheric Gases

The atmosphere is composed of a group of nearly permanent gases, a group of gases of variable concentration, and various solid and liquid particles. If water vapor, carbon dioxide, and ozone are removed, the remaining gases have virtually constant proportions up to a height of 56 *miles*. Table 4 lists the concentrations of permanent constituents of air, and Table 5 lists ranges of concentrations of variable constituents of air. Obviously, the gases most variable in composition play important roles in life support and cycle activities on the Earth.

Table 4. Permanent Composition Of Air.

Constituent gas	Formula	Mass (*amu*)	Volume fraction
nitrogen	N_2	28.02	.781
oxygen	O_2	32.00	.209
argon	Ar	39.94	.009
neon	Ne	20.18	10^{-4}
helium	He	4.00	10^{-4}
krypton	Kr	83.80	10^{-4}
xenon	Xe	131.31	10^{-4}
hydrogen	H_2	2.02	10^{-4}
methane	CH_4	16.04	10^{-4}
nitrous oxide	N_2O	44.01	10^{-4}

Table 5. Variable Composition Of Air.

Constituent gas	Formula	Mass (*amu*)	Volume fraction
water	H_2O	18.01	$0.0 - 10^{-2}$
carbon dioxide	CO_2	44.01	$10^{-4} - 10^{-3}$
ozone	O_3	50.00	$0.0 - 10^{-4}$
sulfur dioxide	SO_2	64.06	$0.0 - 10^{-6}$
nitrogen dioxide	NO_2	46.01	$0.0 - 10^{-8}$

From the above, it is apparent that nitrogen, oxygen, and argon account for 99.99% of permanent gases in the atmosphere. Although these gases are considered invariant, very small changes in space and time may be observed. The uniformity of proportions is produced by mixing associated with atmospheric motion. Above 56 *miles* in altitude, the proportion of the lighter gases increases with height as diffusion becomes more important relative to mixing. The major variable gases in air are caused by combustion, chemical processes in the oceans, and photosynthesis. Solid and liquid particles suspended in air play an important role in the physics of clouds.

The question of atmospheric formation is pertinent. One suggestion is that as celestial bodies acquire more mass, their gravitational fields increase, allowing them to capture gases moving through space. Another tenet presumes that light gases originally present at the formation of a planet escape the gravitational field. And a third idea suggests that gases emitted during geological eruptions are present, held by gravity if heavy enough. The truth probably is a combination of all three.

Some evidence supports a preponderance of the third possibility. The atmosphere of the Earth is scarce in neon, approximately the same molecular weight as water, but abundant in water. Current knowledge of the elements that can be and were generated from natural radioactive decay on the planet, suggests there ought be more neon. Evidently, in the early chaotic stages on Earth, neon atoms drifted off into space. So did water, before volcanic activity replenished supply. The current addition of water to the surface of the Earth is 0.1 km^3/yr. In the past, this rate must have been an order of magnitude greater for the oceans to have been formed in about 4 billion years.

Oxygen, on the other hand, was mostly produced by plant photosynthesis. Oxygen combines readily with many elements at temperatures and pressures common on Earth. Because these elements are abundant on the surface, oxygen is, and has been, rapidly removed from air. The reducing agents of the primordial Earth (ammonia, methane, and water vapor) also spurred the combination of oxygen with other elements, suggesting that little oxygen gas was present in the early atmosphere. So, present oxygen was formed rather recently, mainly by plants. When photosynthetic plants evolved, the oxygen gas added to the atmosphere began to exceed the oxidation rate, and oxygen began to accumulate in the oceans (and further migrate into the atmosphere). It continued to increase in proportion to plant growth and survival. Then about 1 billion years ago, animal life evolved, employing oxygen for respiration and establishing a limit to oxygen accumulation. Thus life forms and life processes changed the atmosphere and oceans, significantly affecting the amount of oxygen in both.

Atmospheric Temperatures

The atmosphere consists of a series of nearly spherical layers characterized by a distinctive vertical temperature distribution up to 60 *miles*, and becoming very hot beyond. The lowest layer, characterized for the most part by decreasing temperature with elevation, is called the *troposphere*. This layer contains about 80% of the total atmospheric mass, and is most closely influenced by evaporation and heat conduction at the surface of the Earth. The troposphere extends some 6 to 11 *miles* upward in the atmosphere. Above the troposphere, extending to 31 *miles* is the *stratosphere*. Temperatures in the upper stratosphere are comparable to Earth temperatures, associated with the absorption of ultraviolet radiation by ozone. Beyond the stratosphere, up to about 50 *miles*, is the next layer, called the *mesosphere*. Temperatures in the mesosphere drop with relative elevation, and rocket data suggests that winds approaching 500 *mi/hr* are not uncommon in this layer. Similarity of temperature distributions in the mesosphere and troposphere suggest similar mixing processes. The *thermosphere*, the next atmospheric layer beyond the mesosphere, exhibits increasing temperature with height, up to 500 *miles*. Temperatures of 1,500 ^oK have been recorded at altitudes of 400 *miles*, a zone where many gases are partially ionized. The diffuse region beyond the thermosphere is called the *exosphere*, or *magnetosphere*. The temperature profile of the atmosphere is given in Figure 5.

Obviously, the amount of sunlight reaching the atmosphere and surface of the Earth are crucial to all atmospheric processes, as well as the amount of sunlight reflected and scattered. The amount of scattered light by oceans or atmospheres is a determinant in their color perception. Color is, of course, a function of light spectrum. White light is composed of red, orange, yellow, green, blue, and violet components. The perceived color of any particular area on Earth may change as one views it, because a cloud is passing overhead, or because the angle of the Sun changes, for example, near sunset. The reason for the blue color of the oceans and the sky is selective light scattering. Blue light, the most energetic and shortest wavelength component, is scattered the most by water particles and atmospheric debris, and red light, the least energetic and longest wavelength component, is scattered the least. Correspondingly, the light scattered by particles and debris is mostly blue, while the residual light is deficient in blue, and predominantly red. Thus, sky and oceans are blue, and sunsets are red. All sunlight is white, but what we see is only that left after scattering and absorption have taken place.

During certain periods, other factors have affected the amount of light received by the Earth. Ice caps, for instance, reflected more light in the past, but changes in the nature of the protective umbrella of the atmosphere have primarily determined the amount of solar radiation reaching the surface of the Earth. Variations in water vapor levels in the atmosphere are linked to temperature changes. As sunlight penetrates the atmosphere, some is absorbed by particles of certain gases in the atmosphere, and then reradiated as infrared radiation, or heat. The same effect occurs when an automobile is parked in the Sun with windows closed. Inside temperatures become very much greater than outside. Glass allows radiation to pass through it. Upon striking the interior, the sunlight is absorbed by the material in the interior, and transformed into infrared.

But other factors, tending to drop Earth temperatures, also enter into the balance. Particulate matter in the atmosphere can and does reflect sunlight. The volcanic dust and ash pumped into the Northern Hemisphere in 1815 by eruption of Mount Pambora in Indonesia canceled summer in the Northern Hemisphere, because the large amount of airborne matter reflected away much more of the sunlight back into space than was normal. Burning fossil fuels, in addition to releasing carbon dioxide, deposit increasing amounts of particulate matter into the atmosphere. The net effect of increasing buildup of atmospheric particulates is a decrease in solar radiation reaching the Earth, and a drop in the average Earth temperature. So reflection of solar radiation and absorption compete. Many are worried about a drop in the temperature of the Earth, if reflection of sunlight is the dominant mechanism. Others worry about temperature increases if absorption is dominant. And of course there are variations in solar radiation over long term cycles due to solar flares, sunspot activity, and changes in the magnetic field of the Earth trapping charged particle. Satellite measurements of the Earth atmosphere suggest cooling to constant temperatures over many decades. Surface measurements suggest heating blaming carbon dioxide at the surface. Satellite measurements are fairly scientific while surface measurements are less so. With that in mind, consider the following regarding global temperature estimates and methods, carbon dioxide and water vapor, and Earth history.

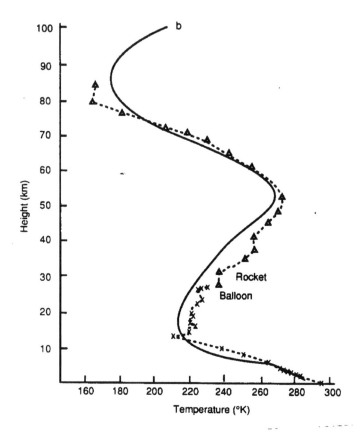

Figure 5. Atmospheric Temperature Distribution

Atmospheric temperatures vary in complicated fashion with elevation. Four distinct layers of monotonic temperature behavior are noted below, called the troposphere, stratosphere, mesosphere, and thermosphere. Beyond 60 miles, temperatures become very hot, in the 1,500 °K range, and the region is called the exosphere.

Global Warming versus Cooling

The subject of global temperatures and changes, proxies, biased and omitted data, statistical methods, long and short term statistical significance and appropriate tests is a complex and controversial subject at best. In light of recent controversies, many rely on estimates of global temperatures using satellite measurements since 1979 because of their scientific precision. In the context of temperature measurements and carbon dioxide, a first look at the Earth's temperature and carbon dioxide history is interesting.

Global temperatures today are at their lowest levels in millions of years, seen in Figure 6. Carbon dioxide levels are similarly lower, seen in Figure 7. The late

Carboniferous to early Permian (315 million years ago) is the only period in the last 600 million years when both atmospheric carbon dioxide and temperatures were as low as they are today. There has been historically much more carbon dioxide in our atmosphere than exists today. During the Jurassic period (200 million years ago), carbon dioxide concentrations were about 1,800 *ppm*. The highest concentrations of carbon dioxide during all of the Paleozoic era occurred during the Cambrian period, nearly 7,000 *ppm*, or about 18 times higher than today. The Carboniferous and Ordovician periods were the only geological periods during the Paleozoic era when global temperatures were as low as they are today. Directly opposite to recent global warming claims, the late Ordovician period was also an Ice Age while maintaining carbon dioxide concentrations nearly 12 times higher than today, that is, 4,400 *ppm*. According to greenhouse theory, Earth then should have been exceedingly hot, but instead, global temperatures were no warmer than today. Clearly, other factors beside greenhouse gases (carbon dioxide, water vapor, methane, and nitrous gases) dominate Earth temperatures and warming-cooling cycles. Keep in mind too that if the surface warms, so should the atmosphere above it by simple heat transfer logic, but that has not been the case from all measuring stations. In fact, the atmosphere above the surface has been cooling slightly from 1979 or so. If the surface really is heating, while the upper atmosphere is cooling, than some sort of heat removal process is taking energy out of the atmosphere. Nothing is plausible nor proposed scientifically nor remotely suggested in technical circles. Plus upper atmospheric temperature measurements use satellites while surface measurements rely on other less precise and reproducible devices for temperature measurements, and seemingly very disparate techniques.

Against historical patterns, recent temperature variations are neither singular nor significant statistically, from both a cooling and warming perspective. The dire claims of nuclear winter in the 1970s due to global cooling were also no more statistically significant than today's claims of catastrophic global warming. Statistical methods applied to rapidly varying data on long time scales must also be carefully chosen to reflect (proper) long term trends. The situation is not unlike the Stock Market. Decades or less, often used for analysis, lead to inappropriate conclusions and incorrect significance against the broader background of century climate behavior, and even longer periods of time. This is seen in Figure 6 depicting average Earth temperatures for the past 20 centuries. Fairly rapid fluctuations on top of both warming and cooling cycles are seen in Figures 6 and 7, and occur both on century and yearly time scales. In such situations, fluctuations far above or below the mean can be expected with high probability, and standard normal (Gaussian) tests (chi squared, student T, F, and derivatives) are not always applicable without modification, and usually other tests are better suited. In the climate arena, this has been noted by experts, and the misuse of normal tests cited appropriately. Another problem, of course, is the mixing of temperature data (satellite, tree rings, ice cores, etc.), with each category requiring different data normalization factors than the others to interpolate findings.

Since 1979, Microwave Sounding Units (MSUs) on polar orbiting satellites have measured the intensity of upwelling microwave radiation from atmospheric oxygen. The intensity is proportional to the temperature in broad vertical layers, as originally correlated with radiosonde (balloon) measurements. Now, satellite units are already calibrated with platinum resistance thermometers before they are launched into orbit. In other words, satellite measurements are uniform, reproducible, reliable, and measure representative temperature distributions across the planet.

Measurement sites are obviously a limited set. Temperature measurements extracted from oxygen microwave emissions need be interpolated from one site to another, often over very dissimilar regions. For instance, a measurement at sea level in the desert may have a near neighbor measurement at an altitude of 14,000 *ft*. One over a hot city may have a near neighbor on ice pack. Over the globe, some 1,600 satellite measurements are taken daily. Given that the surface area of the Earth is near 196,940,400 *square miles*, most of the Earth is not sampled by satellite (nor any other) measurements. This gives rise to large biases, or better put, questionable temperature data for global averaging. Satellite measurements, however, suffer least from these biases.

There are three main surface station based global temperature data sets (GISS, NOAA, CRU), and two satellite based data sets (RSS and UAH). Different agencies use different methods for calculating global temperatures from these five sets. The surface based sets suffer the most from local temperature biases (urban concentrations, missed sites, poor maintenance, selective clustering, absence of colder sites, etc.) and are the least reliable. After *adjustments* have been made to the raw data, temperatures at each station are converted into *anomalies*, that is, difference from an average temperature for a defined period. In the CRU method (also used by IPCC), anomalies are baselined on the average observed in the 1961-1990 period. In the GISS approach, 1976 (one of the coldest years) is used as a baseline, obviously magnifying warming and minimizing cooling departures from the baseline. The Earth is routinely meshed in a series of $5 - 5$ *degree* grids, in these other approaches, and temperatures are arithmetically averaged over all sites (stations) in the cell. Some mesh points have 4 stations reporting, while other mesh points have none. Mesh elements without stations contribute nothing to the global average. Empty sites at colder mesh points and at altitude are not treated correctly in such averaging process, while surface stations in urban areas are usually overweighted.

Briefly, we note the following about interpolation schemes used within caveats above:

- GISS
  GISS adjustments result in more warming than any other data set. These adjustments have been criticized for non-existent warming, stemming from data adjustments with arbitrary cold baseline for computing anomalies.

- NOAA
  NOAA analyses track GISS in general. Like GISS, a cold start year (1976) magnifies NOAA yearly anomalies on the warm side and minimizes anomalies on the cold side. This is well known in most scientific circles.

- CRU
  CRU data contains many empty grid cells, with temperatures interpolated across surrounding cells. The interpolations have been criticized as unrealistic.

- IPCC
  The CRU data used by IPCC is not publicly available, neither raw data nor adjusted data. Refusal to submit CRU and IPCC data to public scrutiny is part of the Climate Gate controversy, along with noted data biases.

- Hockey Stick
  The hockey stick prediction of global temperatures has been already debunked in a number of published analyses. We merely include it for completeness.

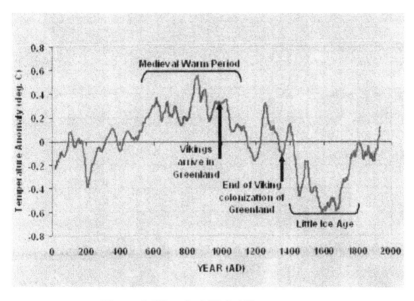

Figure 6. Historical Global Temperatures

Temperatures have varied significantly over the centuries. Global temperatures today are at their lowest levels in centuries. Against historical patterns, recent temperature variations are neither singular nor significant.

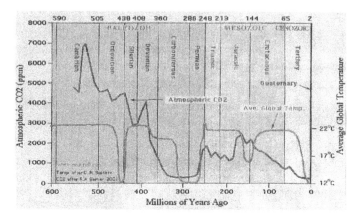

Figure 7. Historical Carbon Dioxide Levels

Carbon dioxide levels have been significantly higher than today with cooler Earth temperatures. The highest concentrations of carbon dioxide during the Cambrian period were 18 times higher than today. The late Ordovician period was also an Ice Age with carbon dioxide levels 12 times higher than present levels.

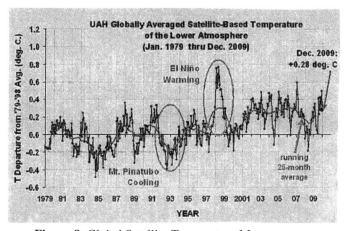

Figure 8. Global Satellite Temperature Measurements

Satellite measurements do not suggest the atmosphere is heating. That is an anomaly if the surface is heating. Contrary, satellite measurements suggest the atmosphere is cooling slightly. If the surface is heating and the atmosphere is cooling, some low altitude energy removal process is occurring. Presently, none are known nor proven scientifically.

- UAH
  We mention the satellite analyses of UAH as closest in approach and temperature averages to other satellite measurements. No *adjustments* are employed in the UAH analyses, unlike all of the above. Satellite data shows no warming from 1979–1997, then El Nino warming 1997–1999, and no warming thereafter according to UAH (Figure 8).

- USNCDC
  The recently funded and constructed United States National Climatic Data Center (USNCDC) in North Carolina also reports from satellite analysis that the planet has cooled as much as 0.6 °C since the high in 1998.

Earth's lower atmosphere contains trace amounts of greenhouse gases (water vapor, carbon dioxide, and methane) which some claim keep the lower layers of the atmosphere very much warmer than otherwise without greenhouse gases. Greenhouse gases must then hypothetically trap much infrared radiation, the radiant heat energy that the Earth naturally emits to outer space in response to solar heating. Actually, because greenhouse gases exist as trace components in the atmosphere, they have small effect on temperatures. Mankind's burning of fossil fuels (mostly coal, petroleum, and natural gas) releases carbon dioxide into the atmosphere, possibly enhancing greenhouse gas concentration. But, as of 2008, the concentration of carbon dioxide in the lower atmosphere was only 45% higher than before the start of the Industrial Revolution in the 1800s. So, it is interesting to note that, even though carbon dioxide is a crucial life support component, there is really precious little of it in the atmosphere. Today only 39 out of every 100,000 molecules of air are carbon dioxide, and it will take roughly another 5 to 10 years of carbon emissions to increase that number to 42. If one computes the thermodynamic properties and heat capacities of the atmosphere with such small contribution from carbon dioxide, impacts of carbon dioxide are totally negligible for heat capacity and transfer. Added to that is the fact that carbon dioxide is not building rapidly, if at all, in the upper troposphere nor stratosphere, nor are temperatures rising therein according to some reports. The question of environmental impact is also one hotly debated, and our comments here should not be construed to suggest continued dumping of carbon, methane, and nitrous gases is without consequence. Rather, the point we make is that these three greenhouse components have little effect on global temperatures in general, and such has been the case for centuries. Water vapor is another story because its concentrations are not trace like carbon dioxide.

Water vapor is by far the most consequential gas in the atmosphere. There is no way to control its levels. All data suggests that water vapor rises and falls with temperature changes, and has done so for centuries. By shear abundance in the atmosphere, water vapor trumps carbon dioxide by many orders of magnitude. Water vapor has the greatest effect on Earth temperatures. Carbon dioxide, methane, and other trace gases in the atmosphere with concentrations below 1,000 *ppm* have virtually no effect on thermal properties of the atmosphere. At 1,000 *ppm*, thermal properties are only impacted at the 0.1% level. Water vapor, seen in Figure 7, is roughly 19,600 *ppm* in the atmosphere. An interesting fact is that recent measurements of carbon dioxide up to many miles in the atmosphere by Mauna Loa show that carbon dioxide, despite recently claimed large increases in surface emissions, is virtually nonexistent as we move up in the atmosphere.

In Table 6 are listed satellite temperature anomalies (LANL) as averaged over the full year from 1979 to the present (column 2). Table 6 compares with other estimates, and shows departures (anomalies) from a running 24 month average, consistent with standard techniques for rapidly varying (monthly) data, that is, Table 6 is a snapshot for cursory comparison of coarse grain data. But even therein, differences in the 1990–2009 running temperatures are evident within the caveats mentioned. The average in Table 6 (column 3) is the average of GISS, NOAA, IPCC, CRU, and Hockey Stick global temperature estimates. Other analyses suggest warming in 1997 to 2009, opposite to the LANL analysis. The cooling from roughly 2000 to 2009 in Table 6 tracks with noted ocean and stratospheric cooling in the same time frame and UAH analysis in Figure 8. Robotics measurements down to 3000 *fsw* in the oceans recorded the cooling, while satellites tracked tropical stratospheric cooling. Additionally, the upper atmosphere over the tropics, generally warmer than adjacent layers, exhibited uncharacteristic cooling over the past 3–5 years.

Moving averages, of course, help to underscore trends in otherwise oscillating data. Additionally, it should be noted that a single estimate for yearly average global temperature is something of a stretch, as Southern Hemisphere temperatures are cooler than Northern Hemisphere temperatures (less land mass and fewer people). Highly industrialized activities are more numerous in the Northern Hemisphere and likely bias all temperature measurements. Prior to 1990, differences are small. From 1990 through 2009, differences from the moving average range 10% to 40% as a rough metric. Statistical significance between LANL and the averages of other compilations is notable, yet significances of both sets against long term trends are negligible.

The periods 1981–1989, 1992–1995, 2007–2009 show cooling to varying degrees in yearly temperatures. The 1987-1989 period shows cooling from the Mt Pinatubo eruption, the 1997-1999 period exhibits warming from a very strong El Nino, and the 2006-2009 period is one of virtually nonexistent sunspot and solar flare activity. From Figures 6 and 8, it is seen that recent warming and cooling trends (1979–2009) are about half those experienced during the Medieval (warm) and Little Ice (cool) Ages. Statistically, recent trends against these earlier periods are not significant, whether using the LANL estimates or the averages in Table 6. Said another way, differences between LANL versus GISS, NOAA, IPCC, and CRU averaged temperatures are interesting, but the warming and cooling trends tracked over the period 1976–2009 are not particularly important nor alarming in either case against century temperature trends. In other words, the data in Table 6 is no more significant than data over millions of years. In fact, the variations over the past centuries subsume variations in Table 6 by large order (see Figure 6). One finds considerable differences among global temperature estimates from all sources. In general, all data suffers from large geographical *holes* in collection sites and nonuniform measurements, excepting the satellite measurements by comparison. Interpolation techniques across measurement sites have been low order accurate. Measurements from cooler regions impact the analysis yielding lower global temperature averages. LANL global temperature estimates for the 1990-2009 period are 10%–40% lower than the average of reporting agencies. Unlike reports from GISS, NOAA, CRU, IPCC, and others, 2009 seems not the warmest year in the past few decades, the Earth has not likely been warming since 1998, and the statistical significance of recent temperature cycles is virtually nonsignificant (both heating and cooling trends). Statistically, differences between LANL estimates and the average of reporting agencies is (χ^2) significant, p =0.80, in Table 6 for anomalies.

To reiterate in a few sentences, we remark:

- from satellite oxygen activation measurements, the lower atmosphere has been cooling since roughly 1998, independent of good or bad surface measurements;
- long and short term heating and cooling cycles over past and present centuries are normal, and present cycles are not statistically significant relative to past cycles;
- carbon dioxide buildup (or depletion) has little to no effect on temperatures on average across the lower atmosphere;
- sunspot and solar flare activities track broadly with temperature cycles and are an area of present investigation relative to Earth temperatures;
- if the Earth were warming, the upper troposphere and stratosphere would be warming, pretty much in lock step, but they have been at constant temperature or cooling for many decades.

Clouds and Lightning

Clouds have been subjects of observation by scientists and poets and painters for hundreds of years, but until this century, their physical properties have been unexplored. Serious attention to clouds began with the observation that water clouds are quite common at very, very cold temperatures, below $-30\,^oC$. In the laboratory, distilled water in small droplets freezes only when cooled below $-40\,^oC$, and there is scatter about this temperature, suggesting stochastic processes. Droplets containing foreign matter (seeds) freeze above $-40\,^oC$, with freezing temperatures varying for substance and droplet size.

Freezing of droplets can be explained on statistical bases. Water molecules in thermal agitation may come into temporary alignment, similar to an ice crystal. Such molecular aggregates may grow, but also be destroyed by random molecular motion. If an aggregate happens to grow to such a size that it is immune to thermal agitation, the whole droplet freezes quickly. The existence of a foreign seed particle makes initial growth of the aggregate more probable, by attracting a surface layer of water molecules on which ice crystals form more readily than in the interior of the droplet. Freezing of the droplet only requires that an aggregate reach critical size, and, therefore, the probability of freezing increases with volume. The probability that at least one foreign particle is present in the assembly also increases with volume, and so, freezing temperature also depends markedly on the volume.

Table 6. Globally Average Temperatures (24 month running average departures)

Year	LANL ΔT (^oC)	Average ΔT (^oC)
1979	0.014	0.014
1980	0.032	0.034
1981	0.052	0.054
1982	-0.001	0.001
1983	-0.016	-0.012
1984	-0.121	-0.110
1985	-0.152	-0.138
1986	-0.164	-0.152
1987	-0.084	-0.071
1988	0.078	0.085
1989	0.059	0.068
1990	-0.043	0.033
1991	-0.003	-0.002
1992	-0.186	-0.156
1993	-0.191	-0.158
1994	-0.117	-0.092
1995	-0.121	-0.094
1996	0.005	0.010
1997	0.218	0.239
1998	0.240	0.254
1999	0.097	0.129
2000	0.054	0.079
2001	0.152	0.189
2002	0.149	0.188
2003	0.130	0.179
2004	0.132	0.180
2005	0.128	0.139
2006	0.092	0.136
2007	0.012	0.129
2008	-0.005	0.085
2009	-0.096	0.009

Suspended solid and liquid particles are present in the atmosphere in enormous numbers, and their concentration rates vary by several orders of magnitude. Sizewise, suspended particles range from 0.005 μm up to some 20 μm in radius. These particles play a crucial role in freezing and condensation processes in clouds. Additionally, suspended particles participate in chemical processes, influence electrical properties of the atmosphere, and, in large concentrations, may be annoying and dangerous.

Clouds experiencing strong updrafts act as electrostatic generators, with the upward moving air carrying small positively charged particles, and the falling precipitation carrying negatively charged particles. Experiments have shown that a separation of charge occurs at the interface between water and ice, or between ice surfaces with temperature and contaminant differences. Upward supercooled water droplets collide with downward soft hail, creating a temperature gradient, and ultimately charge separation in upward and downward moving components of the cloud. Charge separation induces an electrostatic potential, with propensity for discharge from cloud to cloud, or cloud to Earth.

Lightning discharges accompany sufficient buildup of charge density, ρ, across droplets and hail to establish a breakdown electrostatic potential. The rate of charging per unit volume, i, is related to the concentrations of droplets, n, and pellets, N, the collisional efficiency, ε, the relative velocity between pellet and droplet, u, and the pellet radius, r, by,

$$i = \frac{d\rho}{dt} = \pi \varepsilon r^2 nuNe,$$

with e the charge separated per collision. When sufficient charge has separated in time, with electrostatic fields near 30×10^3 *volts/cm*, a breakdown (lightning discharge) occurs, with a total charge transferred in the 20 *coul* range. A thunderstorm of 75 km^3 can build up such a charge separation in about 15 *sec*.

Evaporation of water from land areas maximizes in the tropical zones, but at all latitudes, precipitation exceeds evaporation. Because water vapor stored in the atmosphere is relatively constant over long periods of time, there must be net transport of water from the oceans to the land masses by the atmosphere. Water is effectively transported from the subtropical oceans to the middle latitudes by winds. Similarly, the net radiation absorbed by the atmosphere must be transported to higher latitudes by ocean and wind currents. But because the energy absorbed in the oceans is less than half the total absorbed by Earth and atmosphere, and because the mass of the oceans is more than 100 times the mass of the atmosphere, more heat is carried Poleward by winds than ocean currents. The study of winds which transport heat and moisture Poleward is an interesting one, but not amenable to discussion here. Instead, we merely point out that the hydrosphere and atmosphere are two thermodynamic engines, operating somewhat differently. For the atmospheric engine, the primary heat source may be regarded as tropical land and water surfaces, and the primary heat sink is the upper part of the water vapor atmosphere. In transporting thermal energy from sources to sinks, potential energy of the system tends to decrease with corresponding increase in kinetic energy (winds). For the hydrospheric engine, on the other hand, the primary source is the tropical ocean surface, and the primary sink is the polar ocean. Because source and sink in the hydrospheric engine are at the same geopotential, only weak fluid motions (compared to atmospheric flows) are expected.

Meteorology

The ancient Greeks viewed weather phenomena as the result of the mutual interactions of the four elements, namely fire, air, water, and earth in the four contraries, specifically hot, cold, moist, and dry. Today, the study of individual processes is atmospheric physics, whereas the study of resulting weather conditions, such as temperature, winds, cloudiness, pressure, precipitation, tornadoes, hurricanes (vorticity), frontal systems, and cyclones, is considered meteorology. Prevailing weather conditions at a geographical location is the focus of climatology. Biometeorology is the study of the impact of weather on plants, animals, and humans. Micrometeorology is the study of small scale meteorological phenomena close to the surface of the Earth. Satellite meteorology involves the use of airborne satellites to monitor weather conditions, both on the Earth and other planets. Environmental meteorology is concerned with the impact of weather on the environment. Today, a worldwide network of weather reporting stations (World Weather Watch), under the auspices of the World Meteorological Organization Of The United Nations, exchanges routine weather observations via high speed communications links. The United States network is part of the National Weather Service of the National Oceanographic and Atmospheric Administration (NOAA).

Since 1963, at over 5,000 stations and aboard ships at sea, trained observers (meteorological technicians) routinely make weather observations at *synoptic*, or synchronized, times, actually at 0000, 0600, 1200, and 1800 Greenwich Mean Time (GMT). Weather variables are observed, estimated, or measured exactly. These meteorological variables include:

- temperature (thermometer);
- moisture content (hygrometer);
- atmospheric pressure (barometer);
- horizontal wind motion (anemometer);
- visibility (transmissometer);
- cloud types (visual);
- cloud bases (ceilometer);
- rainfall (rain gauge);
- aerosols, dust, and smog (lidar, radar, and sodar);
- radiation (alpha, beta, and gamma detectors);
- snow depth (visual);
- ground temperature (thermometer).

and others, depending on location. At some 650 stations, at synoptic times of 0000 and 1200 GMT, the free atmosphere is probed with helium filled weather balloons, ascending at controlled rates to an altitude of approximately 30 *km*. Each balloon contains an instrument package containing pressure, temperature, and humidity sensors connected to a radio transmitter. As the balloon ascends, fairly constant signals for the three variables are transmitted at specific frequency. Knowing the balloon ascent rate, and measuring the balloon elevation angle and compass direction, the motion of the balloon can be used to fix wind velocities and directions at various heights. Information is transmitted from the balloon radio on wind soundings (rawinsondes) only on the way up. The balloon will subsequently burst at high altitude and fall back to Earth. Since instruments are generally not recovered, these experiments are costly, and only wealthier nations perform them. Constant level balloons (tetroons) are also employed, and are monitored by remote satellites. Rocket powered instrument packages (rocketsondes) are often fired to heights of 60 *km*, with parachutes deployed at the top of the trajectory to afford constant measuring instrument descent rate.

Commercial aircraft are also instrumented to measure elevation, pressure, temperature, and flight level winds. Aircraft reports (AIREPS) are routinely made at mandatory reporting positions, especially over oceans, and relayed into the weather communication network. Reconnaissance of severe storms and analysis of radioactive particles in the upper atmosphere complement weather data gathering duties of commercial aircraft.

New observational instruments and techniques are evolving rapidly, as a consequence of advances in space technology, computers, communications, electro-optical sensors, and related hardware and software. Conventional and direct measurements of atmospheric properties are being supplemented by remote sensing devices, utilizing active and passive signals from both Earthbound and space platforms.

Active remote sensing systems include radar, lidar, and sodar. Radar is most frequently employed in synoptic observation. Radar consists of high frequency radio waves (.1 *cm* to 10 *cm* wavelength range) which penetrate clouds, but are reflected by precipitation. These microwaves probe the evolution, motion, and structure of precipitation patterns at distances out to several hundred kilometers. Lidar is similar to radar, but uses laser beams, instead of microwaves. Lidar beams are very narrow, and can detect microscopic particulates, aerosols, and dust in the atmosphere. Lidars can even probe turbulent areas with temperature fluctuations. The useful range of lidars, however, is only a few kilometers. Sodars are acoustical devices that emit periodic sound waves. Sound waves, or beeps, are reflected off regions of turbulent temperature fluctuations, providing useful measurements of the thickness of friction surface layers and the diffusive penetration of pollants in urban environments.

Passive remote sensing systems are most commonly placed on orbiting and geostationary satellites. Photographs from satellites are taken with ordinary visible light, showing cloud patterns, water areas, mountains, vegetation, and snow cover, to name a few. Infrared radiometer instruments take pictures day and night. The amount of infrared radiation recorded is a measure of the temperature of the radiating surface, either ground or clouds, thus providing a means to estimate vertical and horizontal temperature of the atmosphere and ocean surface. Other passive measurements from satellites include water vapor, carbon dioxide, ozone, and aerosol content.

Remote sensing brings added dimension to meteorology. Billions of meteorological data entries can be easily processed by high speed digital computers, and made readily available to research and forecast centers in record time. From satellites come global views which show weather patterns in areas so remote that conventional observations have never been made before. From ground or airborne platforms, small scale phenomena can be probed with ever increasing accuracy.

Though the World Weather Watch of participating nations has developed an excellent network for exchanging meteorological information and observations, the fact remains that these measurements are crude and widely separated in time and space. Observational networks are not sufficiently dense to resolve weather phenomena smaller than approximately 500 *km*, and existing computational techniques have difficulty with small scale details, such as fronts, tornadoes, squalls, and small hurricanes. Forecasts beyond a few days are complex, and often fraught with increasing error. Presently, weather forecasts over the Northern Hemisphere and tropics maintain considerable integrity for periods up to 48 *hr*, for weather systems with dimensions in the 1,000 *km* size range (large cyclones and anticyclones). However, small scale features embedded in these systems may cause hour to hour weather variations that are difficult to predict accurately with any degree of skill. The exact location of highly significant weather phenomena, such as severe thunderstorms and tornadoes, heavy snow, sleet, and damaging winds, cannot be predicted accurately beyond a few hours time frame.

For periods of up to 5 days, daily temperature and precipitation forecasts, with moderate accuracy and usefulness, are possible. For periods of 5 days to a month, average temperature only can be predicted with slight accuracy, while skill in predicting precipitation is even slighter. For periods of more than a month, accuracy in seasonal and climate forecasts is minimal. In the Southern Hemisphere, due to reduced number and density of meteorological observations, weather forecasting is less reliable than in the Northern Hemisphere.

All forecasting depends on modern computing technology and robust platforms. The impact of supercomputing on atmospheric and ocean circulation modeling, data collection and analysis, and statistical correlation has been immense.

Geosciences

Geophysics in its broadest sense includes the study of the physical processes and properties of the atmosphere and hydrosphere, as well as solid Earth. Atmospheric physics, meteorolgy, oceanography, and hydrology are branches of geophysics. The branches of solid Earth geophysics include seismology, geodesy, gravitation, geomagnetism and electrodynamics, rheology, and high pressure and temperature physics. Marine geophysics is a subdivision concerned with the properties of the Earth beneath the ocean. Obviously, Earth physics overlaps with geology, chemistry, crystallography, and mineralogy.

The scope of geophysics is immense, but only a tiny segment of cosmology. Gazing out at the sky, one sees scattered points of light in an otherwise dark infinity. Clusters of these points are separated by large distances containing virtually nothing. These points of light, of course, are stars, galaxies, and clusters of galaxies. Galaxies themselves are massive, often more than 100,000 light years across. Millions of galaxies have already been photographed. Closest to Earth, the Andromeda Galaxy is 1,800,000 light years away, as mentioned. If the Universe is infinite, and many suggest that, an infinite number of galaxies is probable.

Galaxies are separated into types, depending on their viewed or perceived shape. Some are spiral, elliptical, barred, and irregular. Our Milky Way Galaxy looks like a whirling roman candle from the top and a wagon wheel from the side, and is 100,000 light years in diameter. Looking out toward the center of the Milky Way on a clear night, Earth observers will note the very dense band of stars filling the skis bandwise, simply the result of viewing space through the Milky Way.

Our Sun, one of the stars of the Milky Way, is not large, more medium sized, and is classified as a Type G star, based on its surface temperature of 6,000 ^oC and composition of mainly hydrogen and helium, serving to fuel thermonuclear burn (fusion) processes. Carbon and nitrogen are also found in appreciable amounts. While viewing these points of light in the sky, observers 400 *yr* ago noted that many of them moved rapidly, while the preponderance remained fixed. Some moving points can be seen with the naked eye, and represent planets, asteroids, and a few comets. Nine planets, Mercury, Venus, Earth, Mars, Jupiter, Saturn, Uranus, Neptune, and Pluto comprise the Solar System, along with much smaller asteroids, such as Ceres.

Earth is the third planet from the Sun, moving with an orbital speed of some 75,000 *mi/hr*, and with solar elliptical (orbit) apogee and perigee of 105 and 102 million miles. From the Moon, 1/81 the mass of Earth and orbiting the Earth every 27 days, the Earth looks like a patchwork of white, blue, and green, due to the predominance of water on the planet. Other planets possess some water, but only in solid phase, ice. Against this cosmological background of immense proportions, the Sun, Moon, and Earth rotate in three body interaction.

Great decisive strides in observing (visually) planetary motions were made by Johannes Kepler in 1609, providing the springboard for later Newtonian mechanics. In *Astronomia Nova*, Kepler recorded the first two of his three laws, and, in *Harmonices Mundi*, stated the third law in 1619:

- the planets rotate about the Sun in elliptical orbits with the Sun at one foci;
- the radius vector from the Sun to a planet sweeps out equal areas in equal times;
- the period squared of planetary orbit is proportional to the third power of the elliptical semimajor axis.

The laws were, with great and skillful computational labor, drawn out of the large body of pretelescopic planetary observations of the master Tycho Brahe in Prague. Using Brahe's data, Kepler struggled with attempting to fit the planetary orbits as circles, then abandoned those attempts following diligent observations of the Martian orbit. Ovals followed with better success, but still the Mars question remained intractable. With ellipses, Kepler was able to finally quantify planetary motion about the Sun. Coupled to Newton's later gravitational synthesis, Kepler's laws stand steadfastly as the foundation stones of modern science.

Geology

Presently, the age of the Earth is estimated at 4.7 billion years, plus or minus a few million years. In that time, cosmic and terrestrial forces have shaped the surface and position of continents and oceans. Geologically, continents and ocean basins are traditionally classified separately. An ocean basin is a vast depression filled with water. A continent is defined as a vast continuous area of land. Computer analyses indicate that the relative positions of the continents, North America, South America,

Asia, Europe, Africa, Antarctica, and Australia, and oceans, Pacific, Atlantic, Indian, Arctic, and Antarctic, have only a one in fourteen chance of being randomly located. In other words, it is highly probable that physical processes have been responsible for their locations. Global plate tectonics, or mantle convection, has emerged in the last 20 years as the single theory predicting continental movement, according to Taylor and Wegener. Their theories are based on the geographical similarities of continental coast lines, bedrock age, heat flow, magnetic band structure, and sediment age and thickness, all correlated in extensive mathematical computer modeling.

With the exceptions of parts of Greenland and Antarctica, the elevations of most prominent islands and continents have been measured. The average land elevation is close to 1,300 ft above sea level. The highest elevation, Mount Everest in the Himalayas, is 29,000 ft above sea level, and the lowest elevation, the Dead Sea in Israel, is 1,300 ft below sea level. The shallowest areas of the oceans are the continental shelves, and the deepest known location is the Challenger Deep in the Mariana Trench, some 35,500 ft below the surface. The mean depth of the oceans is 12,700 ft.

The differences between ocean basins and continents extend beyond comparative topography. Significant differences in rock composition and density, sediment thickness, and related geological properties have been uncovered. One significant similarity, however, is the apparently even average heat flow emanating from both ocean basins and continents. Of course, unusual heat flow characteristics in parts of ocean basins are significant in geotheories. Emanating from the molten core of the Earth is an average heat flux in the range of 0.5×10^{-3} cal/cm^2 to 1.6×10^{-3} cal/cm^2, across continents and ocean basins.

Two descriptors for rock types, simatic and sialic, can be used to differentiate the composition of ocean and continental crust. Simatic rocks contain abundant amounts of the elements iron, magnesium, calcium, silicon, and oxygen. Sialic rocks contain mostly aluminum, potassium, silicon, and oxygen. Both contain similar amounts of sodium. The ocean basins are composed largely of simatic rock, but the continental crusts are less homogeneous, exhibiting a top layer of sialic rock mainly and an underlayer of mixed and then simatic rock. The zones between the crusts of the continents and ocean basins, like the middle layer under the continents, contain appreciable amounts of sodium, aluminum, potassium, iron, magnesium, silicon, and oxygen. These transition rock layers, with intermediate composition, are also termed andesitic rocks. Mapping the distribution of rock types on the Earth has not been a simple chore, because sampling technology has progressed slowly. The Challenger expedition in 1870 collected the first representative ocean floor samples, while the more recent Glomar Challenger expedition was able to drill more than half a mile under the ocean floor.

The continental and ocean basin crusts differ in density by some 10%. The density of the ocean basin crust is about 2.9 g/cm^3, while the average density of the continental crust is some 2.6 g/cm^3. The differences occur because oceanic crust has more iron and magnesium than the continental crust. The relative elevations of continents and ocean basins may be partly related to these density differences, simply because of Archimedes' principle.

The thickness of sediment on the upper part of the crust is highly variable. Sediments in the ocean basins range from 150 *ft* to 3,300 *ft*, while continental sediments range much deeper, from 1,500 *ft* to 9,800 *ft*. Regions where crystalline rock has formed by the cooling of molten material may have no sediment cover. Thickest sediments are found in mountain ranges, like the Rocky Mountains, and in coastal basins, like the lower Mississippi River delta. Drilling and seismic mapping (comparison of sound speed propagation) are the principal means of measuring sediment cover.

Plate Tectonics

A bold theory explaining the origin of ocean basins, and many other geological features of the Earth, emerged in the 1960s, spawning a scientific revolution in geophysics. Called plate tectonics, the theory postulated continental movement on separate mantle-buoyant blocks, or plates. Before 1962, many geologists rejected the idea that continents move, and that the sizes of present ocean basins have changed. Taylor and Wegener proposed mantle convection in 1910, suggesting that movement had occurred, and basing theories on geographical similarities of continental coast lines. In 1963, Matthews and Vine suggested that sea floor spreading might also be occurring, and could be tested by analyzing the magnetic properties of the mid ocean ridges. It is now known that the polarity of the magnetic field of the Earth changes every million years, or so, as recorded in the magnetite of cooled magma making its way up into the crust regions of ocean ridges. Correlating these facts and others, Le Pichon proposed a global plate tectonics model in 1968, which we sketch qualitatively.

For simplicity, the crust of the Earth is divided into six major plates, characteristically the Eurasian, African, Indian, American, Pacific, and Antarctic, as shown in Figure 9. Continents are attached to each of these plates, plates float on the mantle of the Earth, and are free to move around with respect to each other, subject to combined terrestrial, lunar, and solar forces. Plates range in thickness from 43 *miles* to 62 *miles*. In the region of the mid ocean ridges, plates are separating and new crustal rock is moving up to the surface. In trenches, plates are colliding, with one plate sinking down into the mantle. Plates may also slide against each other, such as along California where the Pacific and American plates rub down the San Andreas fault.

Three mechanisms, and combinations, could allow plates to move. Large convection cells, caused by heating deep in the mantle, rise into the mid ocean ridges and sink into the trenches. As plates run over each other, the lower, or sinking, plate cools the mantle causing a downward convection cell. The convection cell induces local displacement of the mantle, and a bulge elsewhere, namely in the mid ocean ridges, ultimately pushing plates apart. Lunar and solar gravitation vary across plates, depending on plate masses and positions, producing relative motion. Where plates separate, deep crustal material would move up and cool. Where plates collide, material would be broken off to drop into the hot mantle, or one plate effectively sheared by the other.

Earlier continental drift and sea floor spreading models postulated that continents and ocean basins move separately from each other, and not on independent mantle-floating plates, thus not coupled in global interaction. The plates in the tectonics model may be entirely ocean basin, like the Pacific plate, may contain ocean basin and continents, like the American plate, or may be predominately continental crust, like the Eurasian plate. It is the motion of the plate which determines continental and/or ocean basin movement, because the continents and basins are attached to the plate.

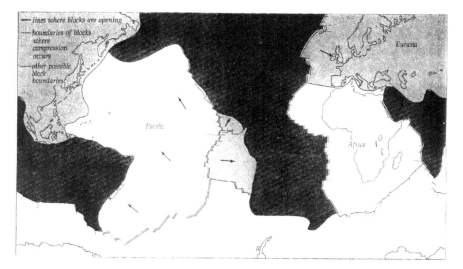

Figure 9. Mantle Plates

Le Pichon suggested the global plate tectonic model in 1968. The crust of the Earth is divided into six major plates, that is, Eurasian, African, Indian, American, Pacific, and Antarctic. Continents and ocean basins both reside on these mantle-buoyant blocks, free to move under combined terrestrial, lunar, and solar forces. Many facts support plate tectonic theories, such as matching coastlines, magnetic bands, bedrock age, sediment thickness, heat flow, earthquake foci, lithology, and fossil correlations.

A number of correlating facts supporting plate tectonic models are evident. Continental coasts and edges of continental shelves fit surprisingly well, especially for South America, Africa, and the Antarctic, as seen on almost any map. Approximately 200 million years ago, all the continents were apparently locked together in a supercontinent, called Pangea, before starting to move apart as time progressed. A simulation is shown in Figure 10, using powerful supercomputers for the reconstruction. Perhaps the most significant supporting evidence is the matching

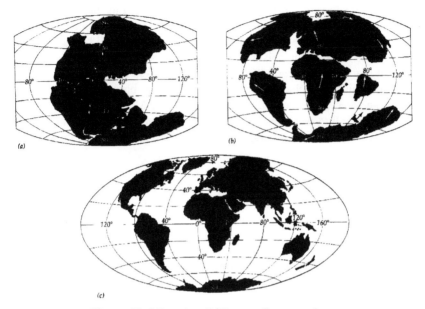

Figure 10. Migration Of Pangea Supercontinent

Some 200 million years ago, all continents were bound into one supercontinent called Pangea, as depicted below in the upper left segment (a). Plate drift and migration gradually pulled Pangea apart, with relative separation 80 million years ago indicated in the upper right segment (b). The present continental and ocean basin configuration is shown below in segment (c). Extensive computer modeling has correlated continental drift theories with Earth observables.

of magnetic band structures on opposite sides of ocean ridges, that is, inferred magnetic polarity and intensity. The reflection match shows spreading on opposite sides at the rate of 1 cm/yr in the mid Atlantic ridge, and 8 cm/yr on the East Pacific rise. At such rate, the whole present Pacific Ocean floor could have formed in less than 200 million years. Cores of bedrock obtained in scattered parts of the ocean basins are all 180 million years old or younger, with oldest found in the northest corner of the Pacific plate, far from actively spreading new crust at the East Pacific rise. The age of sediments overlying bedrock is always younger than the bedrock. Recent sediment is, of course, distributed all over the ocean basin. The thickness of the sediment, and the time span it represents, based mainly on dating of microfossils, increases progressively with distance from the axis of the mid ocean ridges. Heat flow patterns for ocean bottoms indicate low conductivity in the vicinity of trenches, and high conductivity along the ridges, tending to confirm the notion of sinking crust, or deep mantle, at the trenches and rising crust, or shallow mantle, at the ridges. Earthquake foci are located deep in trenches, and shallow in ridges, also supporting sinking and rising materials respectively. Percentages of minerals and mappings of rock fractures in eastern South America and western Africa have been correlated, and similar correlations between rocks in New England, Canada, and the British Isles have been established. Terrestrial fossil correlations between species in Africa, South America, and Antarctica also suggest that a land bridge once linked the continents, since the organisms are incapable of ocean migration.

Recent Mars probes suggest the Red Planet witnessed similar geologic evolution earlier in its history, including mantle convection and plate tectonics. Formed at roughly the same time some 4.3 billion years ago, Mars, about half Earth size, cooled very rapidly several hundred million years ago, lost its atmosphere, and is now geologically dead. Some suggest that present Mars is future Earth.

Oceans and Seawater

Oceans cover 71% of the surface of the Earth, with some 1.4×10^9 km^3 of water contained in the basins. This comprises 97% of all water on the planet, with another 2% in rivers and lakes, 0.9% in snow and glaciers, and less than 0.1% in the atmosphere. The oceans cover approximately 254×10^6 km^2 and weigh some $1,600 \times 10^{15}$ *tons*. The average depth of the oceans is about 4 *km*, but only 1/790 of the total volume of the Earth. The thin film on a basketball after being dunked in water easily represents both the oceans and atmosphere. In this thin film of water and air, exists all life known to man. And many believe all life began in the oceans. Significant elements in the development of life, namely carbon, nitrogen, oxygen, hydrogen, and phosphorous, are present on all planets. As far as we know now, life is present only on Earth. An important fact is that water is present in large amounts (in stable ocean environments for millions of years) only on the Earth. Rivers, lakes, and oceans do not exist on other planets.

Major oceans of the planet are the Pacific, Atlantic, Indian, Arctic, and Antarctic Oceans. Ocean study is oceanography, divided into geological, physical, chemical, and biological branches. The voyages and studies of the Challenger expedition in 1872 spawned the science of oceanography. HMS Challenger was the first steamship to cross the Antarctic Circle in a voyage covering some 70,000 *miles*, probably the most important single expedition ever undertaken to study the sea.

Analysis of the light spectra of the planets in the Solar System suggests that nitrogen, hydrogen, carbon, and oxygen are present on all in varying ratios, but that only Earth possesses water in relative abundance. Water is the most abundant molecule on the surface of the Earth. It is remarkable for a number of reasons. It is called the universal solvent because it dissolves more substances, more often, and in greater amounts, than any other liquid. Virtually everything dissolves in water, though solubilities vary dramatically. Water occurs in all three states, gas, liquid, and solid, and is three times more abundant than all other substances combined. Water possesses the highest surface tension and heat conductivity of all liquids, save mercury, the highest heat capacity, heat of fusion, and heat of vaporization of all common liquids and most solids, and water is virtually incompressible. Water has a relatively low viscosity, transmits sound well, and has a density of 1 gr/cm^3. Water has a profound effect on the surface of the Earth, as the primary erosive and shaping agent.

An automobile trip through our mountain chains offers spectacular views of valleys, plains, peaks, forests, and wildlife. Yet, the composition of 50% of the rocks exposed in these mountain chains contain limestone fossils deposited millions of years ago under marine conditions. Even the Himalayas contain marine fossils. The impacts of the oceans on the Earth are truly impressive, shaping the features of the topography and probably cradling life itself.

Salinity

Water comprising oceans accumulated first in the basins of the Earth, with, as mentioned, 97% of all water on the Earth covering 71% of the surface as seawater. Seawater is salty, averaging some 3.5 *lbs* of salt (mostly sodium chloride and magnesium sulfate) for every 100 *lbs* of seawater, or 3.5%. Much of the salt in the seas came, and still comes, from river runoff, and there is a very slight annual increase in salt content of seawater as rivers continue to denude continents. The buildup is slow, with about 6 million years required to increase the salt content 1%. Early oceans were probably always salty, having been dissolved out of volcanic rock in the ocean basins, and with a primordial atmosphere probably rich in chlorine and hydrogen chloride from volcanic activity. Ninety nine percent of the solid inorganic matter in seawater is chlorine, sodium, magnesium, sulfur (as sulfates), calcium, and potassium.

Ocean salinity varies from place to place. Processes such as evaporization, freezing, salt dissolution, currents, and mixing, which add salt or remove water, increase salinity. Processes that remove salt or add water, such as rain, snow, salt precipitation, runoff from rivers, melting ice, currents, mixing, and rain, decrease salinity. Of these, evaporation and precipitation are the most important. Regions of highest salinity occur where evaporation exceeds precipitation, and regions of lowest salinity occur where precipitation exceeds evaporation. Where these factors are balanced, salinity is constant. In open oceans, variance is minimal. Overall, ocean salinity lies between 3.4% and 3.7%, with some interesting exceptions. The Baltic Sea, with abundant precipitation and runoff, has the lowest salinity, near 1.2%, while the Red Sea, with little entering water and high evaporation, has the greatest salinity, between 4.0% and 4.2%. In the Gulf of Bothnia, off Finland, salinity may drop to 0.5%, while deep pockets of very salty water were found in the Red Sea, near 25%, the saturation point. The saltiest open ocean is the subtropical North Atlantic, with salinity of some 3.75%. The Pacific Ocean is less salty than the Atlantic Ocean because it is less affected by dry winds.

Only near the Poles does the formation of ice and its effect on salinity become important. Salt water under forming ice has higher salinity, because salt tends to separate out of seawater as freezing occurs. Waters in polar regions, particularly in the Antarctic, are more saline than might be expected. Of course, when ice melts, the salinity of adjacent waters decrease, with the net ocean effect averaging out over years to zero. Over time, the salinity of a large body of ocean water at specific temperature changes very slightly. Salinity is thus a conservative property of seawater.

An interesting consequence of dissolved salt in seawater is foaming inhibition. Foaming is the coalescence of many tiny bubbles. Unlike fresh water, which allows bubbles to come together, salt in seawater causes bubbles formed by churning to bounce off one another, preventing coalescence.

Ocean Temperatures

Water has a very high specific heat, warming and cooling very slowly. Ocean water, and the massive amount of heat received as solar radiation, controls most of the climate of the Earth. As massive heat sinks, the oceans can be divided into three layers for temperature characterization, namely, surface, thermocline, and deep, as seen in Figure 11. Surface and deep temperatures vary least, thermocline layer temperatures vary the most. Overall, temperature range with ocean depth is smaller than might be expected, from $-2\,^oC$ to $30\,^oC$, down to 5,000 fsw. In the deep layers, below 3,000 fsw, temperatures are relatively constant and cold, approximately 5 ^oC. Variations in temperature with ocean depth are now thought to be a microstructural effect below the surface layer. Although the areas near the Poles are quite different in actual temperature from areas on the Equator, the regions are similar in profile.

In the deep layer, below 200 to 1,000 m, the water temperature is very uniform and quite cold. No other place on Earth possesses such a narrow temperature range. The total ocean has a temperature range of -2 to $30\,^oC$, a much smaller range than the atmosphere, but at depth even this temperature range is narrowed. The hottest surface temperature of any ocean waters occurs in the Persian Gulf, as high as 36^oC ($96.8\,^oF$) nearshore in the summer. The hot, salty, deep regions of the Red Sea exhibit temperatures as high as 56 ^oC ($132.8\,^oF$) at depths near 2,000 m. Geothermal intrusions, emanating from fractures along ocean rifts, apparently are the cause.

Ocean Currents

The existence of surface currents in the oceans has long been known by mariners, though difficult to see. Early sailors probably first noted them by differences in course attempted and course made. The commanders of Spanish galleons in the Fifteenth and Sixteenth centuries not only knew of prevailing winds in the Atlantic to take advantage for passage, but also the prevailing currents that existed in the sea. Ponce de Leon described the Florida Current in 1513. Benjamin Franklin had a chart of the Gulf Stream drawn to improve the speed of mail delivery between Europe and the Colonies. He made numerous temperature measurements and water color observations on his many trips across the Atlantic to help plot dominant current patterns.

Unlike waves, which at sea cause no water transport, ocean currents do move large volumes of water and mix many layers. The currents described by the Spanish are virtually unchanged today. If the ocean currents are fixed, then so too must be the source of these currents, the wind, noted Edmund Halley (of comet fame) in the late 1600s. Indeed the wind patterns are also fixed.

In the Northern Hemisphere, ocean circulation is clockwise, bringing warm water up from the Tropics on the eastern sides of continents, and cold water down from the polar regions on the western sides. In the Southern Hemisphere, the circulation pattern is reversed, with the same effects on eastern and western sides of continents. These rotational patterns of the ocean flows, and corresponding cyclonic wind patterns, are due to Coriolis forces associated with Earth rotation. And all weather (and associated wind patterns) result from the heating action of solar radiation, particularly in the oceanic basins.

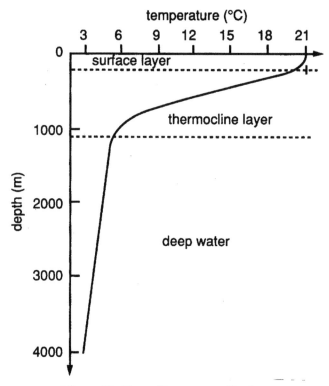

Figure 11. Ocean Temperature Gradient

Average ocean temperature gradients are depicted below. In the surface and deep layers, temperatures are fairly constant. In thermocline layers, temperature gradients (changes) are the largest. Average ocean temperatures obviously decrease with depth. Absorbed solar radiation supplies most of the heat to the oceans. Seasonal variations are the least at the Equator, and greatest in the polar regions.

Although prevailing winds seem unlikely causes of oceanic circulation, because of the perceived variability of winds, such is actually the case. All weather, more correctly climate, results from the heating action of the Sun, causing regions of high and low atmospheric pressure and all winds and storms. Because the relative position of the Earth and Sun does not change from year to year, the heating, and therefore the climate and winds are similar from year to year. With some local variations, the seasonal weather patterns are mostly predictable. The horizontal wind patterns for the globe, that is, the prevailing atmospheric circulations at sea level have been constant for a long time, as seen in Figure 12.

Because the rotation of the Earth piles waters (a few *cm*) on the western edges of the oceans, different types of ocean currents are produced. These surface currents are divided into three categories, namely, Eastern Boundary, Western Boundary, and Equatorial Currents, shown in Figure 13. Currents are connected of course, in that they are all segments of the basic circular (Coriolis) flow patterns in ocean basins due to the rotation of the Earth.

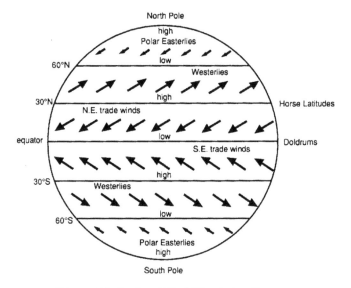

Figure 12. Surface Wind Circulation Patterns

Like ocean currents, wind patterns on the globe follow established pathways. Their relative orientations and directions, like the ocean currents they often drive, have remained the same for centuries. In the simplest sense, wind patterns develop because of unequal heating of various parts of the Earth by the Sun, causing high and low pressure systems in the atmosphere, moving as disturbances in easterly fashion.

Eastern Boundary Currents occur on the east side of oceans (west side of continents), and water runs from the Poles to the Equator. Western Boundary Currents occur on the west side of oceans (east side of continents), and water runs from the Equator to the Poles. Eastern Boundary Currents are slow, about 10 *cm/sec*, and are not deep, maybe near 500 *m*, but they are wide. Western Boundary Currents are opposite, narrow, deep (near 1,000 *m* or better), fast (several *knots*), and move much ocean water around the globe. The Gulf Steam is a well know and studied Western Boundary Current, formed by the confluence of the Gulf Current, Florida Current, and North Atlantic Current. The amount of water flowing in the Gulf Stream is enormous, some 4×10^9 *tons/min*.

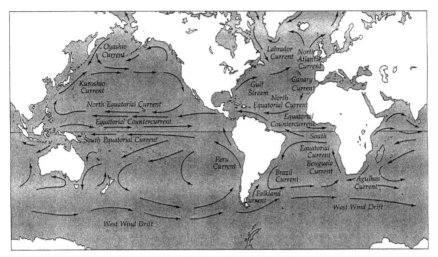

Figure 13. Surface Ocean Circulation

Prevailing winds actually drive global ocean surface circulation. Circulation is clockwise in the Northern Hemisphere and counterclockwise in the Southern Hemisphere. Ocean currents have remained the same for recorded centuries, as determined from marine records and numerous logs over that time span.

Equatorial Currents are also permanent and well established. Like Eastern Boundary Currents, they are slow (0.5 to 1 *knots*), fairly shallow (less than 500 *m*), and wide. There is some seasonal variation to Equatorial Currents, the entire set moving northward in the summer. The South Equatorial Current lies below the Equator, and runs east to west. The Equatorial Countercurrent lies above the Equator, and runs west to east.

Zones

Environments are classified by whatever variable is perceived as significant, albeit physical, chemical, or biological variables. The most common variables for classifying marine environments are depth and light penetration. Four major zones are referenced within these categories, namely littoral, sublittoral, euphotic, and aphotic. Broad characteristics are as follow.

The littoral zone is the area along the shoreline between high and low tide, the most variable and rigorous in the marine environment. Tidal fluctuations produce submarine and subaerial conditions. Waves and longshore currents cause constant movement. Geologic characteristics are also subject to rapid alteration. Human pressure in this zone is very high. And the combinations of all induce major fluctuations in chemical conditions. Water and air temperatures in this zone are close, and fluctuate widely. Ecological relationships between organisms, substrates, and physical and chemical conditions are most complex, a major problem of subtle changes inducing very largescale consequences. The major intertidal environments are rocky shores, sandy beaches, and muddy bays and estuaries.

The sublittoral zone consists of the bottom extending from the low tide area at the shoreline to the edge of the continental shelf (about 200 *m* on average). Physical conditions are determined mainly by the geologic substrate, and by possible wave action and currents. Chemical conditions are largely stable. Temperature at a particular sublittoral area remain constant, except in regions of upwelling where variations of 5 ^oC are possible. Sublittoral temperatures in different geographical regions vary from –2 ^oC in the Arctic to 30 ^oC in the Red Sea. The geology of the zone is as varied as the geology of the continents. Plant and animal life are the most varied and abundant on Earth in this zone.

The euphotic zone is the part of the ocean water and nearshore bottom exposed to solar radiation, especially visible light. Sunlight may penetrate to a depth of 200 *m*. Penetration depth depends on cloud cover, angle of inclination of sunlight to ocean surface, amount of suspended inorganic material, and the population density of planktonic organisms. All life in the ocean depends on sunlight as an energy source. Algae are the most common organisms, and the most essential for the survival of other organisms. Solar energy is used by all plants in photosynthesis to produce carbohydrates, proteins, and lipids that are metabolized by other organisms (animal) in a symbiotic loop. In this zone, sunlight, carbon dioxide, and water are readily available for these processes. Oxygen, a byproduct of photosynthesis, is, of course, essential for animal respiration. Estimates of the amount of oxygen produced by marine plants range from 50% to 90% of the oxygen produced by all plants.

The aphotic zone lies below the maximum depth of sunlight penetration. There is no sharp nor consistent border between euphotic and aphotic zones. The transition may occur at depths anywhere from 100 *m* to 400 *m*, depending on biological, geological, chemical, and physical factors. Physical, chemical, and geological conditions in the aphotic zone vary slowly compared to the continental shelf. Water density increases with depth, but mixing is moderate. The deep zone is known to have lower concentrations of oxygen and carbonate. Temperatures also decrease with depth in slow fashion, with a typical bottom temperature of about 1.6 ^oC. Silicate reactions buffer all chemistry to maintain deep water *pH*. The aphotic zone is not, as many once believed, devoid of life. Three major living modes exist in the zone, namely benthic organisms on, or near, the bottom, wide ranging swimmers which eat surface detritus, and fish predators like giant squid and sharks. Life in the aphotic zone is tightly coupled to life forms in the euphotic zone.

Ocean Trenches and Island Arcs

An interesting feature of the ocean basins are island arcs, because a majority of the active volcanoes are located within them. As the name suggests, the overall pattern of island groups is an arc, and the most common island shape is roughly circular (the result of volcanism). And most often, the concave side of island arcs face a continent, and the convex sides face an ocean basin. Arcs are usually located near the outer edges of a continental shelf, and generally have deep trenches on the oceanic (convex) side. The general pattern oceanward includes the continent, a shallow sea, volcanic island, a trench, and then ocean basin. Geographically, most of the island-trench systems fringe the Pacific, or separate the Pacific from the Indian Ocean, as seen in Figure 14. Exceptions include the West Indies, separating the Caribbean from the Atlantic Ocean, and the South Sandwich Islands at the tip of South America. In the Indo-Pacific province, the Aleutian Islands, Kuril Islands, Japan, Ryukyu Islands, Phillipine Islands, and Malay Archipelago are examples of arc-trench complexes. This distribution is called the *Ring Of Fire* because of active volcanism in the crust of the Earth in trench regions. Rarely is there a year without a spectacular eruption of molten rock, lava flow, clouds of water vapor, and fiery explosions.

Trenches on the convex sides closely parallel the arcuate shape, and are usually named after the island chains they border. Rarely wider than 130 *km*, trenches may be 1,500 *km* long and 10,000 *km* deep. As mentioned, the deepest spot in the oceans is the Mariana Trench, approximately halfway between Guam and the Marianas Islands and Yap and the Carolinas Islands of the western Pacific Ocean. If Mount Everest were placed into the Mariana Trench, the Pacific Ocean would still tower some 2,000 *ft* above it. The bathyscaphe *Trieste*, under Picard and a USN Officer, photographed ripple marks and the tracks and trails of organisms, indicating the presence of currents and oxygen even at great depth in the Mariana Trench.

To explain movement in the crust of the Earth, geologists postulate that mantle materials are near the surface at ridges, suggesting that rocks are found on mid ocean ridges due to mantle crust mixing, that hot material is close to the surface in these areas, and that the distribution of mass is uneven. Volcanic activity is a type of crustal material movement. Gravimeters (pendulums, actually) measure the pull of gravity at any point on the surface of the Earth, and can be used to map the density of surface regions. Over trenches, mass deficiencies relative to surrounding substrates have been catalogued, while mass overloadings of denser material has been found over the islands near the trenches. The island arc region is therefore out of mass balance. An appreciable percentage of earthquakes occurring in the crust are located in the vicinity of arc-trenches. The quakes are usually deep focus, occurring at depths beyond 70 *km* relative to the crust surface (ocean bottom). The crustal imbalance suggested by gravity anomalies and mass imbalance may be partly responsible for the quakes, as earthquakes are shock waves emanating from Earth crust and plate movements. Another possibility is that sinking of crust in the ocean basin causes both gravity anomalies and earthquakes. Because ocean waters cover much of the earthquake (arc-trench) zones, tsunamis frequently originate in the area. A cross section through the island arc system shows the following characteristics:

- the continent slopes normally to the shoreline;
- the continental shelf is composed of sediments from 200 *m* to 1,000 *m* thick; and has some organic reefs in tropical zones;
- volcanic islands;
- trenches;
- decrease in the thickness of crust seaward.

When the origin points of earthquakes (foci) are superimposed on the island arc system, a pattern emerges, as schematized in Figure 15. The shallowest foci are located beneath the trenches, and become progressively deeper toward the continent. A region seaward is relatively free of quakes. The graph of foci is a curved plane extending from the trench to the continent.

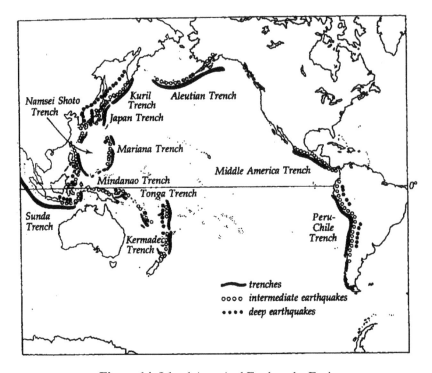

Figure 14. Island Arcs And Earthquake Foci

Island arcs are exciting because a majority of volcanoes reside there. When earthquake foci are superimposed on the arc system, a pattern emerges, as depicted in Figure 15. These foci are usually deep, occurring at depths greater than 75 km below the surface of the Earth.

The mechanisms of ocean trenches and island arcs can be seen in Figure 16. Because magma rises to the surface forming volcanoes, the source of magma must be underneath, probably originating near the intersection of the vertical line descending from the volcano and the zone of the quake foci. This is supported by seismic measurements in the region of intersection, where low velocity seismic waves indicate low density rock (less dense than liquids in general). Some believe the rock is plastic, that is, capable of flowing. Further analysis suggests that the rocks are responding to crustal changes, instead of rigid shifting.

Heat flow emanating from the rocks under trenches is quite low, similar to the flow found in abyssal plains (0.5 to 1.6 $mcal/cm^2$). Near island arcs, heat flow is roughly twice that found in trenches. Although predictable, the general heat flow pattern around the islands is less than might be expected considering the proximity of magma. Apparently, magma is localized at depth and flows to the surface in relatively narrow channels, minimizing heat transfer to surrounding rocks.

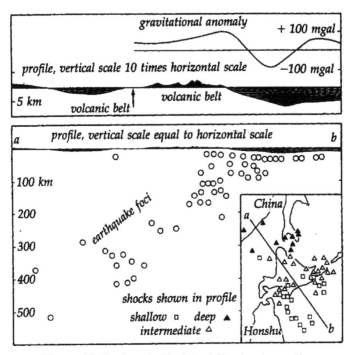

Figure 15. Earthquake Foci And Gravity Anomalies

To explain movements in the Earth's crust, geologists postulate that the mass distribution is uneven. To measure mass density, gravimeters are employed. Over trenches and over island arcs, positive and negative gravity anomalies have been tagged, indicating a mass imbalance. Crustal imbalances around island arcs probably support earthquakes and shock wave propagation.

Ocean Ridges

The mid ocean ridge system is a major submarine topographical feature first charted in 1928 by Kober. Ridges with islands like Hawaii have been known for 200 *yr*, but the discovery of relatively continuous systems extending along ocean bottoms surprised marine scientists. That information was the first step in a revolution of geological thought, culminating in the described tectonic plate theory. A major map of ocean ridges is seen in Figure 17.

Of the shallow earthquakes that occur in the crust, many occur in oceanic ridges. These shallow explosions all occur at depths less than 70 *km* below the surface of the Earth, contrasting with the foci of quakes beneath trenches (all below 70 *km* in depth). Both foci suggest that Earth movements cause the quake, somewhere near the relative surface and with relative surface mass imbalances.

The mineral composition of mid ocean ridges is quite similar. Rocks on Iceland are more similar to rocks on the Pacific-Antarctic ridge than to rocks on Greenland. Generally, rocks are simatic and contain appreciable amounts of iron, magnesium, silicon, and oxygen. Very little sediment has accumulated on ridges or valleys. This seems to indicate that ridge formation is recent, during the last 20 million years or so. Sediment, containing volcanic ash mainly and nothing derived from continents, is a few to 250 *m* thick. Ridges contain mostly young rocks compared to the continents.

Characteristic to most ridges is a rift valley (except the East Pacific rise). Rift valleys have relatively steep sides, flat bottoms, and typically range 200 *m* to 1,000 *m* in depth. Continental cousins can be seen in the Imperial Valley (California) and the East African Valley. They are caused by faulting in which the central block drops with respect to the flanking blocks. The cause of this drop is a tensional force component exerted by the flanking blocks, as seen in Figure 18. Slicing these ridges at approximately right angles are transform faults, indicating that sliding has occurred relative to the north and south sides, with displacements between 10 *km* and 100 *km*. The highest heat flow rates in ocean basins are found in rocks on mid ocean ridges, suggesting that hot material is relatively close to the surface in these areas.

Measurements of the magnetism on both sides of ocean ridges suggested, as detailed earlier, that sea floor spreading was occurring in the region around ocean ridges. Bands of rock with the same magnetic signatures occur as mirror images on both sides of the ocean ridge, with youngest rock closest to the ridge and oldest rock farthest from the ridge zone. These bands exhibit the phenomenon of Pole reversal in the magnetic field of the Earth. Density measurements suggest that low density mantle type material exist near the surface of ridges, and that rocks from the mantle merge with rocks from the crust in upward convective mixing.

Epochal Panoramas

Panoramas of chemical, biological, and geological development in the oceans are schematized in Figures 19–21. Figure 19 depicts ocean chemical cycles (4) globally impacting life on Earth. Figure 20 traces marine animal evolution on geological time scales. Figure 21 offers a taxonomic snapshot of marine life. Interplay, diversity, timescale, and complexity are boundless.

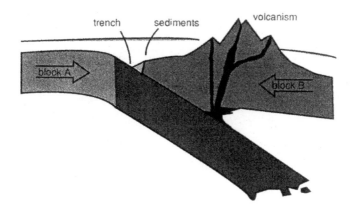

Figure 16. Plate Collision

In regions of trenches, plates are colliding, with one plate sinking down into the mantle, or crumpling into a mountain range. Earthquakes of deep origin are often noted along colliding plate borders, especially along sliding fault zones, such as the San Andreas Fault in California.

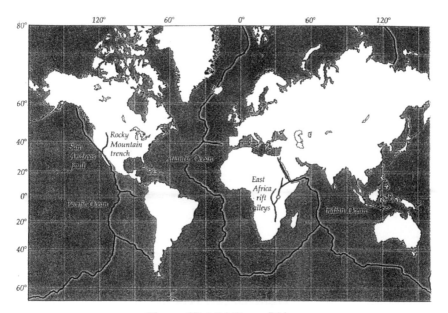

Figure 17. Mid-Ocean Ridges

The mid ocean ridge system is a major submarine topographic feature charted in 1928 by Kober. Ridges with islands, like Hawaii, have been known for 200 years. But the existence of a continuous, linear system of ocean ridges startled marine geologists.

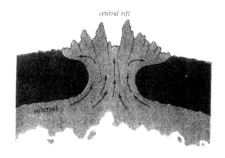

Figure 18. Plate Spreading

In mid ocean ridges, plates separate and new crustal rock moves up into the separation zone. Sea floor spreading is supported by the marching bands of alternating magnetic intensity and polarity on opposite sides of ocean ridges.

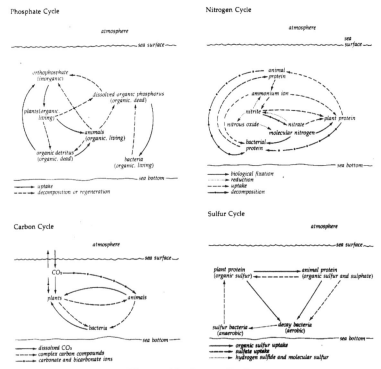

Figure 19. Ocean Cycles.

Life on this planet depends crucially on four chemical cycles, the phosphate, nitrogen, carbon, and sulfur ocean cycles.

Time Unit Began (years ago)	Era or Eon	System or Period	Epoch	Apex Marine Predators
0.01×10^6		Quaternary	Holocene	whales, sharks
10^6		Quaternary	Pleistocene	
10×10^6	Cenozoic	Neogene	Pliocene	
25×10^6	Cenozoic	Neogene	Miocene	
40×10^6		Tertiary — Paleogene	Oligocene	
60×10^6		Paleogene	Eocene	
70×10^6		Paleogene	Paleocene	
130×10^6		Cretaceous		reptiles
180×10^6	Mesozoic	Jurassic		
230×10^6		Triassic		
270×10^6		Permian		
310×10^6		Pennsylvanian		
350×10^6		Mississippian		
400×10^6	Paleozoic	Devonian		placoderms
440×10^6		Silurian		eurypterids, cephalopods
500×10^6		Ordovician		trilobites
600×10^6		Cambrian		
3.5×10^9	Cryptozoic			dominant form unknown
$\sim 4.5 \times 10^9$	Azoic			none

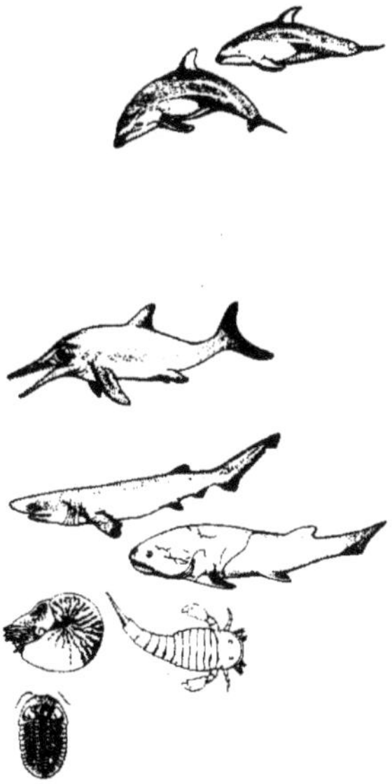

Figure 20. Marine And Geological Time Scales

Developments in oceans and on land span millenniums as far as changes in lifeforms, as contrasted below. Marine and geological epochs are charted across some 4.5 billion years of evolution.

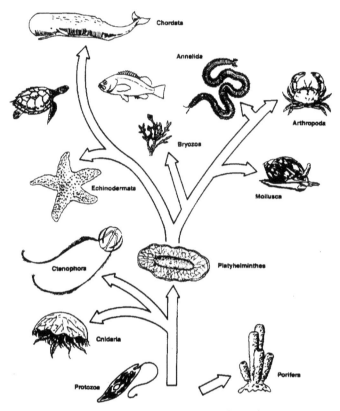

Figure 21. Marine Taxonomy Snapshot

Some well known marine organisms are classified below. Biological taxonomy is a science of very close observations and contrasts.

Keyed Exercises

- *Mark the following statements TRUE or FALSE.*

T	*F̲*	*Rocks on Iceland are similar to rocks on Greenland.*
T̲	*F*	*Simatic rocks contain iron, magnesium, silicon, and oxygen.*
T	*F̲*	*Ocean basins are mainly sialic rock.*
T̲	*F*	*Thickest sediments are found in mountain ranges.*
T̲	*F*	*Once, all continents were bound together in a supercontinent.*
T	*F̲*	*In the Northern Hemisphere, ocean circulation is counterclockwise.*
T̲	*F*	*Prevailing winds are the cause of ocean currents.*
T	*F̲*	*Planets rotate about the Sun in circular orbits.*
T̲	*F*	*Satellite measurements suggest the lower atmosphere is cooling.*
T̲	*F*	*Global temperatures today are at their lowest levels in millions of years.*
T	*F̲*	*The surface of the Earth is divided into 12 plates.*

_T_	F	_Water is virtually incompressible._
_T_	F	_Earthquakes are often noted along colliding plate borders._
T	_F_	_All planets possess water in abundance._
_T_	F	_The HMS Challenger crossed the Antarctic Circle in 1872._
_T_	F	_Particulate matter in the atmosphere reflects sunlight._
T	_F_	_The Sun is mostly helium._
_T_	F	_The Earth is roughly 4.7 billion years old._
T	_F_	_Temperatures in the thermosphere are cold._
_T_	F	_Recent warming and cooling trends are half those of the Ice Age._
_T_	F	_Earth climate is controlled mainly by oceans._
T	_F_	_Recent temperature trends are significant against longer term century cycles._
T	_F_	_The euphotic zone receives little sunlight._
_T_	F	_Island arcs usually have deep trenches on the oceanic side._
_T_	F	_Ocean salinity averages some 3.5% of ocean water._
T	_F_	_Continents are fixed on the Earth surface._
_T_	F	_Plant and animal life are varied in the sublittoral zone._
_T_	F	_Solar flares and sunspots track statistically with warming and cooling data._
T	_F_	_Temperature monitors are most numerous in the Southern Hemisphere._
_T_	F	_Carbon dioxide levels in the Cambrian Era were very high compared to today._
_T_	F	_Water vapor has greater impact on Earth temperatures than carbon dioxide._

- _What is total heat energy, Q, emanating from the core of the Earth if the surface flux, ϕ, is 1.6×10^{-3} cal/min cm^2 and Earth radius, R, is 3959 mi?_

$$Q = 4\pi R^2 \phi, \quad \phi = 1.6 \times 10^{-3} \ cal/min \ cm^2 \times 5.7 \times 10^4 \ cm^2/min \ mi^2 = 91 \ cal/min \ mi^2$$

$$Q = 4 \times 3.14 \times 15.67 \times 10^6 \times 91 \ cal/min = 18 \times 10^9 \ cal/min = 18 \times 10^6 \ kcal/min$$

- _What is the total heat energy, S, bathing the Earth if the solar flux, σ, is 1.98 cal/min cm^2?_

$$S = \left[\frac{\sigma}{\phi}\right] Q = \left[\frac{1.98}{1.6 \times 10^{-3}}\right] \times 18 \times 10^6 \ kcal/min = 22 \times 10^9 \ kcal/min$$

Which dominates Earth's climate?

Solar Radiation

- _What is the charge rate per unit volume, i, for ice pellets of radius, r = 200 microns, moving through water droplets with relative velocity, u = 15 m/sec, at given collisional efficiency, ε = .88, for droplet and pellet densities, n = 1.4 × 10^6 m^{-3} and N = 1.2 × 10^5 m^{-3}, and charge transfer, e = 11 × 10^{-9} coul, at each collision?_

$$\varepsilon = .88, \quad n = 1.4 \times 10^6 \ m^{-3}, \quad N = 1.2 \times 10^5 \ m^{-3}, \quad e = 11 \times 10^{-9} \ coul$$

$$i = \pi \varepsilon r^2 nuNe$$

$$i = 3.1416 \times .88 \times 4 \times 10^{-8} \times 1.4 \times 10^6 \times 1.2 \times 10^5 \times 15 \times 11 \times 10^{-9} \ coul/m^3 \ sec$$

$$i = 3.07 \times 10^{-3} \ coul/m^3$$

If the rate, i, is constant over dt = 10 sec, what is the charge buildup per unit volume, dρ?

$$d\rho = idt = 3.07 \times 10^{-3} \times 10 \ coul/m^3 = 3.07 \times 10^{-2} \ coul/m^3$$

What is the force, F, on a charge, Q = 1.6 × 10^{-9} coul, separated from the cloud of size, V = 10000 m³, a distance, r = 3.5 m?

$$F = \kappa_0 \frac{qQ}{r^2}, \quad \kappa_0 = 8.91 \times 10^9 \ m/f$$

$$q = Vd\rho$$

$$F = 8.91 \times 10^9 \times \left[\frac{1.6 \times 10^{-9} \times 3.07 \times 10^2}{12.25} \right] newton = 3.57 \times 10^2 \ newton$$

What is the electric field strength, E, outside the cloud?

$$E = \frac{F}{Q} = \frac{3.57 \times 10^2}{1.6 \times 10^{-9}} \ volt/m = 2.23 \times 10^{11} \ volt/m$$

- *Match the entries in the first column with the best single entry in the second column.*

(e) Nitrogen, oxygen, argon	(a) Temperatures near 1,500 °K
(m) Troposphere	(b) Weather measurements at 0000, 0600, 1200, 1800
(i) Stratosphere	(c) Diffuse region beyond 500 *miles* upward
(k) Mesosphere	(d) Counterclockwise in Southern Hemisphere
(a) Thermosphere	(e) Over 99% of permanent atmospheric gases
(c) Magnetosphere	(f) Type G star
(l) Baltic and Red Seas	(g) Alternating magnetic bands aside ocean ridges
(f) Sun	(h) Radiation absorption by carbon dioxide and water vapor
(j) Plate tectonics	(i) Ozone absorption od ultraviolet radiation
(d) Ocean circulation	(j) Continental movement on buoyant mantle blocks
(h) Greenhouse effect	(k) Winds approaching 500 *mi/hr*
(b) Synoptic observations	(l) Lowest and highest salinities
(g) Sea floor spreading	(m) Extends 6–11 *mi* upward
(p) Atmospheric pressure systems	(n) Wide, slow, shallow flow
(n) Eastern Boundary Current	(o) Narrow, fast, deep flow
(o) Western Boundary Current	(p) Caused by solar heating
(r) Littoral Zone	(q) Sites of active volcanoes
(s) Aphotic Zone	(r) Along ocean shorelines
(q) Ocean trenches/island arcs	(s) Below maximum depth of sunlight penetration

- *What is the speed of a shallow water wave, $v_{shallow}$, propagating in depth, d = 10 fsw, across the Oso Bay flats at Corpus Christi?*

$$v_{shallow} = (gd)^{1/2} = (32 \times 10)^{1/2} \ ft/sec = 17.9 \ ft/sec$$

- *What is the speed of a deep water wave, v_{deep}, propagating with wavelength, $\lambda = 10\ m$, in the South China Sea?*

$$v_{deep} = (g\lambda/2\pi)^{1/2} = (9.8 \times 10/6.28)^{1/2}\ m/sec = 9.9\ m/sec$$

Wave Motion

All waves transport energy, no matter how complex the interaction with matter. Wave motion pervades all mechanical interaction. Waves can be *transverse*, in which case they oscillate in directions perpendicular to the direction of energy transport, or they can be *longitudinal*, in which case they oscillate in direction of energy transport. Electromagnetic waves in a vacuum are transverse, while acoustical waves in a frictionless media are longitudinal. Water waves are combination of both, possessing transverse and longitudinal components.

Waves are *linear* or *nonlinear*. Amplitudes of oscillation of linear waves are usually scalar quantities, so that the waves can be added, or *superposed*, linearly. Amplitudes of oscillation of nonlinear waves are often vector quantities, so that waves cannot be added, or superposed, linearly. Acoustical waves are linear, while water and electromagnetic waves are nonlinear.

Media supporting wave propagation are *dispersive* or *nondispersive*. Wave speeds, u, in nondispersive media are independent of frequency, f, or wavelength, λ. Wave speeds in dispersive media depend on frequency, or equivalently wavelength. Crests of waves in dispersive media usually propagate near characteristic phase velocity, u, but wave energy transports with the group velocity of the packet, v,

$$v = \frac{\partial \omega}{\partial k},$$

with angular frequency, ω, and wavenumber, k, defined by,

$$\omega = 2\pi f,$$

$$k = \frac{2\pi}{\lambda},$$

and phase velocity, u,

$$u = f\lambda.$$

Specification of ω as a function of k is called a dispersion relationship. Group velocity, v, can be less, or greater, than phase velocity, u. Waves in dispersive media can be linear or nonlinear, transverse or longitudinal (or combination). Water and plasma waves exhibit dispersion, while light waves in a vacuum and acoustical waves in air exhibit nondispersion. In nondispersive

Interference phenomena, or the interaction of different waves, are common to all wave motion, whether linear or nonlinear, transverse or longitudinal, dispersive or nondispersive. When two waves, denoted f and g, with generalized vector amplitudes, **F** and **G**, interact, a third wave, **U**, is produced by superposition (addition), that is, we write,

$$U = \mathbf{F}f(x,t) + \mathbf{G}g(x,t),$$

with x position, and t time. In most applications, the wavefunctions are bounded, so that,

$$|f| \leq 1,$$
$$|g| \leq 1.$$

In principle, the resultant wavefunction, **U**, can then be constructed analytically (closed form), or numerically (open form), with bounds,

$$|\mathbf{F}-\mathbf{G}| \leq |\mathbf{U}| \leq |\mathbf{F}+\mathbf{G}|,$$

Generally, except in simple cases, it is impossible to write explicit expressions for **U** in terms of f, g, **F**, and **G**. The wavefunctions, f and g, are usually complicated, periodically varying in part, space and time functionals, with dependence on wavenumber, k, and angular frequency, ω, that does not separate in form. Linear, nondispersive, plane waves are one simple case, however, where a closed form can be written for the resultant wave,

For linear waves, the amplitudes are scalars, so that,

$$F - G \leq U \leq F + G$$

Making the simplifying assumption that the two plane waves are just sinusoids of different frequency, ω and ω', we can write,

$$U = F\sin(kx - \omega t) + G\sin(k'x - \omega't).$$

obviously another sinusoid with bimodal frequency components. If the amplitudes are equal, that is, $F = G$, a simplification occurs, seen by expanding the sinusoids, with the result,

$$U = 2F\sin\left[\frac{(k+k')x - (\omega+\omega')t}{2}\right]\cos\left[\frac{(k-k')x - (\omega-\omega')t}{2}\right].$$

exhibiting a functional maximum whenever both conditions occur,

$$(k+k')x - (\omega+\omega')t = (2n+1)\pi,$$
$$(k-k')x - (\omega-\omega')t = n\pi,$$

and a minimum in the opposite case, when either condition occurs,

$$(k+k')x - (\omega+\omega')t = n\pi,$$
$$(k-k')x - (\omega-\omega')t = (2n+1)\pi.$$

The resultant wave, U, exhibits classical interference patterns of reinforcement and cancellation in the two cases. All waves, dispersive or nondispersive, linear or nonlinear, transverse or longitudinal, exhibit similar interference patterns of reinforcement and cancellation (*constructive* or *destructive* interference), but with more complicated dependence on time, position, wavenumber, and frequency. Figure 22 depicts the interference pattern for two sinusoids with frequencies of 8π and 10π.

If two sinusoids of the same amplitude and frequency, but traveling in opposite directions, interfere, the resultant wave is called a *standing* wave, because the interference pattern has fixed nodes (zero points of oscillation), given by,

$$U = 2F \sin\ kx \cos\ \omega t,$$

with these fixed nodes occurring at the phase points,

$$kx = n\pi.$$

Waves propagating continuously (without breakup and reformation) in a media generate interference patterns described above. If waves breakup, reform, and propagate anew, the interference pattern is more complicated, and the process is termed *diffraction*.

Diffraction refers collectively to the scattering of a wave train into many small wavelets, and the subsequent recombination of the wavelets into a new wave train. Passage of a wave train through a small aperture, through a scored grating, or by a knife edge falls into this category. Propagation of waves into regions of geometrical shadow is another example. The passage of water waves past a narrow breakwater, light through a ruled lens, and X-rays off crystalline lattices is diffractive.

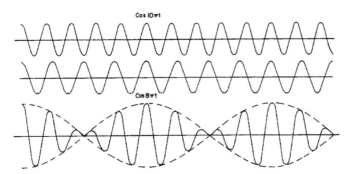

Figure 22. Wave Interference Pattern

Two sinusoids of equal amplitude, F, interfere as shown below, using frequencies 8π and 10π sec^{-1}. Reinforcement and cancellation of the two waves occurs according to,

$$U = 2F \sin\left[\frac{(k_8 + k_{10})x - 18\pi t}{2}\right] \cos\left[\frac{(k_8 - k_{10})x - 2\pi t}{2}\right]$$

with F the amplitude, and k_8, k_{10} wavenumbers for the sinusoids.

In diffraction, when reconstructing initially scattered waves, phase relationships between recombining wavelets are important, because it is the difference between the phases of recombining wavelets that causes interference patterns of constructive and destructive wave interaction, called diffraction patterns. For light, diffraction patterns are seen as alternating areas of light and dark intensity. The angular extension of a diffraction pattern is on the order of λ/d, with λ the wavelength, and d the relevant transverse dimension of the diffracting object. For $d \gg \lambda$, the angular width of the diffraction pattern becomes small, and not of importance. This is the realm of geometrical propagation, where waves travel in straight lines. In the other case, $d \ll \lambda$, scattering and diffraction become more important effects, a regime outside of simple rectilinear wave propagation.

The mathematical treatment of diffraction is forbidding, fortunately, the simple example of a diffraction grating is the most instructive. If light is normally incident on a thin ruled piece of glass, with rulings separated by a distance, d, scattered wavelets will reform and propagate radially outward from each rule. Along a line (envelope) oriented at angle, θ, to the normal to the grating, all wavelets are in phase, and the resultant wavefront exhibits sharp maxima whenever adjacent pathlength differences are integral numbers of wavelengths, n, that is,

$$n\lambda = d\sin\theta.$$

The diffraction pattern can be seen on plane surfaces in back of the grating, as alternating bands of bright and dark images of the diffracting surface, that is, bands for gratings, concentric circles for small apertures.

Diffraction gratings are widely employed to disperse white light into spectral components. Typically, these gratings are fashioned into plane or concave mirror surfaces, with a large number of parallel grooves. Groove frequencies vary from 20 to 3,600 per *mm*. Incident light is diffracted by the grooves, but for given wavelength, is only visible in directions for which all groove wavelets interfere constructively. For any angle of incidence, ϕ, the grating equation can be generalized,

$$n\lambda = d(\sin\theta + \sin\phi).$$

Figure 23 shows a typical diffraction pattern for arbitrary angle of incidence. X-rays are diffracted by regular three dimensional crystalline lattices. Denoting the lattice separation, d, the condition for constructive interference of X-rays is similar to a grating,

$$n\lambda = 2d\sin\theta,$$

with θ the angle between beam and reflecting lattice plane. Light passing through a small circular aperture is diffracted. For radius of opening, a, the intensity per unit solid angle, $\partial I/\partial \Omega$, is,

$$\frac{\partial I}{\partial \Omega} = \left[\frac{ka^2}{\pi}\right]\left[\frac{2J_1(ka\theta)}{ka\theta}\right]^2,$$

with θ measured from the normal to the opening, and J_1 the Bessel function of first order. The circular diffraction pattern has a strong central maxima, followed by a first minima at $\theta = 0.66\lambda/a$, and subsequent maxima, falling off rapidly in intensity, and minima.

Holography, or wave front reconstruction, is one of the more important applications of optical diffraction. Holographic photography differs from regular photography in that holographic cameras record light reflected from every point on the object, not just the light forming an image on the photographic plane. The hologram consists of a hodgepodge of specks, blobs, blurs, and whorls, bearing no resemblance to the object. Nevertheless, the hologram contains in special code, and decipherable only upon application of diffraction theory, all the information about an object that would be contained in a regular photograph, plus other information that cannot be recorded in a photograph. Applications of holography span information storage, image processing, metrology, and biomedical analysis.

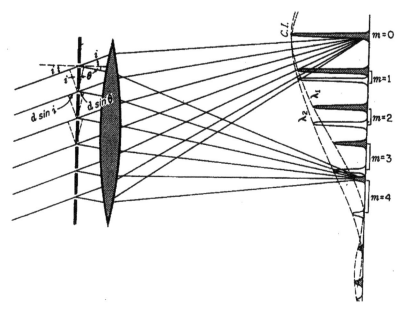

Figure 23. Diffraction Spectra

Light diffracted from a grating with ruled separation, d, incident at angle, φ, interferes constructively at angles, θ, such that,

$$n\lambda = d(\sin\theta + \sin\phi)$$

with λ the wavelength of incident light.

Waves interact with matter in many complex ways. Consider a floating block of wood, and surface water waves incident upon it. The block is set into vertical oscillations by the passage of the wave, and the vertical oscillations produce a circular wave traveling outward from the block in concentric circles. One describes the phenomena as isotropic scattering of incident energy. If the block is very small, or the wave very long, the block rises and falls with the surface of the water, and little energy is scattered. If the block is very large, or the waves very short, the block is motionless, and the wave is reflected. Reflection, however, is clearly a special case of scattering. For a particular block, energy scattered might be considered a function of wavelength, and then, total energy scattered in all directions reaches a maximum for a particular *resonant* wavelength. These observations pervade all types of wave motion and interactions with matter, be they acoustical, electromagnetic, gravitational, thermal, plasma, or water waves.

Water Waves

The mathematical description of water waves, or surface waves as they are generically classed in fluids, is one of the earliest successes of hydrodynamics. Assuming zero fluid viscosity, incompressibility, and an initial rest condition for the fluid, complicated hydrodynamic relationships can be simplified, by casting the flow equations as driven by an impulsive hydrodynamical force. Although the resulting relationships are linear, surface wave dynamics are certainly not so simple, nor are the boundary and applied impulse conditions.

Surface water waves result from the interaction of gravity, surface tension, and wind shear. Neglecting the viscosity and compressibility of water, gravity and surface tension act as restoring forces, wanting to maintain the surface flat in the presence of any disturbance. Such simplifications provide a linear basis for analysis of water motion, requiring wave slopes that are smaller than unity. Under simple impulse, such as the wind, fluid particles trace elliptical orbits, approaching nearly horizontal motion at horizontal boundaries, and circular motion far from them. Amplitudes for such fluid oscillations decrease exponentially at depth, d, with inverse scale length, k, the wavenumber,

$$k = \frac{2\pi}{\lambda},$$

and λ the wavelength. Components of the water wave propagate perpendicularly to the wave crests with phase velocity, u, given by,

$$u^2 = \left[\frac{g}{k} + \frac{\gamma k}{\rho}\right] tanh\ kd,$$

where g is the acceleration of gravity, γ is the surface tension of water, and ρ is the water density. Short waves, with $k^2 > g\rho/\gamma$, are primarily affected by surface tension, and are called *capillary* waves. Long waves, with $k^2 < g\rho/\gamma$, are controlled by gravity, and are termed *gravity* waves. In contrast to elastic and electromagnetic waves, surface wave velocities vary generally with wavelength, λ, and are thus dispersive. Short waves are highly dispersive, tending to dissipate energy over distance, with characteristic group velocity, w,

$$w = \frac{\partial (uk)}{\partial k},$$

while long waves propagate in less dispersive modes, almost with phase velocity, u.

Approximate expressions for the velocities of capillary and gravitational waves can be extracted in appropriate limit. For small argument, kd, that is, $kd < 1$, we have,

$$tanh\ kd \approx kd - \frac{(kd)^3}{3}.$$

Then, for long waves, with $k^2 < g\rho/\gamma$, we obtain,

$$u^2 \approx gd = v_{shallow}^2,$$

employing oceanographic descriptor, $v_{shallow}$, for gravitational waves. For short waves, with $k^2 > g\rho/\gamma$, employing the approximation after differentiation, we similarly find,

$$w^2 \approx \frac{g}{k} = v_{deep}^2,$$

using oceanographic descriptor, v_{deep}, for capillary waves.

Shallow waves (long wavelengths) ultimately break on a beach, while deep waves (short wavelengths) are dispersive, compared to shallow waves, and become shallow waves before they break on a beach. Shallow water waves occur in depths less than one half their wavelength, while deep water waves occur in depths greater than one half their wavelength.

Deep water waves change to shallow water waves as depth decreases, initiating an interesting fluid phenomena. As ocean bottoms become shallow, waves begin to experience drag. If swell crests are 20 ft apart, waves will feel bottom at a depth of 10 ft (half of the wavelength). As this occurs, wave speed, $v_{shallow}$, decreases, causing crests to pile up on each other. The top of the decelerating waves move faster than the dragging bottom, causing curling of the top. Traveling further, the crest leans too far forward, topples, and breaks into foam and surf. For short periods of time just before breaking, the crest velocity may be twice the wave speed. Waves generally break when the depth of the water is 4/3 the wave height. Breaking waves are divided into two categories, spillers and plungers. Spillers roll in evenly for some time, as the bottom smoothly decreases in depth with flat ramp. Plungers break rapidly over short distances, pounding the beach. Plunging occurs when deep water waves change rapidly to shallow water waves, and spilling occurs when deep water waves change into shallow water waves very gently. The primary factor is the nature of the bottom.

Water wave motion can be likened to the light phenomena of refraction, reflection, and diffraction. When deep water waves enter shallow regions at an angle, they are refracted, or bent, as they feel bottom, caused by a reduction in wavelength with decrease in depth. Waves fronts approaching the shore bend so as to more nearly fit the shore. Water waves can also be diffracted into shallow zones behind steep-sided obstacles. Such diffracted waves have been observed in a harbor, bay, or inside a breakwater, and will be smaller than the source waves creating them. Diffraction patterns of choppy sea have been observed for miles downwind of Pacific atolls, perhaps serving as a means to navigation for early Polynesian mariners. Waves striking a shore may not break if the bottom depth is deeper than 4/3 the wave height, instead they can be reflected with very little energy loss. Reflected and incident waves may interfere, so that crests and troughs will coincide, cancelling or reinforcing each other at times.

Fluidization

Fluidization of solids by liquids is a process intermediate between the flow of solids through fluids, and the flow of fluids through solids. When a fluid is passed upward through a bed of granular solids, such as surge through rock and coral debris, a pressure drop accompanies the flow across the bed. When this pressure drop approaches the weight of the bed per unit cross sectional area, the individual granules become disengaged from one another, and the bed begins to resemble a liquid in the state of boiling. It appears that the bed has been *fluidized*. When the particles remain mostly localized, the granular system is a fixed bed. In a moving bed, the particles remain in contact but move as a whole. In a turbulent bed, particles of different size continually mix and change relative position.

The pressure drop, ΔP, necessary for threshold fluidization is given by,

$$\Delta P = L\,(1 - \varepsilon)(\rho_s - \rho_f),$$

with ε the porosity, solid and fluid densities, ρ_s and ρ_f, and bed length, L. Commercially, fluidization plays an important role in catalytic cracking and reduction of heavy petrochemicals. Underwater, swell rolling over coral and rock debris produces interesting fluidization patterns as water waves touch ocean bottoms.

Seiches

Continuous winds and barometric changes across large, partially enclosed bodies of water, such as Lake Erie, establish standing wave patterns across the axis of the body. These long waves rhythmically oscillate off opposite ends of the basin, producing *seiches*, with periods of 14–16 *hours*. Water at leeward and windward ends may rise and fall 8-10 *ft*. If winds shift, the surface will oscillate, alternately rising and falling at each end. Oscillations and wavelengths depend upon the depth and size of the basin.

In ocean bays, seiching is linked to the arrival of long wavelength storm swells and flow. After initial disturbance, seiching continues at a natural frequency determined by the harbor or bay. A seiche in Lake Michigan in 1954 abruptly raised the water level in and around Chicago some 10 *ft*, resulting in the loss of 7 lives. Seiching is more common across inland water basins than oceanic bays and harbors.

Wind and Waves

Tides are the result of combined gravitational and centrifugal forces, but waves are produced when energy is imparted to the surface of water. To produce large waves, high velocity winds must move in the same direction over a wide area for a reasonably long period of time, like hours. A 20 *knot* wind, blowing for at least 10 *hr* along a minimum distance (fetch) of 80 *miles*, will generate some waves with a average height of 11 *ft*. A 50 *knot* wind, blowing for 3 days over a fetch of 1,500 *miles*, will produce some large waves over 110 *ft* in height. The largest wave ever measured occurred during a storm in 1933, reckoned by a US Navy tanker to be 132 *ft* in height. On the average, though, most ocean waves are about 9 *ft* in height.

As winds abate, or waves leave a storm zone, they change, sort themselves out, and become known as *swell*. Swell generally moves faster than the storm centers that created them, which is the reason that waves from a storm may reach shore well ahead of the storm. The shortest waves tend to die out shortly after leaving the storm region, because of destructive interference with each other. The remaining waves of all sizes tend to lose height and sort themselves out according to wavelength. A common figure for speed of swell with a period of 10 *sec* is about 37 *mi/hr*. The longer wavelength component waves move more rapidly than the shorter ones, and arrive at land sooner. This means that as the newly formed swell moves from a storm region, the wave train spreads out. The farther from a storm region, the longer it takes for the wave train to pass any given point. Waves generated below the Equator may take two weeks to reach Alaska. A wave breaking on the California coast may have been formed in the Antarctic, or north of Hawaii, while those hitting New Jersey may have originated in the South Atlantic, or Iceland. Once out of the storm area where energy loss is greatest, swell crosses open ocean with very little energy loss, until expending itself on beaches in a rush of white water.

Energy expended by crashing waves is tremendous, something like 34,000 *hp* per mile of coastline for waves 5 *ft* in height. In Oregon, a 135 *lb* rock was thrown into the air 152 *ft* before nesting in the roof of a lighthouse. In Scotland, a piece of cement weighing 1,300 *tons* was torn loose and moved by waves, requiring wave pressures of some 6,000 lb/ft^2. Nearly all wave energy is lost on breaking. Because the energy of a wave is released in such a short period, energy density is actually much greater than the storm creating the wave.

Ocean surface waves are divided into deep and shallow wave categories. Shallow waves are the ones that hit the beaches, and deep water waves are the source of shallow water waves. Waves longer than 1.75 *cm* are controlled by gravity and inertia, while waves smaller than 1.75 *cm* are controlled by surface tension. Shallow water waves, or long waves, occur in water whose depth is less than one half the wavelength. Deep water, or short waves (even though these may have a longer wavelength), occur where the depth is greater than one half the wavelength. The speed of shallow water waves, $v_{shallow}$, depends only on the depth of the water, while the speed of deep water waves, v_{deep}, depends only on the wavelength,

$$v_{shallow} = (gd)^{1/2},$$

$$v_{deep} = \left[\frac{g\lambda}{2\pi} \right]^{1/2},$$

for wavelength, λ, and water depth, d.

Tides

Unlike waves which are highly variable, tides come and go relentlessly every day. Tides not only affect oceans, but ponds, lakes, land, and even people experience tidal forces, caused by the combined gravitational attraction of the Sun and Moon. Tides in the Great Lakes measure some 2 *in*, while the continents rise and fall 1.5 *ft*. The atmosphere itself bulges 7 *miles* under tidal flow. Corresponding to the rise and fall of tides, the weight of an adult is increased and decreased some 2 *g*. Solar tides are caused by the Sun, and lunar tides are caused by the Moon. Although the Moon is much smaller than the Sun, it is so much closer that lunar tides are much greater than solar tides. Bulges nearest the Sun, or Moon, are caused by gravitational attraction, while bulges opposite are caused by centrifugal reaction to the gravitational bulge. The continual oscillation of water caused by tidal motion can be considered a very long, shallow wave, with wavelength half the circumference of the Earth, and period of 12.5 *hr*. The crests and troughs of the wave are high and low tides, and the wave moves with a speed of 660 *ft/sec*. Points on the hydrosphere experience two high and two low tides daily. Tidal energies are enormous, near 2×10^9 *kilowatt yr*, and the tidal swing between high and low water can reach 50 *ft*, seen in the Bay of Fundy in Canada. But, because ocean basins are shaped differently, tides vary widely across the globe. Off Tahiti, tidal swings are less than 1 *ft*. Highest tides occur when the Earth, Moon, and Sun are in a straight line (spring tide), while the lowest tides occur when the Sun and Moon are at right angles to each other (neap tides).

Near land, the horizontal and vertical flow of water caused by tides becomes apparent. The effects of local winds or weather cause tidal anomalies that at times are more pronounced that the tide itself. Storm surges, associated with low pressure, cause local bulges in the hydrosphere, which, when coupled to tidal flow, can produce very high water along shore lines. Hurricanes and cyclones are the more notable examples of storm surges. Changing tides can set up currents, especially in constricted areas. The current under the Golden Gate Bridge in San Francisco during a change in tides is 6 *knots*, about the same as the East River in New York. In the Straits of Georgia, tidal currents may reach 10 *knots*. Ships crossing the English Channel as the tide comes in can ride 6 *hr* of favorable current to the Straits of Dover, and then continue with the outgoing tidal current to the North Sea.

It has been estimated that friction between the tides and the ocean bottom as water flows back and forth is slowing the rotation of the Earth by about 1 *sec* every 120,000 *yr*. A recent calculation also indicated the total use of the tidal flow (2×10^9 *kilowatts/yr*) would slow this rotation by some 24 *hr* in 2,000 *yr*. Certainly, such meddling of tides is not realistic, but the notion of tidal power stations is not out of the question.

Bores

One of the most striking effects is the tidal *bore*, occurring during spring tides in long estuaries with slowly diminishing depth. As tides enter the the estuary, they are slowed by the constrictive opening. Additional water entering at a constant rate catches up with the initial water flow, resulting in a foaming, churning wall of water moving up the estuary. Most of the rivers of the world do not develop tidal bores, but some that do are spectacular. The bore of the Amazon moves upstream for over 300 *miles* at a speed near 12 *knots*, with a roar heard for 15 *miles*. Tidal bores in the Tsientang Kiang estuary in China attain heights of 25 *ft*, driving all boaters out of the water until passage. Upon passage, boaters can ride the bore upstream.

Some simple energy balances can be applied to bore propagation, case shown and depicted graphically in Figure 24. Assume that a bore of height, h_2, and propagating at speed, v, overtakes a channel of height, h_1, and then moves with speed, u, pushing on channel flow continuously, so that,

$$vh_2 = u(h_2 - h_1)$$

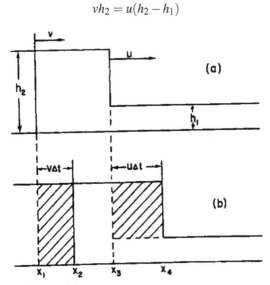

Figure 24. Bore Propagation In A Channel

Bore propagation up a shallow channel or estuary is simply a matter of waves piling up on top of each other, shown below. Simple application of energy and momentum conservation suggests that bore propagation speed, u, takes the form,

$$u^2 = \frac{gh_2(h_1 + h_2)}{2h_1}$$

Tidal bores can sometimes reach 25 ft in height.

Energy impulse-momentum change (conservation) requires,

$$(\rho h_2 u \Delta t - \rho h_1 v \Delta t)v = \frac{1}{2}(\rho gh_2^2 - \rho gh_1^2)\Delta t$$

so simplifying, we see,

$$u^2 = \frac{gh_2(h_1 + h_2)}{2h_1}$$

as the relationship for the combined (bore-channel) propagation speed.

Tsunamis

Tidal waves, or *tsunamis*, are not caused by tides, but rather by sudden movement in the crust of the Earth, such as an earthquake, fault slip, underwater landslide, avalanche, or resonance in a submarine trench that sets adjacent water in motion. To initiate a seismic wave, the surface of water may only have to fall a few inches. Tsunamis are very long waves, with wavelengths of 150 *miles*, traveling at speeds near 472 *mi/hr*, almost the speed of a jet plane. A seismic activity may produce a packet of three or four waves about 15 *minutes* apart, with the first not the most severe. At sea, these waves may only be a couple of feet above the surface, so a person at sea may be completely unaware of their existence. As the waves approach the shore, however, they are slowed down and water piles up rapidly. Rising 66 *ft* above flat shores, they pulverize coasts in a wall of water. The Chilean earthquake in 1960 generated the greatest tsunami of modern times, caused by motion of a major underwater fault. Waves reaching Japan a day later were 17 *ft* high. The Krakatoa volcanic eruption in 1883, coloring sunsets with dust for years all around the globe, generated a seismic marine disturbance some 33 *ft* in height.

An unnatural explosion, such as a thermonuclear bomb, may also generate tsunamis. There was some concern that the world's first thermonuclear detonation at Eniwetok Atoll in the Marshall Islands might also trigger a tsunami akin to that of the Krakatoa volcano. Eniwetok is similar to the island of Krakatoa, and the calculated energy of the thermonuclear release is similar in magnitude to the volcanic eruption. The famous explosion did generate a tsunami, but only a small one. The bomb crater did not broach the outer edge of the Atoll reef, and did not come in contact with the sea.

Cyclonic Flows and Vorticities

An easy way to envision cyclonic flows and vorticities in the atmosphere (and oceans too for that matter), is to contrast a straight cut across a CD with a penknife when the CD is fixed, and then when it is rotating. Cutting from edge to center when the CD is fixed produces a straight cut. When rotating, the cut is not straight across the CD, but rather curved. The CD moves as the penknife cuts across it, and a curved mark results. So, too, the air atmosphere as winds and ocean water as currents experience a deflection on a curved path as the Earth rotates. These deflections are the Coriolis effects quantified earlier. The combination of all factors creates clockwise gyres of the oceans and winds in the Northern Hemisphere, and counterclockwise gyres of the same in the Southern Hemisphere. Intense gyres and vorticities in the atmosphere spawn hurricanes and typhoons over the oceans, and tornadoes and cyclones over land masses. Hurricanes are very large swirling masses of moist air forming over the water in warm (Equatorial) regions, but away from the Equator where they can begin their spinning motion (Coriolis deflection). They occur in the North Atlantic, Gulf of Mexico, Caribbean, and southeastern part of the North Pacific. In the western North Pacific, this same storm is called a typhoon. Because of a greater expanse of feeding warm water in the western Pacific, typhoons are often larger and more intense than hurricanes. Tornadoes are much smaller funnel shaped cyclonic disturbances, formed over land masses. Although tornadoes spawn the most violent winds on Earth, their overall speeds on the Earth's surface are slow, and their lifespans are relatively short. Tornadoes are sometimes called cyclones in other parts of the world. Over water, tornadoes are called waterspouts, and are significantly fewer in number than land cyclones.

A cyclonic flow is a low pressure area in the atmosphere where winds spiral inward. Cyclonic flows may cover an area half as large as the United States. Tornadoes are special, intense cyclonic flows spanning 300 to 8,000 feet in diameter. Cyclonic flow development is supported by the warm waters of tropical and subtropical climates, as well as well as updrafting in violent thunderstorms over land and water.

A hurricane is a powerful, whirling storm that measures 200 to 300 *miles* in diameter. Winds near the center blow at speeds of 75 *mi/hr*. Many hurricanes have caused widespread death and destruction. Hurricanes develop from easterly waves in the tropical zones, actually long, narrow regions of low pressure in the ocean trade winds. Easterly waves may grow into tropical depressions, with winds up to 31 *mi/hr*, and then into tropical storms, with winds up to 74 *mi/hr*, and finally into hurricanes. Hurricane winds swirl about an eye, a calm area in the center of the storm about 20 *miles* in diameter with few winds and clouds. Storm clouds, called wall clouds, surround the eye. The strongest winds and heaviest rains occur in the wall clouds, with winds sometimes reaching 180 *mi/hr*.

In the Northern Hemisphere, hurricane winds blow around the eye in counterclockwise motion, and blow in clockwise motion in the Southern Hemisphere. Hurricane eyes travel at speeds of 10 to 15 *mi/hr*, fairly slow moving. Most hurricanes move westward at first, becoming stronger and larger as they progress. Then, they turn from the Equator and pick up more speed. If they reach temperate latitudes, hurricanes eventually turn east (extratropical storms then), and end as weak storm centers over cool oceans. However, many hurricanes hit landfall, depositing strong winds and heavy rainfall as they move inward from coastal regions. As the hurricane eye reaches land, the rain stops and the air becomes calm, for a while. Less than an hour, or so, later, the eye passes and wind and rains return. Overall, the hurricane weakens as it moves over land because its source of energy, evaporating warm water, has been removed. Friction of the rougher land surface also slows the winds, but heavy rains continue. Associated with the passage of a hurricane over the coast can be a large rise in water levels, a phenomenon called the *storm surge*, often as disastrous as the winds and flooding.

In the United States, most hurricanes affect areas in the Gulf of Mexico and Atlantic Ocean. On average, about 6 to 8 hurricanes develop annually in these regions, most of them in September. As many as 15 have occurred in a single year. During the hurricane season in the United States (June to November), meteorologists keep a close watch on the Atlantic, Pacific, Gulf of Mexico, and Caribbean, collecting such information as air pressure, temperature, and wind speeds. Using this information, they track potential storms with satellites, airplanes, and radar, warning communities in the path of the storm.

Hurricane Floyd, more than 600 *miles* wide and bigger than the entire state of Florida, pounded the Bahamas in 1999, and then swept northward along the southeast coast of the United States. With maximum wind speeds of 155 mi/hr, Floyd was only 1 mi/hr short of a C5 hurricane, the highest and most serious designation assigned by the National Weather Service. The last C5 hurricane to strike the United States was Camille in 1969, killing more than 250 people on the Gulf Coast and in Virginia.

Akin to hurricanes, typhoons are violent, low pressure storms that occur in the western Pacific and Indian Oceans. Typhoons begin near the Equator, and move westward, as do hurricanes, gathering size and intensity. The circular winds around the center (eye) often reach 150 mi/hr. Moving ashore, typhoons impact landfalls with heavy rains and powerful winds. As with hurricanes, a rush of seawater, the storm surge, often accompanies a typhoon moving landward.

Tornadoes (and cyclones) are miniature hurricanes (typhoons) formed mostly over land, but under very different circumstance and way. Tornadoes are produced inside powerful thunderstorms, which in turn are created near the junction between warm moist air and cold dry air. Conditions spawning tornadoes exist when this moist, warm air gets trapped beneath a stable layer of cold dry air by an intervening layer of warm dry air a stratified sandwich called an inversion. If the system cap is disturbed by a front or upper atmospheric disturbance, the moist, warm air rises and punches through the stable air holding it down. Rising, the warm air also spirals, energized with latent heat released by condensing water vapor. Aided by shear winds at different levels, the rotating updraft gains energy and speed, culminating in a tornado. Width range is 150 ft to 1 *mile* roughly, with maximum winds near 300 mi/hr (F5). Groundspeed of tornadoes can approach 60 mi/hr, and tornadoes may touch the ground a few hundred feet, or rage along for a hundred miles.

Although tornadoes occur throughout the world, including India and Bangladesh, they are most intense and devastating in the United States. Tornadoes strike anytime of day, but are most frequent in the afternoon and evening, after solar heating has produced hot, moist air during the day. On average, the United States experiences some 100,000 thunderstorms each year, spawning about 1,000 tornadoes. The National Weather Service estimates that 42 people are killed each year by tornadoes. Tornadoes release much energy. One with wind speeds of 200 mi/hr releases energy at a rate of 1 billion *watts*, about equal to the output of a pair of large nuclear reactors. But the thunderstorms that spawn tornadoes are even more powerful, releasing 40 trillion *watts*, some 40,000 more powerful than a tornado.

Tornado Alley is the name given to the swatch of land traversing diagonally from eastern Idaho to western Louisiana, an alley where cool dry Canadian air clashes with warm moist Gulf air, precipitating conditions favorable to tornadic thunderstorms. But tornadoes are common in Alabama, Arkansas, Florida, Georgia, Illinois, Indiana, Iowa, Kansas, Mississippi, Nebraska, South Dakota, and Wisconsin. A swarm of tornadoes ripped Oklahoma in May, 1999, killing 43 and destroying thousands of homes. The National Oceanic and Atmospheric Administration (NOAA) reported that 45 twisters hit Oklahoma and 14 hit Kansas in that time frame of destruction.

Reports also suggested that the impacts of these tornadoes were bomblike in destructive quality, virtually leveling buildings.

A waterspout is a weak (usually) tornado over water. They are most common along the Gulf Coast and southeastern States. In the western United States, waterspouts occur with cold fall or late winter storms, when tornadoes are least suspected to develop. Also associated with thunderstorms are downbursts, downward flowing wind that sometimes comes blasting out of a thunderstorm. Damage can be as bad as tornado damage, since the wind can be as strong as an F2 tornado, but debris is blown straight away from a point on the ground, not lofted airborne and transported downwind by the vortex.

Storm Surges

Another spontaneous phenomena, the storm surge, is often disastrous to areas adjacent to the seas. Effectwise, it can be similar to a tsunami, but the phenomena is different. A tsunami often appears in a region experiencing good weather, and if advance warning is not given, there would only be a few minutes warning at best. Storm surges occur during bad weather, and result from a combination of factors. First are the tides themselves. Second, intense storms, such as hurricanes, can raise the level of the sea surface locally. These large storms are characterized by regions of low atmospheric pressure, causing a bulge in the sea surface. Coupled with high winds in one direction for many hours, these forces can pile water up on the shore causing considerable flooding and surging water, possibly lasting one or two tidal cycles.

The gale that swept down from the North Sea across England and piled water on the Dutch coast on February 1, 1953, was such a storm surge. Almost 1,800 people drowned as 80,000 *acres* of dike rimmed, low lands were flooded. Considering all factors, it has been estimated that probability of such a superstorm is 1 in 400 *yr*. The Galveston Flood of 1900 was also a storm surge. Hurricane force winds of 193 *km/hr* pushed normal 0.7 *m* tides up over 5 *m*, and with 8 *m* storm waves virtually destroyed the city. A storm surge in the Ganges River in India picked an American freighter up and set it down 1 *mile* inland. On November 12, 1970, a massive bulge of water, coupled to a large typhoon, struck and buried the populated coast of East Pakistan, killing over 500,000 people in the worst natural catastrophe since the Yellow River Flood in China in 1887.

Prevailing Atmospheric Highs and Lows

The heating of the Earth's surface varies with time of the year, depending on the angle of the Earth's attitude with respect to the Sun and solar rays. Because this relative angle changes throughout the year, weather patterns, specifically areas of prevailing high and low atmospheric pressure (*highs* and *lows*) must change. But as the heating cycle each year is reasonably constant, a series of seasonally permanent (prevailing) highs and lows are set up across the planet. These are not to be confused with the wandering highs and lows that cause everyday weather, though they are ultimately linked to the big seasonal highs and lows. With seasonal shifting of these areas of pressure, oceanic surface currents do shift somewhat. On the western edges of continents, these small current shifts result in dramatic weather changes between summer and winter.

During January, an immense low pressure system is docked in the North Pacific. In the summer, this low is replaced by a high, more to the east in location. These two systems determine the overall yearly weather of much of the West Coast of the United States. Wintertime, the counterclockwise winds of the low, laden with moisture from contact with water warmed by the Kuroshio Current, blow in and over the Pacific Northwest, Canada, and Alaska. This warm moist air gives the Pacific Northwest, west of the coastal ranges, its cloudy, rainy, but temperate winters. Such a rainy season is termed a *monsoon*, often incorrectly associated only with tropical regions. With summer comes the formation of the high, and winds move in a different direction, off land. These winds are now dry and warm, giving the area its dry and warm summers. Thus, a monsoon is really a seasonally reversing wind pattern, caused by seasonal variation in prevailing atmospheric pressure. This pattern is not the same all over the globe, as the summers of all of Southeast Asia and India, for example, have wet onshore winds and resultant rainy seasons. Along the West Coast, monsoonal effects stretch from Alaska to San Diego.

Another important effect linked to wind reversal is *upwelling*. Off the West Coast, winter winds drive water onto the coast, making surface levels higher than normal, some 3 *cm*. In summer, winds are moving down the coast, and surface water near the coast is pushed at an angle to the right of wind direction, but offshore to be sure. Deep cold water moves up to replace the outward surface transfer, in a process termed upwelling. Upwelling is important because it brings nutrient rich waters to the surface and enhances biological activity. With vertical transfer of water by this means, and coupled others, the surface waters would be stripped of nutrients sustaining life. The mixing also means that the water is actually colder off the West Coast in summer than winter. Only when the winds abate for a few days, is the surface water warm enough for pleasant swimming.

The northward flow of the cold nutrient rich Humboldt Current along the westside of South America, coupled with upwelling from southerly winds, furnishes a supply of nitrates and phosphates supporting perhaps the world's most abundant populations of marine life. The Peruvian fishing industry depends on the Humboldt Current and upwelling, as do millions of fish eating birds, whose droppings of guano are the basis of the hugh Peruvian fertilizer industry. Symbiotic is the term applied to the coupling of currents, winds, and biological activity.

But, periodically (like every 7 *yrs*), the offshore winds drop in intensity, and warm Equatorial waters move in to displace the cold waters of the Humboldt Current, and the entire picture changes. Called *El Nino* (the boy child) in referring to the Christ child because the phenomenon occurs during the Christmas season, the warm waters and rapid depletion of nutrients cause massive plankton and fish kills. Tons of dead fish pile up on beaches, and the oxygen content of the water is quickly lowered. With the death of fish, thousands of birds also die. The past two years, 1998 and 1999, have been linked to wind driven changes in coastal water temperatures, bringing us to a fuller discussion of El Nino, and its coupled cold water sister intrusion, called *La Nina* (the girl child).

El Nino and La Nina

El Nino is a major disruption of the ocean-atmosphere system in the tropical Pacific having important consequences for global weather. Among consequences are increased rainfall across the southern tier of the United States, and Peru, attendant destructive local flooding, drought in the western Pacific, and devastating brush fires in Australia. Impacts, however, are global, since the oceans fuel atmospheric energy transfer and circulation patterns dictating weather. El Nino occurrences in 1911, 1932, 1939, 1941, 1951, 1958, 1965, 1986, 1991, 1993, and 1994 were observed. And occurrences in 1891, 1925, 1953, and 1997 were relatively severe.

Observation of water temperatures, currents, and winds in the tropical Pacific provide clues to the formation of El Nino. Normally, trade winds blow east to west across the tropical Pacific, piling water about 0.5 *m* higher at Indonesia than at Ecuador. The sea surface is often 8 ^oC warmer in the western Pacific, compared to temperatures off South America, due to upwelling of cold water from deeper levels in the eastern Pacific. Normally oceanic thermoclines separating warm from cold water are near 50 *m*, but deepen during El Nino. Rainfall increases in the rising air over the warmer waters, while the eastern Pacific remains relatively dry. During El Nino, the trade winds relax in the central and western Pacific, leading to warmer waters and a depression of thermoclines in the eastern Pacific, down to near 150 *m*. The reduced upwelling of nutrient rich water has a negative effect on all life and processes in the euphotic zone, affecting all levels of the food chain. Rainfall follows the warm water eastward, with flooding in Peru and California, and drought in Indonesia and Australia. The eastward displacement of the atmospheric heat source overlaying the warmest waters results in large changes in global atmospheric circulation, forcing changes in weather regions far removed from the tropical Pacific.

La Nina is characterized by fairly cold ocean temperatures in the Equatorial Pacific. During La Nina, easterly trade winds strengthen remarkably, inducing a very strong (cold) upwelling in the eastern tropical Pacific. Surface temperatures fall some 4 ^oC compared to normal. Eastward moving atmospheric and oceanic waves first help to bring cold water to the surface through a complex series of events still under study. As these easterlies strengthen, the upwelling intensifies in bootstrap fashion. La Nina conditions, like El Nino, last from 9 to 12 months, with some episodes lasting 2 years. La Nina was observed in 1903, 1906, 1909, 1916, 1924, 1928, 1938, 1950, 1954, 1964, 1970, 1973, 1988, and 1995, with La Nina half as frequent as El Nino since 1975.

Global climate impacts from La Nina tend to be opposite those of El Nino. At higher latitudes, effects of both are seen most clearly in the wintertime. During El Nino years, winter temperatures are warmer than normal in the North Central region, and cooler than normal in the Southeast and Southwest. During La Nina years, winter temperatures are warmer than normal in the Southeast, and cooler than usual in the Northwest.

El Nino and La Nina occur on average every 3-5 *yrs*, with more recent spacings on the order of 2–7 *yrs*. Surface temperatures in the central and eastern tropical Pacific diverge from normal in roughly bell curve fashion, with El Nino and La Nina at opposite ends (tails). Some believe there are really only two states, El Nino or La Nina, with the average something between them. According to some experts, El Nino has been present 31% of the time, and La Nina has been present 23% of the time. The frequency of El Nino has increased in recent decades, a shift possibly linked to global warming and climate change.

El Nino and La Nina impact global weather and storm formation, according to recent studies. Hurricane activity in the Gulf and Caribbean basins is thought to increase during La Nina. The position of the jet stream changes dramatically during El Nino and La Nina. During El Nino, the jet stream is oriented west to east over the northern Gulf of Mexico and Florida. During La Nina, the jet extends from the central Rockies to the eastern Great Lakes. Since tornadoes are more likely along the jet stream, severe weather and tornadic activity are likely to be further north and west during La Nina, compared to El Nino.

Jet Stream

The *jet stream* is a wobbly river of fast flowing air at high altitudes above the Earth, generally flowing in an easterly direction. Jet streams by definition flow faster than 57 *mi/hr*, but the term is applied to all upper level wind flows. Usually the jet separates cold polar air to the north from warm tropical air to the south. During major cold outbreaks, the jet stream often dives south, into the Gulf of Mexico. During unusually mild winters and during summer, the jet stream retreats northward into Canada. At middle latitudes (roughly between 20° and 60°), air in the upper troposphere tends to move in relatively narrow, fast bands (streams) that wobble back and forth flowing eastward. Two jets are often present, a polar jet (30° to 60°), and a subtropical jet (20° to 30°). At times, the polar jet splits into two branches, or one or both jet streams lack continuity or definition.

The jet stream is usually thousands of kilometers long, stretching the length of countries, and is caused by differences in surface temperatures on the Earth. Its path is determined by the greatest temperature differences found near the surface, usually occurring where cold polar air masses clash with warm tropical ones. On collision, high speed winds develop in the upper atmosphere due to rising lower air. Jets are always strongest in the winter for this reason. As air masses move, so does the jet stream. Flow patterns on a global scale follow in lowest order from Bernoulli's law, linking temperatures, pressures, fluid flow densities, and heat exchange in a macroscopic energy balance. Whatever the boundary conditions on the flow patterns, the strongest jets and highest winds develop along the greatest temperature gradients, with flow speed scaling linearly with temperature gradient (zero order). Jet stream flow speeds top out near 155 *mi/hr*, though usually in 90 *mi/hr* range. However, the atmosphere is a very complicated place, and generalizations are often difficult.

Jets powerfully influence synoptic weather patterns (a few thousand kilometers across lasting a day up to a week). As air races through the stream column, some parts of the flow pattern tend to converge, increasing the weight of air on the surface of the Earth, which in turn increases pressure on the surface below (high pressure system). Moreover, convergence within the jet stream tends to also force air beneath the stream downward. As air descends in the atmosphere, the pressure on it increases and compresses it, thereby warming the sinking air. The warming sinking air evaporates any existing clouds, or prevents cloud formation in the first place. Such areas generally experience clear weather. However, air in other parts of the stream pattern tend to diverge, reducing the total weight of air above the surface of the Earth and lowering surface pressure (low pressure system). Divergence of the flow pattern tends to lift the air beneath the jet to replace the diverging part. Rising air encounters lower atmospheric pressure, so the rising air expands and cools. If the rising air cools enough, clouds form in it, which in turn may produce precipitation (rain). Large scale divergence of high speed winds aloft induces large scale lifting of air in the troposphere, and extended regions of cyclonic warm and cold air (warm and cold fronts), easily spotted on satellite images, and often extending thousands of miles (fronts).

As the jet stream races eastward, the sinuous wobbles developed in the stream flow due to temperature gradients tend to shift slowly eastward too. The smaller the wobble, the faster it propagates eastward. Large wobbles often stall, sometimes stopping completely. The regions of convergence and divergence within the jet stream, and the patterns of clear and stormy weather associated with convergence and divergence, correlate with certain parts of the wobble. As wobbles propagate eastward, so do patterns of clear and stormy weather, somewhere on the order of 20 *mi/hr* to 30 *mi/hr*.

Keyed Exercises

• *Mark the following statements TRUE or FALSE.*

T	F	*A waterspout is a tornado over water.*
T	F	*Tornado Alley is a zone where Canadian air clashes with Gulf air?*
T	*F*	*Tsunamis are caused by tides?*
T	F	*Water waves are not linear waves.*
T	*F*	*Diffraction refers to the continuous propagation of wave wavelets.*
T	F	*Fluidization involves solids and fluids.*
T	*F*	*Seiches are moving wave patterns in closed basins.*
T	*F*	*Ocean waves shorter than 1.75 cm are controlled by gravity and inertia.*
T	*F*	*Tides are caused primarily by the Sun.*
T	F	*Bores are caused by tides moving upstream.*
T	*F*	*Cyclonic flows in the atmosphere are linear and smooth.*
T	F	*La Nina is characterized by cold ocean temperatures in the Equatorial Pacific.*

• Match the entries in the first column with the best single entry in the second column.

(d) Tsunami	(a) Propagates in long estuary
(h) Fluidization	(b) Due to gravitational and centrifugal forces
(e) Linear wave	(c) Exhibits interference pattern
(g) Nonlinear wave	(d) Caused by underwater earthquake
(i) Seiche	(e) Has scalar amplitude
(f) Storm surge	(f) Caused by hurricane
(a) Bore	(g) Has vector amplitude
(b) Tide	(h) Suspended particles appear to be boiling
(c) Wave diffraction	(i) Water level oscillation in closed basin
(k) Deep water wave	(j) Long wavelength, gravitational wave
(j) Shallow water wave	(k) Short wavelength, capillary wave
(o) Jet stream	(l) Very cold upwelling
(q) El Nino	(m) Produces most intense winds on Earth
(l) La Nina	(n) Tropical storm 300 *miles* in diameter
(m) Tornado	(o) High speed, upper level air flow
(n) Hurricane	(p) Switching of prevailing highs and lows
(r) Upwelling	(q) Westerly abatement in tropical Pacific
(p) Monsoon	(r) Cold nutrient rich surface waters

• What is the speed, u, of a tsunami (tidal wave), wavelength, $\lambda = 150$ miles, and frequency, $f = .31\ hr^{-1}$, slamming into Guam?

$$u = \lambda f = 150 \times .31\ mi/hr = 465\ mi/hr$$

• Light, of wavelength λ, is incident at an angle of $\phi = 45^o$ on a grating scored at a separation, $d = 3\lambda$. At an observation angle, $\phi = 60^o$, how many diffraction fringes, n, occur?

$$n\lambda = d(\sin\theta + \sin\phi)$$

$$d = 3\lambda, \ \sin\phi = \sin 45^o = .707, \ \sin\theta = \sin 60^o = .866$$

$$n = 3(\sin 45^o + \sin 60^o) = 3(.707 + .866) = 4.7$$

• Two sinusoids traveling at the same wave speed, v, and with the same amplitudes, differ in frequency, f, by a factor of 2. What are the conditions for functional maxima to occur in space, x, and time, t?

$$\omega = 2\pi f, \ \omega' = 2\pi f' = 4\pi f$$

$$\lambda = \frac{v}{f}, \ k = \frac{2\pi}{\lambda} = \frac{2\pi f}{v}, \ \lambda' = \frac{v}{f'} = \frac{v}{2f}, \ k' = \frac{2\pi}{\lambda'} = \frac{4\pi f}{v}$$

$$(k+k')x - (\omega+\omega')t = (2n+1)\pi, \ (k-k')x - (\omega-\omega')t = n\pi$$

$$\frac{fx}{v} - ft = \frac{2n+1}{6}, \ ft - \frac{fx}{v} = \frac{n}{2}$$

- *If the angular frequency, ω, of a complex water wave is a quadratic function of wavenumber, k, so that, $\omega = 40\pi^2 k^2 + 2\phi\pi$, what is the corresponding group velocity, v, of the wave packets?*

$$v = \frac{\partial\omega}{\partial k} = \frac{\partial(40\pi^2 k^2 + 2\phi\pi)}{\partial k} = 80\pi^2 k$$

What is the corresponding phase velocity, u?

$$f = \frac{\omega}{2\pi}, \quad \lambda = \frac{2\pi}{k}$$

$$u = f\lambda = \frac{\omega}{k} = 40\pi^2 k + \frac{2\phi\pi}{k}$$

- *What is the pressure drop, ΔP, necessary to activate fluidization in a coral bed of length, $L = 2.6$ ft, assuming porosity, $\varepsilon = .68$, in the coral debris, and coral density some 1.05 times denser than sea water ($\rho_{sea} = 64$ lbs/ft³)?*

$$Ł = 2.6 \ ft, \quad \varepsilon = .68, \quad \rho_{sea} = 64 \ lbs/ft^3, \quad \rho_{cor} = 1.05 \times 64 \ lbs/ft^3 = 67.2 \ lbs/ft^3$$

$$\Delta P = L(1-\varepsilon)(\rho_{cor} - \rho_{sea}) = 2.6 \times .32 \times 3.2 \ lbs/ft^2 = 2.66 \ lbs/ft^2$$

- *If a tidal driven bore of nominal height, $h_2 = 3$ ft, systematically roars up a channel of depth, $h_1 = 1$ ft, what is the (combined) flow speed, u?*

$$h_2 = 3 \ ft, \quad h_1 = 1 \ ft$$

$$u = \left[\frac{gh_2(h_1 + h_2)}{2h_1}\right]^{1/2} = \left[\frac{32 \times 3 \times 4}{2}\right]^{1/2} ft/sec = 13.8 \ ft/sec$$

Under these conditions, what is the initial bore speed, v, before pileup of channel waters?

$$vh_2 = u(h_2 - h_1)$$

$$v = u\frac{(h_2 - h_1)}{h_2} = 13.8 \times \frac{2}{3} \ ft/sec = 9.3 \ ft/sec$$

- *When bore and channel heights are nearly equal, $h_2 = h_1 = h$, what is the propagation speed, u, and what kind of wave does such bore approximate?*

$$u^2 = \frac{2gh^2}{2h}$$

$$u = (gh)^{1/2} \ (shallow \ water \ wave)$$

• *Match the following characteristics to El Nino (EN) and/or La Nina (LN):*

Absence of strong westerly winds in the eastern Pacific?

EN

Warmer subtropical waters?

EN

Colder subtropical waters?

LN

Fires in Australia?

EN

Strengthening easterly trade winds?

LN

Cooler winter temperatures in the Southwest and Southeast?

EN

Occur every 3-5 yrs on average?

EN, LN

Occur more often since 1975?

EN

Warmer winter temperatures in the Southeast?

LN

Reduced upwelling?

LN

Impact global climate?

EN, LN

More northern and western tornadic activity?

LN

Present 31% of the time?

EN

- *Match the following to diverging (D) and/or converging (C) jet stream flow patterns.*

Flow patterns satisfy Bernoulli's law?

D, C

Causes wandering high pressure systems?

C

Tends to lift air?

D

Produces precipitation?

D

Warming sinking air?

C

Wobbles sinuously?

D, C

Due to surface temperature gradients?

D, C

- *Match the following cyclonic flow characteristics to hurricanes and typhoons (H) and/or tornadoes and cyclones (T).*

Center winds blow at 75 mi/hr?

H

Rotate counterclockwise in the Northern Hemisphere, clockwise in the Southern Hemisphere?

H, T

Develop mainly over land?

T

Draw energy from warm waters?

H

Range 150 ft to 1 mile in diameter?

T

Waterspout?

T

Calm centers with few clouds?

H

Spawned by thunderstorms?

$$T$$

Generate storm surges?

$$H$$

Maximum winds of 300 mi/hr?

$$T$$

Have spiraling inward winds?

$$H, T$$

Energized by condensing water vapor?

$$T$$

Hundreds of miles across?

$$H$$

Mostly occur June through October?

$$H$$

Experience Coriolis deflection?

$$H, T$$

- *If the jet stream is traveling, v, at 155 mi/hr, how long, t, does it take to cross the USA assuming a straight line flow pattern and width of the USA, l, equal to 2,600 mi?*

$$t = \frac{l}{v} = \frac{2,600}{155} \, hr = 16.7 \, hr$$

- *If the jet stream wobbles into circular subflows with radii, r, approximately 200 mi from center of the flow, what is the centripetal acceleration, a, experienced by the jet stream?*

$$a = \frac{v^2}{r} = \frac{155^2}{200} \, mi/hr^2 = \frac{24025}{200} \, mi/hr^2 = 120.1 \, mi/hr^2$$

Part 2

PRESSURE, DENSITY, AND BUBBLES

Atomistics and Elementals

The concept that one or a few elementary substances could interact to form matter was originated by Greek philosophers in the Sixth Century, BC. The atomic hypotheses, indispensable to our understanding of chemical elements, originated with the philosopher Leucippus and follower Democritus in the Fifth Century, BC. These two interacting concepts of elements and atoms are unsurpassed in their importance to the development of science and technology.

Aristotle accepted from earlier philosophers that air, water, earth, and fire were elements, and he added a fifth, the ether, representing the heavenly bodies. Although all matter was formulated from these elements, the elements themselves represented qualities and were nonmaterial. Centuries later, as alchemists found new transformations, three more were added to the list, namely, sulfur, mercury, and salt. These were thought to represent the quantities of combustibility, volatility, and incombustibility. This view prevailed for about 2000 *yrs.*

In 1661, on the heels of Democritus, Robert Boyle developed a chemical atomic theory, giving definition to chemical elements as certain primitive and simply unmingling bodies. Boyle also deduced the ideal gas law from experiments in the laboratory. A century later, Lavoisier composed a list of elements based on experimentally verifiable definition, that is, a chemical substance is one that cannot be decomposed into simpler structures by chemical means. The list was some 30 elements long, and was based on some careful studies of decomposition and recombination. The list included some stable compounds, such as silica and alumina, which defied decomposition with existent technology, and also heat and light. The Greek notion was still lingering.

Continued work by Lavoisier led to the law of definite proportions, which states that in any given compound, the elements always occur in the same proportions by weight no matter how the compound is synthesized. This was generalized to the law of equivalent weights, or that weight which will combine with or replace a unit of standard weight from a standard element, such as hydrogen.

Two centuries later, in 1808, John Dalton postulated an atomic theory that incorporated atomic weight as distinguished from equivalent weight (but including equivalent weight as a supercase) and was capable of explaining empirically derived and observed laws of chemical combination. Dalton postulated:

- all atoms of a given element are identical but different from the atoms of another element;
- compounds are formed from these elemental atoms;
- chemical reactions result from the atoms being arranged in new ways;
- if only one compound can be formed from X and Y, then that compound contains one X and one Y atom.

The fourth assumption (incorrect as we know) suggested that nature is more simple than real. Lussac, Avogadro, and Cannizzaro later corrected Dalton's fourth assumption, merely by interjecting nX and mY atoms in the chemical reaction stream. Mendeleev, in 1865, using these assumptions constructed the first Periodic Chart, with 65 elements in the list.

Mendeleev made an important discovery while looking for relationships among these elements. The properties of the elements are periodic functions of their atomic weights. This periodic law allows the arrangement of elements in the table in order of increasing weight, such that the table contains columns and rows of elements with similar properties, by row and/or column (Periodic Table). For the first time in history, it was shown that the chemical elements form an entity in their interrelationships, and seemingly undiscovered elements with predictable properties could be sought to fill holes in the table. In modern times, the Periodic Table has been filled, so to speak, for $Z \leq 94$ in the natural world. However, particle accelerators and cosmic probes continue the search for *superheavies*, with a number of short lived elements already added to the Table (californium, einsteinium, fermium, rutherfordium, hahnium, nobelium, curium, berkelium, and others).

Today, very high speed computers can simulate the motion of atoms and molecules in space and time for assumed forces of attraction and repulsion between them. This particular brand of high speed molecular simulation is called molecular dynamics (MD) and is in the forefront of materials and drug design. Important physical and chemical properties can be extracted from the simulations using millions of atoms and molecules. Calculations can last for many hours on multiprocessor computers with gigaflop speeds, that is, a billion operations per second. Operations are addition and subtraction of decimal numbers, with division and multiplication a series of continuous subtractions and additions which are tallied.

Atoms themselves are no longer the fundamental building blocks of matter, nor are constituent protons and neutrons. Neutrons and protons, and indeed other elementary particles like mesons, are composed of smaller, seldom measured particles called quarks. Quarks are thought to have strange properties, spin states, and electric charge that limit their interactions selectively. Quarks and bound states of quarks are an active avenue of research requiring very high energy particle accelerators and powerful computing resources.

Binding Energy

Individual atoms in the free state give up some of their mass-energy to form bound states. This is consistent with the theory of relativity. This is true for nuclear, chemical, electromagnetic, and gravitational fields binding particles, or conglomerates of particles, together. The binding energy, Δm, is also called the *mass defect* and is simply the difference between the bound conglomerate mass, M, and the free masses of all constituent particles,

$$\Delta m = M - \sum_{i=1}^{N} m_i$$

$$\Delta mc^2 = \Phi$$

with N the total number of particles in the assembly, and m_i their free masses. The mass defect is always negative denoting that mass-energy has been given up to a binding potential, Φ, attracting all particles into a single conglomerate. The conversion from mass to energy is $931.1\ MeV/amu$, with M and m_i given in atomic mass units, *amu*. A simple example can be seen in the following way.

The mass of copper, Cu^{29}, is $62.9137\ amu$. The copper nucleus is composed of 29 protons and 34 neutrons, with proton atomic weight $1.00728\ amu$ and neutron atomic weight $1.00867\ amu$. Neglecting all electrons because their masses are very small compared to the nuclear mass, we have,

$$\Delta m = 62.9137\ amu - (29 \times 1.0073 - 34 \times 1.0087)\ amu = -0.5922\ amu = -551.4\ MeV$$

If electrons are added, the mass defect is more negative by some 1–$2\ MeV$.

In the world of particle physics, the amount of mass that is lost by elementary particles such as quarks in binding together to form protons, neutrons, mesons, and their anti-particles is enormous, often thought to be well over half their rest mass. Quarks are thought to be the constituent particles that make up the observed spectrum of observable particles and resonances. Quarks in the free state have never been observed, of course, up to now, but the search continues using very high energy particle colliders. Estimates of quark masses (and there are more than one type) range from $300\ MeV$ all the way up to $91,000\ Mev$. If standard protons and neutrons have observable masses of roughly $1,000\ Mev$, quarks with masses larger than that must be giving up considerable amounts of mass-energy to binding.

Pressure

Clearly pressure and density are fundamental concepts at the lowest level of description. Both stem from Feynman's conjecture that the *atomic hypothesis*, namely all things are made of atoms moving in perpetual motion, is the most succinct statement we can make about scientific knowledge. Atoms have mass, occupy space, collide with each other, and can repel or attract each other. That atoms have mass, occupy space, and move in collisional paths is a microscopic statement that matter has density, exerts pressure, and links temperature to measure collisional speeds.

Macroscopically, such a fundamental conception exhibits itself in the equation of state of a solid, liquid, or gas. The equation of state relates pressure, density, and temperature in one relationship. That atoms attract or repel one another is the basis of chemical, atomic, and elementary particle reaction kinetics.

Atoms may certainly stick together (attract into bound states), forming larger molecules that also have mass, occupy space, and move in collisional paths. Molecules may also attract or repel other atoms and molecules. Or they may directly interact producing new species after binding or colliding. And the process continues along the same path to larger fundamental blocks. Molecules, may synthesize into macromolecules, and so on. Soon the process results in matter on perceivable state and scale (liquid, gas, or solid). The atomistics view is totally compatible with our level of perception and we can measure down to the atomistic level.

But, if we lived in a smaller world (subatomic), we might point to the substructure of electrons, neutrons, and protons comprising atoms. And then we would suggest that quarks, partons, and gluons, thought to be the building blocks of subatomic particles are the objects of the succinct statement applied to atoms. And then the structure of these components might be further divided.

Both pressure and density are intuitive, fundamental concepts, elucidated and measured at early times in our scientific history by the Greeks, Romans, Babylonians, Egyptians, and probably others, well before atomic hypotheses. Pressure, P, is simply the force, F, per unit area, A, that is,

$$P = \frac{F}{A}$$

and is equal in all directions (scalar quantity, while force itself is formally a vector quantity). As will be seen, pressure in gases results from molecular collisions with surroundings. Pressure from extended matter results from the collective forces applied across boundaries of fluids and solids.

Density

Density ρ, similarly is mass, m, per unit volume, V,

$$\rho = \frac{m}{V}$$

and suggests how tightly packed matter can exist. Weight density, ρg, is weight per unit volume, differing from mass density by the acceleration of gravity, g. Both are used interchangeably in applications. Objects denser than a fluid will sink in that fluid, and objects less dense than a fluid will float. Sinking objects have *negative* buoyancy, while floating objects have *positive* buoyancy. Objects with the same density as the fluid have *neutral* buoyancy, and can be moved about without sinking or rising. Relative buoyancy obviously depends on fluid and object densities. Table 7 list densities of known, naturally occurring, elements as function of atomic number, Z, and atomic mass, A.

Table 7. Densities Of Elements

Element	Z	A	$\rho\ (g/cm^3)$	Element	Z	A	$\rho\ (g/cm^3)$
H	1	1.008	.0009	Cd	48	112.41	8.65
He	2	4.003	.0017	In	49	114.82	7.28
Li	3	6.940	.53	Sn	50	118.70	6.52
Be	4	9.013	1.85	Sb	51	121.76	6.69
B	5	10.82	2.45	Te	52	127.61	6.24
C	6	12.01	1.62	I	53	126.91	4.93
N	7	14.08	.0013	Xe	54	131.30	.0059
O	8	16.00	.0014	Cs	55	132.91	1.87
F	9	19.00	.0017	Ba	56	137.36	5.52
Ne	10	20.18	.0009	La	57	138.92	6.19
Na	11	22.99	.971	Ce	58	140.13	6.78
Mg	12	24.32	1.74	Pr	59	140.92	6.78
Al	13	26.98	2.70	Nd	60	144.27	6.95
Si	14	28.09	2.42	Pm	61	145.01	7.23
P	15	30.98	1.82	Sm	62	150.35	7.70
S	16	32.06	2.07	Eu	63	152.08	5.22
Cl	17	35.46	.0032	Gd	64	157.26	7.95
Ar	18	39.94	.0018	Tb	65	158.93	8.33
K	19	39.10	.87	Dy	66	162.51	8.56
Ca	20	40.08	1.55	Ho	67	164.94	8.76
Sc	21	44.96	2.52	Er	68	167.27	9.16
Ti	22	47.90	4.58	Tm	69	168.94	9.35
V	23	50.95	5.96	Yb	70	173.04	7.01
Cr	24	52.01	7.10	Lu	71	174.99	9.74
Mn	25	54.94	7.22	Hf	72	178.53	13.32
Fe	26	55.85	7.86	Ta	73	180.95	16.62
Co	27	58.94	8.91	W	74	183.86	19.28
Ni	28	58.71	8.86	Re	75	186.22	20.53
Cu	29	63.54	8.94	Os	76	190.24	22.48
Zn	30	65.38	7.14	Ir	77	192.18	22.42
Ga	31	69.72	5.91	Pt	78	195.09	21.37
Ge	32	72.60	5.36	Au	79	197.02	19.39
As	33	74.91	5.73	Hg	80	200.61	13.55
Se	34	78.96	4.79	Ti	81	204.39	11.85
Br	35	79.92	3.12	Pb	82	207.21	11.35
Kr	36	83.82	.0037	Bi	83	209.03	9.75
Rb	37	85.48	1.53	Po	84	210.06	9.24
Sr	38	87.63	2.54	At	85	211.12	10.24
Y	39	88.92	5.52	Rn	86	222.13	.0010
Zr	40	91.22	6.43	Fr	87	223.09	
Nb	41	92.91	6.45	Ra	88	226.05	5.04
Mo	42	95.95	10.21	Ac	89	227.13	
Tc	43	98.02		Th	90	232.09	11.32
Ru	44	101.12	12.23	Pa	91	231.12	15.43
Rh	45	102.91	12.53	U	92	238.07	18.91
Pd	46	106.42	12.22	Np	93	237.52	
Ag	47	107.88	10.52	Pu	94	239.12	19.73

Solids and fluids possess essentially fixed density under nominal pressure changes, but gases, and flexible objects containing gases, change density rapidly under pressure change. Relative buoyancy also changes rapidly as object density varies. For contained gases, density and buoyancy changes result from changes in volume. The body itself, and equipment specifically worn by divers, contain air spaces that can expand and contract under pressure changes. The lungs, wet and dry suit, and buoyancy compensator (BC), for instance, respond readily to pressure change, inducing commensurate buoyancy change. Since salt water is denser than freshwater, it exerts a greater buoyant force than fresh water. Buoyancy changes in fresh and salt water thus differ as object density changes.

Buoyancy changes occur when divers descend and ascend, move between fresh and salt water and/or different elevations. Buoyancy is lost relative to the surface when wet suit divers descend. Since fresh water is less dense than salt water, buoyancy is lost in fresh water relative to salt water. Similarly, since ambient pressure at altitude is less than at sea level, wet suits expand at elevation, increasing buoyancy. Effects can be quantified by Archimedes' and Boyle's laws. In all cases, effects ultimately relate to the densities of constituent fluid media.

Archimedes' Principle

According to Archimedes many centuries ago, any object displacing a volume, V, of fluid of density, ρ, is buoyed upward by a force, B, equal to the weight of the displaced fluid. From what we know about pressure in a fluid, this fact can be deduced easily.

Imagine a uniform block, of height, h, and cross sectional surface area, A, so that its volume, V, is

$$V = Ah.$$

Submerging the block in a fluid of density, ρ, in an upright position, we can add up all the pressures on the block to determine the buoyant upward force, B. The sum total of all pressures on faces is zero, since every force on every face is balanced by an equal force on the opposite face. At the top of the block, a downward force, F_d, is exerted by the

$$F_d = \rho g A d,$$

with d the depth of the submerged top face of the block. At the bottom of the block, an upward force, F_u, is exerted by the fluid,

$$F_u = \rho g A (h+d).$$

The difference of the two forces, B, is the buoyant (upward) force,

$$B = F_u - F_d = \rho g A h = \rho g V,$$

or Archimedes' principle.

Wetsuits expand and compress, while fresh water is less dense than salt water. Both affect diver buoyancy because of Archimedes principle and Boyle's law. Consider the wetsuit effect first.

Wetsuits

Gas bubbles in wetsuits are subject to Boyle's law as external pressure changes, though the response is something less than 50% of the volume change predicted by the gas law. To estimate the buoyancy increase due to wetsuit expansion at elevation, we compute the effect using Archimedes principle and Boyle's law directly, and then scale the result by the factor 0.50, as a figure of merit. Denoting the volume of the wetsuit on the surface at sea level, v_0, and the corresponding volume at altitude, v_h, we have by the gas law,

$$33 \, v_0 = P_h \, v_h,$$

with P_h surface pressure at altitude. The theoretical buoyancy change (gain), ΔB_{alt}, at altitude is given by,

$$\Delta B_{alt} = \rho g (v_h - v_0),$$

with ρ the actual water density. Using the above gas law, it follows that,

$$\Delta B_{alt} = \rho g v_0 \left[\frac{33}{P_h} - 1 \right].$$

Making the assumption that the wetsuit offsets the weight belt, somewhere near 10% of diver body weight, w,

$$\rho g v_0 = .10 \, w,$$

and that the expansion of the wetsuit is some 50% of maximum, we obtain,

$$\Delta B_{alt} = .050 \, w \left[\frac{33}{P_h} - 1 \right].$$

Approximating ambient pressure at altitude,

$$P_h = \frac{33}{\alpha} \approx 33 \, (1 - 0.0381h),$$

$$\alpha = exp \, (0.0381h),$$

with h the elevation in multiples of 1,000 ft, we find,

$$\Delta B_{alt} \approx .0017 \, wh,$$

as the approximate buoyancy gain, good to few percent up to 7,000 ft. Figure 25 plots buoyancy increase against altitude.

Fresh and Salt Water

Application of Archimedes principle directly to a diver submerged in fresh and salt water at sea level yields the fresh water buoyancy loss, ΔB_{sea}. Denoting total diver plus gear weight, W, and the corresponding volume of water displaced at sea level in salt water, v, we have for neutral buoyancy,

$$W = \rho g v,$$

with ρ sea water density. The difference in buoyant forces acting upon an object of displaced volume, v, in fresh water and salt water is the buoyancy change (loss),

$$\Delta B_{sea} = \rho g v(\eta - 1) = W(\eta - 1),$$

with η the fresh water *specific* density (ratio of fresh water to salt water density). Taking $\eta = 0.975$, there results,

$$\Delta B_{sea} = -.025W,$$

with the minus sign denoting a buoyancy loss. The buoyancy loss for given diver weight is shown in Figure 26.

Seed and Bubble Response

Under changes in ambient pressure, bubbles will grow or contract, both due to diffusion and Boyle's law. The change under Boyle's law is straightforward. Denoting initial and final pressures and volumes with subscripts, i and f, we have,

$$P_i V_i = P_f V_f$$

with bubble volume,

$$V = \frac{4}{3}\pi r^3$$

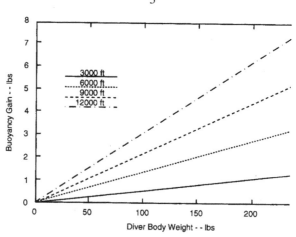

Figure 25. Wetsuit Buoyancy Gain At Altitude

Accounting just for altitude pressure reduction, wetsuit buoyancy gain, Δw, at the surface at altitude, relative to the surface at sea level, can be computed from the relationship,

$$\Delta w = 0.50 f w \left[\frac{33 - P_h}{P_h} \right]$$

with P_h ambient surface pressure at elevation, h, in multiples of 1,000 ft,

$$P_h = 33 \, exp \, (-0.038h)$$

diver body weight, w, and weight belt fraction of diver weight, f.

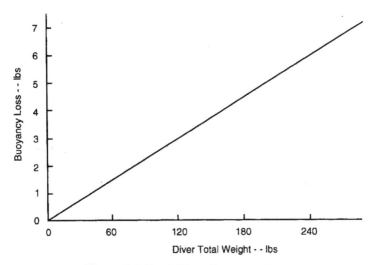

Figure 26. Fresh Water Buoyancy Loss

Fresh water is less dense than salt water. Simple application of Archimedes' principle yields buoyancy loss, ΔW, in terms of diver total weight, W,

$$\Delta W = -0.025 \; W$$

merely reflecting the density difference between fresh and salt water. Salt water density is 64 lbs/ft³, and fresh water density is 62.4 lbs/ft³.

for r the bubble radius. The above supposes totally flexible (and permeable) bubble films or skins on the inside, certainly not unrealistic over small pressure changes (laboratory experiments). Similarly, if the response to pressure changes of the bubble skins is a smooth and slowly varying function, the above is also true in low order. Obviously, the relationship reduces to,

$$P_i r_i^3 = P_f r_f^3$$

for the simple radial response to pressure change.

But in the case of structured, impermeable membranes, capable of offsetting constrictive surface tension, the response to Boyle's law is modified,

$$\xi_i P_i V_i = \xi_f P_f V_f$$

with ξ structure functions depending on pressure, P. For thin, permeable, and elastic bubble skins, $\xi = 1$. For all else, $\xi \neq 1$. For cases of gels studied in the laboratory, as an instance, surfactant stabilized micronuclei do not behave like ideal gas bubbles with thin elastic films. Instead under compression-decompression, their behavior is always less than ideal. That is to say, volume changes under compression or decompression are always less than computed by Boyle's law, similar to the response of a wetsuit described above.

Such behavior is implicit in bubble models like the VPM and RGBM somewhat, accounting for permeable and impermeable response under pressure changes. Or one may employ equation-of-state relationships for bubble coatings. During a rapid compression from initial ambient pressure, P_i, to increased pressure, P, seeds and micronuclei are subjected to crushing compression which decreases radial size. This produces increased tolerance to supersaturation in blood and tissues since smaller nuclei form macroscopic (unstable) bubbles less readily than larger ones. The greater the crushing pressure, $\Delta P = P - P_i$, the greater the supersaturation required to excite a given number of bubbles in the body. A given distribution of nuclei in the body has, for each ΔP, a critical radius, r_i, as seen earlier. Nuclei with radii less than r_i will not grow into bubbles, while nuclei with radii greater than r_i will be excited into growth. Said another way, all nuclei larger than r_i for any compression-decompression schedule, ΔP, will evolve into macroscopic bubbles while the rest will not. But just how excited micronuclei grow requires a model for the behavior of effective surface tension under compression-decompression.

According to the VPM (lab experiments), the corresponding change in critical radius, r, following compression, ΔP, in the *permeable* region, satisfies the relationship,

$$\Delta P = 2(\gamma_{max} - \gamma)\left[\frac{1}{r} - \frac{1}{r_i}\right]$$

with γ_{max} the maximum compressional strength of the surfactant skin, γ the surface tension, and r_i the critical radius at P_i. When P exceeds the structure breakpoint, P_{max}, an equation appropriate to the *impermeable* region must be used. Denoting the crushing pressure differential, $\Delta P_{max} = P - P_{max}$, the VPM requires,

$$\Delta P_{max} = 2(\gamma_{max} - \gamma)\left[\frac{1}{r} - \frac{1}{r_{max}}\right] + P_{max} + 2P_i + P_i\left[\frac{r_{max}}{r}\right]^3$$

$$r_{max} = \left[\frac{P_{max} - P_i}{2(\gamma_{max} - \gamma)} + \frac{1}{r_i}\right]^{-1}$$

is the radius of the critical nucleus at the onset of impermeability, obtained by replacing P and r with P_{max} and r_{max} above. The allowed tissue supersaturation, $\Delta\Pi$, is given by,

$$\Delta\Pi = 2\frac{\gamma}{\gamma_{max}r}(\gamma_{max} - \gamma)$$

with, in the permeable region,

$$r = \left[\frac{\Delta P}{2(\gamma_{max} - \gamma)} + \frac{1}{r_i}\right]^{-1}$$

and, in the impermeable region,

$$r^3 - 2(\gamma_{max} - \gamma)r^2 - \frac{P_i}{\varsigma}r_{max}^3 = 0$$

for,

$$\zeta = \Delta P_{max} - P_{max} + 2P_i + \frac{2(\gamma_{max} - \gamma)}{r_{max}}$$

Thus, allowed supersaturation is a function of three parameters, γ, γ_{max}, and r_i. They can be fitted to exposures and lab data. Additionally, nuclei regenerate over times scales, ω, such that,

$$r = r_0 + [1 - \exp{(-\omega t)}](r_i - r_0)$$

with r_0 the critical radius at initial time ($t = 0$). The fourth parameter, ω^{-1}, is on the order of days.

Hyperbaric Chambers

Hyperbaric chambers are used to treat a number of maladies with different high pressure gases, maladies such as wounds, gangrene, DCI, and multiple sclerosis (MS). Often the treatment mixture is oxygen (or mostly oxygen), and the treatment process is called hyperbaric oxygen therapy (HBOT). This is particularly true for wounds, gangrene, and MS. With DCI, treatment includes mixtures of nitrogen, helium, and oxygen blended in proportions to avoid oxygen toxicity and inert gas narcosis. The combination of increased ambient pressure and elevated levels of oxygen help to dissolve bubbles and also wash out inert gases.

Oxygen, when breathed under increased atmospheric pressure, is a potent drug. Hyperbaric oxygen, if administered indiscriminately, can produce noticeable toxic effects. Safe time-dose limits have been established for hyperbaric oxygen, and these profiles form the basis of treatment protocols. The past 10 to 15 years have seen the introduction of disease specific hyperoxic dosing. Emergency cases, such as carbon monoxide poisoning or cerebral arterial gas embolism (AGE) may only require one or two treatment schedules. In cases where angiogenisis is the primary goal, as many as 20 to 40 visits to the hyperbaric chamber may be requisite. The precise number of treatments often depends upon the clinical response of the patient. Transcutaneous oximetry can often provide more exacting dose schedules, improving treatment and cost effectiveness. With the exception of DCI and AGE, periods of exposure last approximately 2 hours. Treatments may be given once, twice, or occasionally three times daily, and provided in both inpatient and outpatient settings.

Several beneficial mechanisms are associated with intermittent exposure to hyperbaric doses of oxygen. Either alone, or more commonly in combination with other medical and surgical procedures, these mechanisms serve to enhance the healing process in treatable circumstances.

Hyperoxygenation provides immediate support to poorly perfused tissues in sections of compromised blood flow. The elevated pressure within the hyperbaric chamber results in a 10 to 15 fold increase in plasma oxygen concentrations. Translated to arterial oxygen tensions, values near 1,500 to 2,000 *mmHg* are observed, thereby producing a 4 fold increase in the diffusion length of oxygen from functioning capillaries. While this form of hyperoxygenation is only temporary, it does buy time and maintain tissue viability until corrective measures or new blood supply are established.

Neovascularization represents an indirect and delayed response to hyperbaric oxygen therapy. Therapeutic effects include enhanced fibroplast division, neoformation of collagen, and capillary angiogenisis in areas of sluggish vascularization, such as radiation damaged tissue, refractory osteomyelitis, and chronic ulceration in soft tissue.

Antimicrobial inhibition has been demonstrated at a number of levels. Hyperbaric oxygen induces toxin inhibition and toxin inactivation in clostridial perfingens (gas gangrene). Hyperoxia enhances phagocytosis and white cell oxidative killing, and has been shown to support aminoglycocide activity. Recent studies suggest that prolonged antibiotic screening follows application of high pressure oxygen.

Phase reduction, application of Laplace's and Boyle's law to separated gases in tissue and blood, forms the basis of hyperbaric treatment of decompression sickness and arterial gas embolism, as known for more than a century. Commonly associated with divers and diving, AGE is a frequent iatrogenic event in modern medicine, resulting in significant morbity and mortality, and remains grossly underdiagnosed. The process is enhanced gas diffusion from free phases to the venous blood flow for elimination through the lungs. Increasing pressure increases the outgassing gradient, and shrinks gas phases by Boyle contraction.

Vasoconstriction is an important spinoff of hyperbaric oxygen, manging intermediate compartment syndrome and other acute ischemias, as well as reducing interstitial edema in grafted tissues. Studies in burn wound applications indicate a significant decrease in fluid resuscitation requirements when HBOT is added to wound therapy.

Reperfusion injury attenuation is a recently discovered mechanism associated with hyperbaric oxygen. Leukocyte deactivation has been traced to high concentrations of oxygen in the blood, with the net effect the preservation of tissues that might otherwise be lost to ischemia-reperfusion injury. Reperfusion injury occurs with direct hypoxia and inappropriate activation of leukocytes.

Keyed Exercises

- *Mark the following statements TRUE or FALSE.*

T	<u>F</u>	*Atoms are the fundamental building blocks of matter.*
<u>T</u>	F	*All atoms of a given element are identical.*
<u>T</u>	F	*The Greeks thought air, water, earth, and fire were fundamental.*
<u>T</u>	F	*Simulation of fundamental properties of matter is called molecular dynamics.*

T	F	The binding energy of two particles can exceed their rest masses.
T	F	Objects denser than a fluid will sink in the fluid.
T	F	Quarks and anti-quarks have not been observed in the free state.
T	F	Most of the elements in the Periodic Table are short lived.
T	F	The mass defect is always negative in sign.
T	T	The equation of state connects pressure, density, and temperature.

- What is the mass defect, Δm, of carbon dioxide, CO_2, with molecular weight 44.0095 amu?

$$M = 44.0095 \ amu, \ \sum_{i=1}^{44} m_i = (22 \times 1.0073 + 22 \times 1.0087) \ amu = 44.3520 \ amu$$

$$\Delta m = 44.0095 \ amu - 44.3520 \ amu = -0.2570 \ amu$$

If electrons are included with mass 0.0005 amu, what is the mass defect, Δm?

$$\Delta m = -0.2570 \ amu - 22 \times 0.0005 \ amu = -0.2680 \ amu$$

- From Table 7, what is the mass, m, of 1500 cm^3 of iron (Fe)?

$$\rho_{Fe} = 7.86 \ g/cm^3, \ m = \rho_{Fe} V = 7.86 \times 1500 \ g = 11.8 kg$$

What volume, V, does 600 g of calcium (Ca) occupy?

$$\rho_{Ca} = 1.55 \ g/cm^3, \ V = \frac{m}{\rho_{Ca}} = \frac{600}{1.55} \ cm^3 = 387 \ cm^3$$

What is the gram molecular weight, G, of osmium (Os), and density, ρ_{Os}?

$$A_{Os} = 190.24, \ G = A_{Os} \ g = 190.24 \ g, \ \rho_{Os} = 22.48 \ g/cm^3$$

- What is the pressure of a column of seawater, $d = 33 \ fsw$, assuming density, $\rho = 64 \ lbs/ft^3$?

$$P = \rho g d = 64 \times 33 \ lbs/ft^2 = 2112 \ lbs/ft^2 = 14.6 \ lbs/in^2$$

What is the pressure of a column of fresh water, $d = 34 \ ft$, assuming density, $\rho = 62.4 \ lbs/ft^3$?

$$P = \rho g d = 62.4 \times 34 \ lbs/ft^2 = 2121 \ lbs/ft^2 = 14.7 \ lbs/in^2$$

- A 448 lb winch gear, displacing a volume, $V = 2 \ ft^3$, rests on a hard sea bottom at 99 fsw. What surface volume of air, V_{sur}, is needed to inflate lift bags to bring the gear to the surface?

$$d = 99 \ fsw, \ \rho = 64 \ lbs/ft^3, \ w = 448 \ lbs$$

$$V_{lift} = \frac{w}{\rho} = \frac{448}{64} \ ft^3 = 7 \ ft^3$$

$$V_{sur} = V_{lift} \left[1 + \frac{d}{33} \right] = 4 \times 7 \ ft^3 = 28 \ ft^3$$

- A buoy weighing 48 lbs occupies, $V = 3 ft^3$. What fraction, ξ, of its volume will float above water?

$$V = 3 \ ft^3, \ \xi = \frac{V - V_{dis}}{V}$$

$$V_{dis} = \frac{w}{\rho} = \frac{48}{64} \ ft^3 = .75 \ ft^3$$

$$\xi = \frac{3 - .75}{3} = .75$$

- A 75 kg diver journeys to a mountain lake at 1,830 m. What is the surface wetsuit buoyancy, Δw, increase?

$$\Delta w = .0029wh, \ h = \frac{1830}{1000} \times 3.28 = 6, \ w = mg$$

$$\Delta w = .0029 \times 75 \times 9.8 \times 6 \ newton = 12.7 \ newton$$

- What is the salt water to fresh water buoyancy loss, ΔW, for a salvage diver plus gear of mass, $m = 90 \ kg$?

$$W = mg$$

$$\Delta W = -.025 \ W = -.025 \times 90 \times 9.8 \ newton = -22.5 \ newton$$

- What are composite partial pressures, p_i, for 80/10/10 trimix breathing gas at ocean depth of 400 fsw ($f_{He} = .80, \ f_{O_2} = .10,$ and $f_{N_2} = .10$)?

$$p_i = f_i \ (33 + 400) \ fsw \quad (i = He, O_2, N_2)$$

$$p_{He} = .80 \times 433 \ fsw = 346.4 \ fsw$$

$$p_{O_2} = .10 \times 433 \ fsw = 43.3 \ fsw$$

$$p_{N_2} = .10 \times 433 \ fsw = 43.3 \ fsw$$

- A pearl diver plus all gear weigh 128 lbs, and are buoyed up in the water with a force of 124 lbs. What does the pearl diver weigh, ΔW, in the water?

$$\Delta W = 128 - 124 \ lbs = 4 \ lbs$$

If a BC provides lift, how much additional lift, ΔB, is necessary to float the pearl diver at neutral buoyancy?

$$\Delta B = \Delta W = 4 \ lbs$$

- How much fresh water, V, does a 200 lb lift bag displace?

$$\rho = 62.4 \ lbs/ft^3, \ W = 200 \ lbs$$

$$V = \frac{W}{\rho} = \frac{200}{62.4} \ ft^3 = 3.2 \ ft^3$$

- *A fully inflated BC displaces, V = .78 ft³, of sea water. What is the lift, B, provided by the BC?*

$$B = \rho g V$$

$$B = 64 \times .78 \ lb = 49.9 \ lb$$

- *A fully clad diver displaces, V = 3.5 ft³, of fresh water. What is the buoyant force, B, on diver and gear?*

$$B = \rho g V$$

$$B = 62.4 \times 3.5 \ lb = 218 \ lb$$

If diver plus gear weigh, W = 200 lb, how much add additional weigh, ΔW, must be added to the belt for neutral buoyancy?

$$\Delta W = B - W = (218 - 200) \ lb = 18 \ lb$$

- *Mark the following statements TRUE or FALSE.*

<u>T</u>	F	Oxygen breathed at high partial pressures can be a drug.
T	<u>F</u>	Hyperbaric chambers are only used to treat divers.
T	<u>F</u>	Decreasing pressure shrinks gas bubbles.
<u>T</u>	F	Hyperbaric oxygen induces toxin inhibition.
T	<u>F</u>	Elevated chamber pressure produces reductions in plasma concentrations.
<u>T</u>	F	HBOT can be a useful treatment for arterial gas embolism.
<u>T</u>	F	Bubble growth is best controlled by increasing ambient pressure.
T	<u>F</u>	Reperfusion injury occurs with direct hyperoxia.
T	<u>F</u>	Vasoconstriction is an important spinoff of nitrogen high pressure in diving.

- *Using EOS data in Table 10 by taking $\xi \propto r_s$, if a bubble of volume 3 μm at a depth of 99 fsw is released to the surface at sea level pressure, what is the surfacing volume?*

$$P_i = 132 \ fsw, \quad V_i = 3 \ \mu m, \quad \xi_i = 0.53, \quad P_f = 33 \ fsw, \quad \xi_f = 0.80$$

$$V_f = \frac{\xi_i P_i V_i}{\xi_f P_f} = \frac{.53 \times 132 \times 3}{.80 \times 33} \ \mu m = 7.95 \ \mu m$$

- *In gel experiments, if the critical radius, ε, is inversely proportional to the crushing pressure differential, ΔP, what happens to the critical radius if the crushing differential is tripled?*

$$\Delta P_f \varepsilon_f = \Delta P_i \varepsilon_i, \quad \Delta P_f = 3\Delta P_i$$

$$\varepsilon_f = \frac{\varepsilon_i}{3}$$

Metrology and Calibration

Capillary gauges employ pressure ratios to register depths, using a sea level ratio calibration point, while bourdon and oil filled gauges measure direct pressure and subtract off sea level atmospheric pressure to register depths. Submersible tank gauges also measure pressure directly, and subtract off atmospheric pressure. Mechanics are straightforward, as follows, taking the capillary gauge first.

Capillary Gauges

In any fluid, capillary gauge readings are dependent on the volume of compressed air in the tube. Out of the fluid, at atmospheric pressure, P_h, the volume of the tube occupied by air, v_{max}, is maximum. At actual depth, d, the volume of the tube, v, occupied by air is less (because of compression). At depth, d, the total pressure, P, is simply,

$$P = P_h + \eta d,$$

with η the fluid specific density. By Boyle's law, the volumes are related,

$$(P_h + \eta d)v = P_h v_{max},$$

for any specific density, η, and any surface pressure, P_h. Capillary gauges are calibrated for sea level atmospheric pressure, $P_0 = 33 \ fsw$, and in salt water, $\eta = 1$, at some depth, δ, so that the volume ratio reduces,

$$\frac{v_{max}}{v} = \left[\frac{33 + \delta}{33} \right].$$

In any other fluid, at actual depth, d, the corresponding gauge reading, δ, can be obtained by substituting the calibration relationship into the above, and simplifying, with the result,

$$\delta = \left[\frac{33}{P_h} \right] \eta d.$$

For fresh water, $\eta = 0.975$, as noted, and atmospheric pressure, P_h, at elevation, h, decreases exponentially. Capillary gauge readings versus depth are plotted in Figure 27 for various altitudes.

Bourdon and Oil Filled Gauges

Other gauges measure absolute ambient pressure and mechanically subtract off surface pressure to give a reading. Thus, at depth, d, a bourdon or oil filled gauge in fluid of specific density, η, senses ambient pressure, P, subtracts off a constant, X, and registers a mechanical response, Y,

$$Y = \eta d + P_h - X,$$

If calibrated at depth, δ, in salt water, $\eta = 1.0$, for sea level atmospheric pressure, $P_0 = 33\ fsw$, then,

$$Y = \delta + 33 - X$$

Substituting equations yields the gauge reading, δ, in any fluid, η, at actual depth, d, for any surface pressure, P_h,

$$\delta = \eta\ d + P_h - 33,$$

in analogy to a capillary gauge. Bourdon and oil filled gauge readings at elevation are plotted against actual depth in Figure 28. Mechanically, submersible pressure (tank) gauges work the same way.

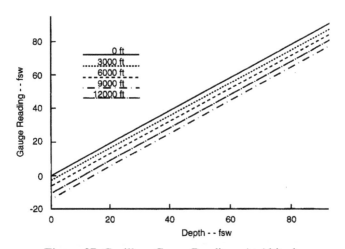

Figure 27. Capillary Gauge Readings At Altitude

Capillary gauges read equivalent sea level depth at altitude (always greater than actual depth), facilitating direct table entry with the gauge reading. In terms of actual depth, d, the gauge reading, δ, is simply,

$$\delta = \eta\ \left[\frac{33d}{P_h}\right] = \beta d$$

with η specific density, P_h atmospheric pressure, and all depths and pressures measured in fsw. Scaling is thus linear.

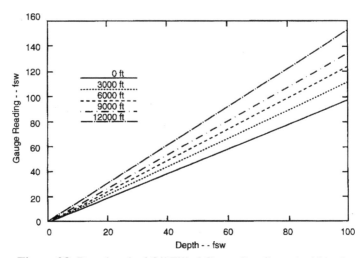

Figure 28. Bourdon And Oil Filled Gauge Readings At Altitude

Bourdon and oil filled gauges register depths at altitude that are less than actual depth, d. The gauge reading, δ, takes the form

$$\delta = \eta d + P_h - 33$$

for surface pressure, P_h, and specific density, η. The scaling is linear, as with capillary gauges.

Submersible Tank Gauges

Submersible gauges read tank pressure directly. Knowing the rated tank pressure, P_r, and rated gas volume, V_r, permits rapid estimation of air remaining in the tank for breathing. The rated tank pressure is the maximum recommended pressure for the tank upon filling. The rated tank volume is the amount of gas, initially at standard temperature and pressure, compressed to the rated tank pressure. For instance, the standard steel 72 ft^3 tank, is rated at 2,475 lbs/in^2, meaning that, $V_r = 72\ ft^3$, and that, $P_r = 2,475\ lbs/in^2$.

From Boyle's law, we can write for any tank pressure, P, and remaining breathing volume, V, denoting the actual tank volume, V_t, and standard pressure, P_0, usually 1 *atm*,

$$PV_t = P_0V,$$

and we also know at rated pressure, P_r, and volume, V_r,

$$P_rV_t = P_0V_r.$$

Dividing the above two equations yields the ratio,

$$\frac{P}{P_r} = \frac{V}{V_r},$$

which permits direct estimation of remaining air volume, V, for submersible gauge reading, P, and specified P_r and V_r. The ratio, P_r/V_r is called the *tank constant*, using any convenient set of units.

Compressibility and Cubical Expansion

Under pressure and temperature changes, all matter undergoes expansion or compression. The coefficient of volume change, κ, under pressure change, at constant temperature, T, is called the *isothermal* compressibility,

$$\kappa = -\frac{1}{V}\left[\frac{\partial V}{\partial P}\right]_T,$$

and the coefficient of cubical expansion, β, measures the volume change under temperature change, at constant pressure,

$$\beta = \frac{1}{V}\left[\frac{\partial V}{\partial T}\right]_P,$$

and these quantities can certainly be measured experimentally for any material. The corresponding thermal coefficient, ζ, measures change of pressure, P, with temperature, T, at constant volume, V, and is simply related to κ and β through,

$$\zeta = \left[\frac{\partial P}{\partial T}\right]_V = -\left[\frac{\partial V}{\partial T}\right]_P\left[\frac{\partial V}{\partial P}\right]_T^{-1} = \frac{\beta}{\kappa}.$$

For solids and liquids, β, κ, and ζ are very small, virtually constant over small ranges of temperature and pressure. For gases, the situation is different. Ideal gases, from the equation of state, simply have,

$$\kappa = \frac{1}{P},$$

$$\beta = \frac{1}{T},$$

so that compressibility and expansion coefficients depend inversely on pressure, P, and temperature, T. The thermal coefficient is similarly given by,

$$\zeta = \frac{P}{T} = \frac{nR}{v}.$$

Activities Rate

Regulator function exploits air compressibility to deliver air to the lungs at any ambient pressure. Filled with compressed air at ambient pressure, the lungs can function underwater in the same manner as on the surface, inflating and deflating normally. However, underwater, assuming the same metabolic consumption rate for given activity, the diver uses more air to fill the lungs than on the surface, because the air is compressed. At sea level, we consume air at a rate, χ_0. Relative to χ_0, the underwater rate is greater. At elevation, the surface consumption is less than χ_0.

Variation in consumption rate with ambient pressure is a gas density effect (regulator function), while variation in rate with activity is a metabolic effect (oxygen requirement). Figure 29 graphs surface consumption rates at altitude for corresponding sea level consumption rates. Table 8 lists nominal consumption rates at sea level for various activities, in water and on land. Certainly these activities rates vary with individual, temperature, physical condition, body morphology, lung capacity, drag, mental state, metabolism, and so on.

Table 8. Activities Air Consumption Rates At Sea Level.

Land/Water Activity	Sea Level Consumption Rate χ_0 (ft^3/min)
Reclining/Floating Horizontally	.6
Standing/Floating Vertically	.8
Walking/Light Treading	1.0
Jogging/Slow Swimming	1.3
Running/Moderate Swimming	1.6
Sprinting/Cold Arduous Diving	2.0

Effective Consumption

Compared to the sea level surface consumption rate, the altitude surface consumption rate is reduced by the ratio of ambient pressure to sea level pressure, α. Quite obviously the surface rate at altitude, decreases inversely with elevation. Underwater rates, of course, continue to increase with pressure. Thus at depth, reductions in surface pressures at altitude have increasingly lesser effect on consumption rates, an effect also seen in wetsuit bouyancy with increasing pressure.

Denoting the altitude surface consumption rate, χ_h, the consumption rate, χ, at depth, d, and implied elevation, α, scales directly with the pressure, that is, neglecting the 3% density difference between salt and fresh water for simplicity,

$$\chi = \chi_h \left[1 + \frac{d\alpha}{33} \right].$$

The total pressure, P, satisfies a similar relationship in terms of surface pressure, P_h,

$$P = P_h + d = \frac{33}{\alpha} + d = \frac{33}{\alpha} \left[1 + \frac{\alpha d}{33} \right].$$

At any altitude, consumption rates increase rapidly with depth, offsetting reduced surface rates. The surface rate at altitude, χ_h , is related to the surface rate at sea level, χ_0, by the relationship,

$$\chi_h = \frac{\chi_0}{\alpha} \approx \chi_0 \left(1 - 0.038h \right),$$

for h the usual elevation in multiples of 1,000 ft.

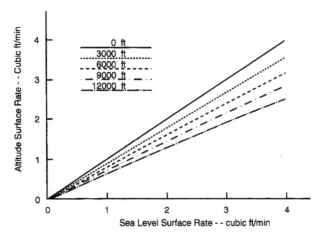

Figure 29. Consumption Rates at Altitude

Air (breathing mixture) consumption rates at elevation are less than at sea level for the same depth, d, because the density of regulator inspired air (breathing mixture) is less than at sea level. Defining the sea level consumption rate, χ_0, the altitude surface consumption rate, χ_h, is given by,

$$\chi_h = \chi_0 \left[\frac{P_h}{33} \right] = \frac{\chi_0}{\alpha}$$

so that the consumption rate, χ, at actual depth, d, is accordingly written,

$$\chi = \chi_h \left[1 + \frac{\alpha \eta d}{33} \right]$$

Variation of consumption rate with altitude is a density effect (regulator function), while variation in consumption rate with physical activity is a metabolic effect.

High Pressure Cylinders

High pressure cylinders are mostly made from steel and aluminum, although prototypes of stainless steel and fiber wound composites have appeared. Carbon steel, used in early tanks, has been replaced with chrome molybdenum steel. Aluminum is alloyed with other metals, such as magnesium and titanium. Steel tanks were introduced in the late 1940s, and aluminum tanks became popular in the 1970s, though the first were imported from France in 1950. Cylinders carry compressed gases for underwater breathing, and are rated according to maximum working pressure, and the corresponding volume occupied by the breathing gas at 1 *atm*. Table 9 summarizes tank characteristics for a number of rated steel and aluminum cylinders. Steel tanks are generally heavier and exhibit negative buoyancy when filled with air. Aluminum tanks are lighter and tend to exhibit positive buoyancy before all tank air is depleted. To recover the buoyancy characteristics of steel tanks, aluminum tanks of the same size must have thicker walls, thus increasing their weight, but not their displacement.

Table 9. Cylinder Specifications.

material	Volume (ft^3)	Pressure (lbs/in^2)	Length (in)	Diameter (in)	Weight (lbs)	Buoyancy (lbs)
steel	15	3300	13.80	4.00	7.5	-1.30
aluminum	14	2015	16.60	4.40	5.4	3.22
aluminum	50	3000	19.00	6.90	21.5	2.25
steel	50	1980	22.50	6.80	20.8	2.43
steel	72	2475	25.00	6.80	29.5	3.48
aluminum	72	3000	26.00	6.90	28.5	3.60
aluminum	80	3000	26.40	7.25	33.3	4.00
aluminum	80	3000	27.00	7.25	34.5	4.12
steel	95	3300	25.00	7.00	39.1	-6.11

Pressures in a tank cylinder increase as temperature increases, decrease as temperature decreases. Denoting the initial pressure and temperature, P_0 and T_0, and the final pressure and temperature, P and T, we have, assuming an ideal gas,

$$\frac{P_0}{T_0} = \frac{P}{T},$$

or,

$$P = \frac{T}{T_0}P_0,$$

Put another way, the change in pressure, ΔP, satisfies,

$$\Delta P = P - P_0 = P_0 \left[\frac{T}{T_0} - 1\right].$$

The pressure change depends linearly on the temperature ratio, T/T_0, increasing or decreasing as T increases or decreases.

Regulators and Rebreathers

Regulators, rebreathers, and compressors move gases from one reservoir to another at different pressure, and often, temperature. Regulators and rebreathers simply reduce gases at high pressure to low pressure, and compressors elevate gases at low pressure to high pressure. In both cases, gas flows involve high pressures and turbulent flows, for which steady state dynamics are a low order approximation, particularly as time scales decrease. The essence of regulator, rebreather, and compressor flow dynamics can be extracted from a simple high pressure flow model, namely, a fixed reservoir with connecting flow, treating the air as an ideal gas. In zero order, for adiabatic flow, and in the absence of shaft work and elevation changes, the flow temperature change, dT, and velocity change, dv, are related,

$$\frac{dv}{dT} = \frac{1}{v}\frac{\gamma R}{1-\gamma},$$

with universal gas constant, R, and $\gamma = 5/3$. With this approximation for laminar flow, the volume flow rate, J, in a hose of length, dl, with cross sectional radius, r, is given by,

$$J = \frac{\pi r^4}{8\eta} \frac{dP}{dl}$$

for dP the pressure drop in dl, and η the viscosity of the fluid (gas).

Crucial to the operation of rebreathers is a constant and continuous mass flow of breathing gas, subject to oxygen metabolic requirements and depth. Mass balance simply requires that the flow into the breathing bag equals the amount used by the body plus that exhaled into the breathing bag or exhalation bag. Denoting the breathing gas flow rate, F, the metabolic oxygen (consumption) rate, m, the source oxygen fraction, f_{O_2}, and inspired (breathing bag) oxygen fraction, i_{O_2}, mass balance is written,

$$f_{O_2}F = i_{O_2}F + (1 - i_{O_2})m$$

The source flow rate, F, and oxygen fraction, f_{O_2}, depend on nozzle and mixture. The metabolic rate, m, depends on workload, and the inspired fraction, i_{O_2}, is uniquely determined with the other three specified. Or, for requisite inspired fraction, i_{O_2}, and metabolic rate, m, the source rate, F, and oxygen source fraction, f_{O_2}, can be fixed within limits. Workload rates, m, range, 0.5–20.5 l/min, while source flows, F, depend on depth, cylinder and nozzle, with typical values, 5–16 l/min. As seen, the source oxygen fraction, f_{O_2}, is uniquely determined by the maximum depth, d_{max}, and maximum oxygen pressure (typically 1.6–1.4 atm). Always, inspired oxygen partial pressures are kept between hyperoxic and hypoxic limits, roughly, 0.16–1.6 atm. At depth, d, the source flow rate, F, decreases according to,

$$F = \frac{F_0}{1 + d/33}$$

for F_0 the surface rate, unless the flow is depth compensated.

All RBs strive for fairly constant oxygen partial pressure, p_{O_2}, or oxygen mix fraction, f_{O_2}, or something in between for dive depth limits, through a combination of injectors, sensors, and valves. High operational oxygen partial pressures coupled to lower inert gas partial pressures minimize decompression requirements, obviously, but oxtox concerns are raised. For fixed oxygen partial pressure, p_{O_2} in atm, the oxygen fraction, f_{O_2}, depends on depth, d, and altitude, h,

$$f_{O_2} = \frac{p_{O_2}}{\alpha^{-1} + \eta d/33}$$

For fixed oxygen fraction, f_{O_2}, oxygen partial pressure varies,

$$p_{O_2} = f_{O_2}(\alpha^{-1} + \eta d/33)$$

In both cases, the total inert gas fraction, f_i, is always given by,

$$f_i = 1 - f_{O_2}$$

and varies little when f_{O_2} is relatively constant. Additionally, for fixed diluent fractions of helium and nitrogen, δ_{He} and δ_{N_2}, the breathed helium and nitrogen fractions, f_{He} and f_{N_2}, are also in both cases,

$$f_{He} = f_i \frac{\delta_{He}}{\delta_{He} + \delta_{N_2}}$$

$$f_{N_2} = f_i \frac{\delta_{N_2}}{\delta_{He} + \delta_{N_2}}$$

In the following, we confine discussion to sea level, and in salt water, that is, $\alpha^{-1} = 1$ and $\eta = 1$, and consider CCRs, and then SCRs.

Pure oxygen CCRs are fairly simple devices, employing just oxygen in the breathing mixture. Obviously, there are no inert gas decompression requirements on pure oxygen. Oxtox (CNS and full body), however, is a major concern on oxygen CCRs. In such a device, the volume of gas in the breathing loop is maintained constant, and oxygen added to compensate for metabolic consumption and increasing pressure. On ascent, breathing gas need be vented if not consumed metabolically. Oxygen CCRs inject pure oxygen into the breathing loop, so that, $f_{O_2} = 1$, with corresponding oxygen partial pressure (atm),

$$p_{O_2} = (1 + d/33)$$

for sea level activities. Because of oxtox concerns, oxygen CCRs are limited for diving, somewhere in the 20–30 fsw range in keeping p_{O_2} below 1.6 atm.

Mixed gas CCRs allow deeper excursions than pure oxygen CCRs by diluting the breathing mix with inert gases, notably nitrogen and helium. Fresh oxygen is injected into the breathing loop only as needed to compensate for metabolic oxygen consumption. Partial pressures of oxygen are measured in the loop with oxygen sensors, and oxygen is injected to maintain constant oxygen partial pressure, called the *set point*. Operationally, mixed gas CCRs are simpler to use than their sisters, mixed gas SCRs. Efficiency and safety concerns obviously track directly to oxygen sensors. Mixed gas CCRs maintain constant oxygen partial pressures, p_{O_2}, with a combination of diluents and pure oxygen. The oxygen fraction, f_{O_2}, varies with depth,

$$f_{O_2} = \frac{p_{O_2}}{1 + d/33}$$

and the breathed total inert gas fraction, f_i, makes up the difference,

$$f_i = f_{He} + f_{N_2} = 1 - f_{O_2}$$

for the general case of helium and nitrogen diluents. The oxygen, helium, and nitrogen breathed gas fractions, f_{O_2}, f_{He}, and f_{N_2} vary continuously with depth, d. If the (fixed) diluent helium and nitrogen fraction are denoted, δ_{He} and δ_{N_2}, the breathed helium and nitrogen fractions become,

$$f_{He} = (1 - f_{O_2})\gamma_{He} = f_i\gamma_{He}$$

$$f_{N_2} = (1 - f_{O_2})\gamma_{N_2} = f_i\gamma_{N_2}$$

with diluent ratios, γ_{He} and γ_{N_2},

$$\gamma_{He} = \frac{\delta_{He}}{\delta_{He} + \delta_{N_2}}$$

$$\gamma_{N_2} = \frac{\delta_{N_2}}{\delta_{He} + \delta_{N_2}}$$

Partial pressures at depth for the inert gases are then simply,

$$p_{N_2} = f_{N_2}(1 + d/33)$$

$$p_{He} = f_{He}(1 + d/33)$$

and the oxygen partial pressure, p_{O_2}, is constant.

A semiclosed circuit rebreather (SCR) is very similar to a CCR and operates with an overpressure relief valve to vent gas in maintaining ambient pressure in the loop. A metering valve is necessary to assess metabolic oxygen consumption and breathing gas injection rates. A number of injection systems exist and all are designed to compensate for metabolic oxygen consumption. Three of interest include the constant ratio injection, constant mass flow injection, and the respiratory volume injection systems.

SCRs in the constant ratio injection category have an oxygen and diluent gas source. Diluent injection varies with depth and oxygen injection links to a mass transport control system. The injection strategy approaches constant p_{O_2} performance in the breathing loop. In this case, the fraction, f_{O_2}, varies with depth,

$$f_{O_2} = \frac{p_{O_2}}{1 + d/33}$$

and breathed total inert gas fraction, f_i, makes up the difference,

$$f_i = f_{He} + f_{N_2} = 1 - f_{O_2}$$

as before for mixed gas CCRs. Retaining diluent fractions, δ_{He} and δ_{N_2}, breathed helium and nitrogen fractions remain,

$$f_{He} = f_i\gamma_{He}$$

$$f_{N_2} = f_i\gamma_{N_2}$$

Partial pressures at depth for the inert gases are still,

$$p_{N_2} = f_{N_2}(1 + d/33)$$

$$p_{He} = f_{He}(1 + d/33)$$

With a constant mass flow injection SCR, a set gas mixture point controls a constant flow of diluent into the loop. Exhaust is vented through an overpressure relief valve. A single diluent source is employed, while in constant mass flow SCRs, both oxygen partial pressure and oxygen fraction are more variable than in all other RB devices. For depth ranges anticipated, minimal and maximal values of oxygen fraction, f_{O_2}, can be determined from the mass balance equation and used for dive planning contingencies, such as oxtox and decompression, from the above set of equations.

The respiratory volume injection SCR is a variant of the constant mass flow device. The injection rate of diluent is coupled to the diver's breathing rate, maintaining an almost constant fraction, f_{O_2}, in loop oxygen. Single diluent source is again used. Operationally, a fairly constant f_{O_2} results, and oxygen partial pressure, p_{O_2}, varies with depth,

$$p_{O_2} = f_{O_2}(1 + d/33)$$

and breathed total inert gas fraction, f_i, makes up the difference,

$$f_i = f_{He} + f_{N_2} = 1 - f_{O_2}$$

as above. With same diluent fractions, δ_{He} and δ_{N_2}, breathed helium and nitrogen fractions are roughly constant too,

$$f_{He} = f_i \gamma_{He}$$

$$f_{N_2} = f_i \gamma_{N_2}$$

Breathed inert gas partial pressures vary at depth,

$$p_{N_2} = f_{N_2}(1 + d/33)$$

$$p_{He} = f_{He}(1 + d/33)$$

and the oxygen partial pressure, p_{O_2}, varies as indicated above.

To achieve such ends in flow programming, RBs are extremely complex systems. Extensive diver training and technical knowledge are keynoted in RB diving and usage. Nonetheless, RB divers are growing in numbers across technical and recreational segments.

Steady Flow

The most general statement about mass flow continuity takes the form,

$$\frac{\partial \rho}{\partial t} + \nabla \cdot (\rho \mathbf{v}) = 0$$

for mass density, ρ, and velocity, $\mathbf{v}$. Certainly, within this conservation statement, a variety of turbulent and nonturbulent flow regimes are possible. Most often flows are turbulent (as seen above). For incompressible flow without circulation, the velocity field (vector), $\mathbf{v}$, satisfies two additional constraint equations,

$$\nabla \cdot \mathbf{v} = 0$$

$$\nabla \times \mathbf{v} = 0$$

the so called steady state condition. The above (with some mathematical finesse), lead to streamline results for pressure, p, density, ρ, elevation, z, and velocity, v,

$$p + \frac{1}{2}\rho v^2 + \rho gz = \gamma$$

with g the acceleration of gravity, and γ a flow constant.

Yet, to a lower order (nonturbulent) in flow regimes, a steady state approximation to fluid flow dynamics can be stated very simply in terms of energy balances. Denoting initial and final states of a flowing fluid (gas or liquid), i and f, in a system capable of doing external work, W, and exchanging heat, Q, application of the first law yields for the differential increase of total energy, U, of the system,

$$U = Q - (W + p_f V_f - p_i V_i)$$

for p pressures and V volumes. Assuming that the total energy, U, of the flowing system consists of internal energy of the fluid, mu, kinetic energy, $1/2mv^2$, and potential energy, mgz, the balance takes the simple form,

$$Q - (W + p_f V_f - p_i V_i) = m(u_f - u_i) + \frac{1}{2}m(v_f^2 - v_i^2) + mg(z_f - z_i)$$

where z is the position, v is the flow speed, and u is the specific internal energy of the fluid. The representation above is also known as Bernoulli's generalized law. Its importance is well established in that it is the governing relationship for flight, that is, a pressure reduction on the top side of a wing or airfoil, relative to the pressure on the bottom side, results in hydrodynamical lift (then flight). It is also the basic governing relationship for blood flow in the arterial and venous circulation of the body.

Another example is flow through a nozzle, discussed earlier. If the work, W, and heat exchanged, Q, are zero (certainly an idealization), as in air exhausting from the valve of a scuba tank, the initial and final (exiting) flow velocities depend only on initial and final enthalpies, h, with

$$h = mu + pV$$

so that,

$$mv_f^2 = mv_i^2 + 2(h_i - h_f)$$

at the same elevation, z. More generally, the work, W, and heat exchanged, Q, are not zero, and so we see,

$$mv_f^2 = mv_i^2 + 2(h_i - h_f) + 2(Q - W)$$

which applies to tank cooling or heating in exhausting or filling a breathing mixture. Both cases assume laminar flow. In perspective, we also recall for incompressible and adiabatic fluid flow with no shaft work,

$$p_i + \frac{1}{2}\rho v_i^2 + \rho g z_i = p_f + \frac{1}{2}\rho v_f^2 + \rho g z_f = \gamma$$

and γ the *streamline* (constant) in phase space, for

$$\rho = \rho_i = \rho_f$$

because the fluid is incompressible. Historically, such is Bernoulli's law, and follows easily from the above mass-energy conservation laws.

General Flow Conservation

In the above, special features and cases of certain flow regimes were discussed. Three broad statements about fluid flow take the form of continuity equations for mass, momentum, and energy, and are basically conservation laws for fluids. The above rest upon these three differential statements.

Conservation of mass for fluid flow is written,

$$\frac{\partial \rho}{\partial t} + \nabla\cdot(\rho \mathbf{v}) = 0$$

for ρ local fluid density, and $\mathbf{v}$ local fluid velocity. Momentum conservation is more complicated, taking the form,

$$\rho\left[\frac{\partial \mathbf{v}}{\partial t} + (\mathbf{v}\cdot\nabla)\mathbf{v}\right] = -\nabla P + \mathbf{F}$$

with pressure, P, and total force, $\mathbf{F}$. Finally, the energy conservation statement is,

$$\frac{\partial}{\partial t}\left[\frac{1}{2}\rho v^2 + \varepsilon\right] + \nabla\cdot\left[\frac{1}{2}\rho v^2 + \varepsilon\right]\mathbf{v} = W.$$

with internal energy, ε, and external energy source, W. A relationship connecting pressure, P, internal energy, ε, and density, ρ, the equation of state (EOS) described earlier, closes the above flow relationships, permitting exact numerical solution for arbitrary boundary conditions and flow regimes.

The above set are posed in the fixed (Eulerian) reference frame, through which the fluid moves. Another frame, moving with the fluid (Lagrangian), is often more suitable for numerical application, particularly when vortices, subscale disturbances, and turbulence are present. Flow dynamics in regulators (high speed, nozzle deflection, eddying) fall into the latter category, and numerical simulations often rely on Lagrangian analysis in the moving fluid stream. Transformation to the Lagrangian frame in the above set is most simply accomplished using the advective derivative, D/Dt, related to the Eulerian time derivative, $\partial/\partial t$, via,

$$\frac{D}{Dt} = \frac{\partial}{\partial t} + \mathbf{v} \cdot \nabla$$

as the temporal operator in the moving (Lagrangian) frame.

Keyed Exercises

- *What is the relative buoyancy, ΔB, of an empty 95 ft^3 steel tank rated at 3300 lbs/in²?*

$$\Delta B = -6.11 \ lbs$$

What is the approximate tank volume, V?

$$r = \frac{d}{2}, \quad d = 7 \ in, \quad l = 25 \ in$$

$$V = \pi r^2 l = \frac{\pi d^2 l}{4} = \frac{3.14 \times 49 \times 25}{4} \ in^3 = 962 \ in^3 = .56 \ ft^3$$

What does the tank weigh, w?

$$V = .56 \ ft^3, \quad \rho = 64 \ lbs^3/ft, \quad \Delta B = -6.11 \ lbs$$

$$w = \rho g V - \Delta B = 64 \times .56 + 6.11 \ lbs = 42.5 \ lbs$$

- *A mole of air in a tank at 300 °K is released to the atmosphere and registers an average temperature drop of 30 °K. What is the mean square speed change, vdv, of the exiting gas?*

$$\frac{dv}{dT} = \frac{1}{v} \frac{R\gamma}{1-\gamma}$$

$$\gamma = \frac{5}{3}, \quad R = 8.317 \ j/gmole \ °K, \quad dT = -30 \ °K$$

$$vdv = dT \left[\frac{R\gamma}{1-\gamma}\right] = 30 \times \left[\frac{8.317 \times 5/3}{2/3}\right] m^2/sec^2 = 623.7 \ m^2/sec^2$$

If the mean square speed change is roughly half the velocity squared of the exiting gas, what is the average velocity, v?

$$\frac{v^2}{2} = vdv = 623.7 \ m^2/sec^2$$

$$v = (2vdv)^{1/2} = (2 \times 623.7)^{1/2} \ m/sec = 35.3 \ m/sec$$

- *The air pressure in a scuba tank drops from 2475 lbs/in² to 1500 lbs/in² in 8 min. What is the air consumption rate, χ?*

$$\chi = \frac{2475 - 1500}{8} \ lbs/in^2 \ min = 121.9 \ lbs/in^2 \ min$$

If the tank is rated at 72 ft³, what is the consumption rate, χ, in ft³/min?

$$121.9 \ lbs/in^2 \ min \times \frac{72 \ ft^3}{2475 \ lbs/in^2} = 3.5 \ ft^3/min$$

- *How long, t, will a tank containing, $V = 34$ ft³, of air last at 33 fsw for an EOD specialist swimming against a 6 knot very cold current in the ocean?*

$$P_0 = 33 \ fsw, \quad \chi_0 = 2 \ ft^3/min, \quad \chi = \chi_0 \left[1 + \frac{d}{P_0} \right]$$

$$\chi = 2 \times \left[1 + \frac{33}{33} \right] \ ft^3/min = 4 \ ft^3/min$$

$$t = \frac{V}{\chi} = \frac{34}{4} \ min = 8.5 \ min$$

- *What is the air consumption rate, χ, at depth, $d = 46$ ft, and elevation, $z = 6,500$ ft, for sea level surface consumption rate, $\chi_0 = .95$ ft³/min, in fresh water?*

$$\chi = \frac{\chi_0}{\alpha} \left[1 + \frac{d\eta\alpha}{P_0} \right]$$

$$\chi = \frac{.95}{1.28} \times \left[1 + \frac{46 \times .975 \times 1.28}{33} \right] \ ft^3/min = 2.03 \ ft^3/min$$

- *If a hookah unit pumps a surface rate, $\chi_0 = 5$ ft³/min, of air, what rate, χ, will it deliver at depth, $d = 20 fsw$, on a reef?*

$$\chi = \chi_0 \frac{P_0}{P_0 + d} = 5 \times \frac{33}{53} \ ft^3/min = 3.13 \ ft^3/min$$

- *What fill rate at 9,000 ft elevation will a high speed compressor deliver if its rated output is 10 ft³/min at sea level?*

$$\chi_0 = 10 \ ft^3/min, \quad h = 9$$

$$\alpha = exp \ (-0.038 \times 9) = 1.41$$

$$\chi = \frac{\chi_0}{\alpha} = \frac{10}{1.41} \ ft^3/min = 7.09 ft^3/min$$

- At an altitude, $z = 1,300$ m, what reading, δ, will a capillary gauge register at actual depth, $d = 18$ m, in fresh water?

$$\delta = \alpha \eta d, \quad h = \frac{1300}{1000} \times 3.28 = 4.26$$

$$\alpha = exp\,(-0.038 \times 4.26) = 1.19, \quad \delta = 1.19 \times .975 \times 18 \; msw = 20.3 \; msw$$

What does a bourdon (oil filled) gauge read, δ ?

$$P_0 = 10 \; msw, \quad P_{4.26} = 8.4 \; msw$$

$$\delta = \eta d + P_h - P_0 = .975 \times 18 + 8.4 - 10 \; msw = 15.9 \; msw$$

- A tank rated 80 ft^3 at 3000 lb/in^2, registers a pressure, $P = 1420 \; lb/in^2$ on a sub gauge. What is the remaining air volume, V ?

$$V = V_r \frac{P}{P_r}$$

$$V = 80 \times \frac{1420}{3000} \; ft^3 = 37.8 \; ft^3$$

What is the tank constant, κ?

$$\kappa = \frac{P_r}{V_r} = \frac{3000}{80} \; lb/in^2 \; ft^3 = 37.5 \; lb/in^2 \; ft^3$$

- What is the inspired oxygen fraction, i_{O_2}, for a rebreather delivering 7.6 l/min of 50/50 nitrox to a Navy SEAL needing 1 l/min oxygen for metabolic consumption off the coast of Kuwait?

$$i_{O_2} = \frac{f_{O_2}F - m}{F - m}$$

$$f_{O_2} = .50, \quad F = 7.6 \; l/min, \quad m = 1.0 \; l/min$$

$$i_{O_2} = \frac{.5 \times 7.6 - 1.0}{7.6 - 1.0} = \frac{2.8}{6.6} = .42$$

If ambient pressure doubles, what is the nozzle flow, F_d, and inspired oxygen fraction, i_{O_2}?

$$F_d = F \frac{P}{2P} = \frac{7.6}{2} \; l/min = 3.8 \; l/min$$

$$i_{O_2} = \frac{.5 \times 3.8 - 1.0}{3.8 - 1.0} = \frac{.9}{2.8} = .32$$

Doppler Effect

A change in the observed frequency of sound, light, and other waves, caused by relative source-observer motion, is known as the Doppler effect. One example is a change in train whistle pitch upon approach and retreat. The observed frequency, f', is higher than the source frequency, f, as source and observer approach each other, and lower as source and observer retreat from each other.

For sound waves that propagate with characteristic velocity, u, in a medium (air, water, tissue), the Doppler shift depends on both source velocity, v_s, and observer velocity, v_o. The number of sound waves per second arriving at the observer can be estimated by simply counting the waves emitted per second by the source, and the change per second in the number of waves in flight from source to observer,

$$f' = f\,\frac{u - v_o}{u - v_s},$$

with source and observer velocities measured along the direction from source to observer (longitudinal component). If the observer is at rest, obviously,

$$\Delta f = f' - f = f\,\frac{v_s}{u - v_s},$$

as the usual case. If the observer is moving, and the source is at rest,

$$\Delta f = f' - f = -f\,\frac{v_o}{u}.$$

Definition of the sound speed, u, derives from the pressure derivative with respect to density,

$$u^2 = \frac{dP}{d\rho},$$

which, in the adiabatic limit of no heat flow, reduces to,

$$u^2 = \frac{Y}{\rho},$$

$$Y = -V\frac{dP}{dV},$$

with Y the *bulk modulus* of the material. For ideal gases, $Y = 5/3\,P$, but in solids and liquids, the bulk modulus must be determined.

A gas bubble will scatter sound waves in tissue by virtue of differences in bubble and tissue density, ρ, and bulk modulus, Y. First attempts to detect gas in tissues using ultrasound were designed to measure attenuation in fundamental frequency by scatter or reflection of the sound signal passed across the tissue region under investigation. Such techniques have the advantage that they can localize the gas region. However, both transmission and reflection techniques suffer from the heterogeneous nature of tissue, both in density and bulk modulus. Such an approach, called the pulse echo technique, has given way today to Doppler methods of detecting moving bubbles.

Moving Bubbles

Doppler devices used to monitor bubbles in the circulation, or trap speeders with radar detectors, are simple. High frequency waves, emitted by a sending crystal of a Doppler probe, easily travel through body tissue, with a portion reflected back towards a receiving crystal. Tissue moving toward or away from the sending unit will reflect part of the source signal with a frequency shift determined by the velocity of the reflecting medium. Integrated Doppler systems discard the unshifted portion of the reflected signal, and only analyze the shifted portion. Shifted signals fall within the human audibility range. In the veins, bubbles reflect more of the signal than flowing blood, with chirps and pops superimposed on continuous flowing blood background sounds. Detected bubbles are graded from 0 to 4, roughly no bubbles to 1,000 or more per minute.

Doppler probes are inserted into leg and arm veins, pulmonary arteries (heart to lung), and even the heart ventricles. Bubbles detected in veins or ventricles are traveling from tissues to the lungs. They may, or may not, be associated with free phases at joints, or in the spinal column, causing DCS at these sites. Doppler prediction of DCS falls in the 10% to 15% success range, even for high grade bubbles (3–4 Doppler grade). While less than totally predictive, the preponderance of high Doppler grade bubbles for a dive profile renders the profile suspect at least. Following a typical nonstop dive to the limits, Doppler bubble levels tend to peak in an hour, or two. Recent studies by the Divers Alert Network (DAN) at Duke University reported that some 18% of recreational dives produced some level of Doppler bubbling, on tables or decompression meters.

Acoustical signals in the *megahertz* frequency range are typically employed in Doppler analysis. The size and velocity of reflecting bubbles in the flowing media are crucial factors in the reflected return signals. Where flow rates are the highest, the smallest bubbles can be detected with Doppler technology. Roughly, entrained bubbles in the 20–40 μm diameter range are detectable in flows ranging 50–60 cm/sec, as seen in Figure 30, using 5 *megahertz* acoustical signals.

Operational Diving

The past twenty years, or so, have witnessed a number of changes and additions to diving protocols and table procedures, such as shorter nonstop time limits, slower ascent rates, discretionary safety stops, ascending repetitive profiles, multilevel techniques, both faster and slower controlling repetitive tissue halftimes, lower critical tensions (*M*-values), longer flying-after-diving surface intervals, and others. Stimulated by Doppler technology, decompression meter development, theory, statistics, or safer diving concensus, these modifications affect a gamut of activity, spanning bounce to multiday diving. As it turns out, there is good support for these protocols on operational, experimental, and theoretical grounds, and a comprehensive model addressing these concerns on firmer basis than earlier models is certainly possible, having been proposed by numbers of investigators.

Spencer pioneered the use of Doppler bubble counting to suggest reductions in the nonstop time limits of the standard US Navy Tables, on the order of a repetitive group or two at each depth in the USN Tables (1–4 *fsw* in critical tensions), basing recommendations on lowering bubble counts at shorter nonstop time limits. Others have also made similar recommendations over the past 15 years.

Smith and Stayton noted marked reductions in precordial bubbles when ascent rates were cut from 60 *fsw/min* to 30 *fsw/min*. In similar studies, Pilmanis witnessed an order of magnitude drop in venous gas emboli (VGE) counts in divers making short, shallow, safety stops following nominal bounce exposures at the 100 *fsw* level, while Neumann, Hall, and Linaweaver recorded comparable reductions in divers making short, but deeper, stops after excursions to 200 *fsw* for longer times.

An American Academy of Underwater Sciences (AAUS) workshop on repetitive diving, recorded by Lang and Vann, and Divers Alert Network (DAN) statistics suggest that present diving practices appear riskier under increasing exposure time and pressure loading, spawning development of ancillary safety measures for multidiving. Dunford, Wachholz, Huggins, and Bennett noted persistent Doppler scores in divers performing repetitive, multiday diving, suggesting the presence of VGE in divers, all the time, under such loadings.

Ascent rates, safety stops, decompression computers, and altitude diving were also the subject of extensive discussion at workshops and technical forums sponsored by the American Academy of Underwater Sciences (AAUS) and the Undersea and Hyperbaric Medical Society (UHMS) a few years back, as summarized by Lang and Vann, Lang and Egstrom, and Sheffield, Results of discussions culminated in a set of recommendations, folded within standard Haldane table and meter procedures, even for exposures exceeding neither time limits nor critical tissue tensions. More recently, the question of deep stops has been a subject of considerable discussion, particularly from the technical diving side where deep stops are standard operating procedures on mixed gases for OC and RB activities. Fuller discussion follows in the context of accumulated (Data Bank) dive profiles mated to deep stop (bubble) models using maximum likelihood statistical techniques. Suffice it to say here that both deep stops and shallow stops can be effected within the same statistical risk, but deep stops are always deeper and overall decompression time is always shorter. In the common parlance, deep stops control the bubbles earlier, while shallow stops treat the bubbles less efficiently over longer time spans. Shallow stops have been the foundation of decompression diving for over 100 years, but that is now changing as more and more technical divers use deep stop software, tables, and computers based on modern dual phase gas transport models. Part 7 covers some diveware of interest to the technical diver in more detail.

Keyed Exercises

- *Match the entries in the first column with the best single entry in the second column.*

(f) Spencer	(a) Divers Alert Network
(h) Smith and Stayton	(b) American Academy of Underwater Sciences
(a) DAN	(c) Higher repetitive bubble scores
(g) Doppler	(d) Deep stop bubble count reduction
(d) Neumann	(e) Shallow safety stops
(b) AAUS	(f) Reduced NDLs
(e) Pilmanis	(g) reflected sound
(c) Bennett	(h) slow ascent rates

- *Shallow safety stops are made*
  ( ) at the surface
  (x) in the 10–20 fsw zone
  ( ) at 1/2 the bottom depth

- *Deep stops are made*
  (x) consistent with bubble dynamics
  ( ) to minimize dissolved gas elimination
  ( ) at 1/2 the depth of the first decompression stop

- *A gas bubble will scatter sound waves in the body*
  ( ) because of surface tension
  (x) because of differences in bubble and tissue densities
  ( ) both of the above

- *Acoustical signals for Doppler monitoring in the body*
  ( ) propagate with ultraviolet frequency
  ( ) reflect best in the flowing blood
  (x) range in megahertz frequency

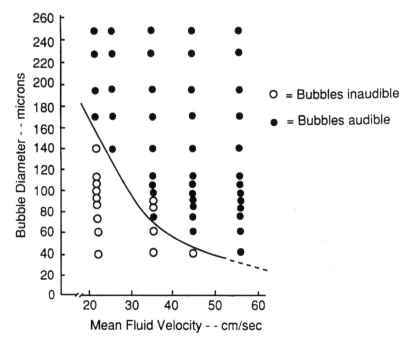

Figure 30. Moving Doppler Bubble Diameter and Speed

Bubble detection by measuring frequency shift in acoustical signal is dependent on reflecting bubble speed. The graph below details minimum detectable bubble diameter for various entraining fluid velocities, using an acoustical signal of 5 megahertz.

The upshot of these studies, workshops, discussions, and tests are a set of discretionary protocols, not necessarily endorsed in all diving sectors, but which might be summarized as follows:

- reduce nonstop time limits a repetitive group, or two, below the standard US Navy limits;
- maintain ascent rates below 60 *fsw/min*, preferably slower, and requisitely slower at altitude;
- limit repetitive dives to a maximum of three per day, not exceeding the 100 *fsw* level;
- avoid multiday, multilevel, or repetitive dives to increasing depths;
- wait 12 *hr* before flying after nominal diving, 24 *hr* after heavy diving (taxing, near decompression, or prolonged repetitive) activity, and 48 *hr* after decompression diving;
- avoid multiple surface ascents and short repetitive dives (spikes) within surface intervals of 1 *hr*;
- surface intervals of more than an hour are recommended for repetitive diving;

- safety stops for 2–4 *min* in the 10–20 *fsw* zone are advisable for all diving, but particularly for deep (near 100 *fsw*), repetitive, and multiday exposures;
- do not dive at altitudes above 10,000 *ft* using modified conventional tables, or linear extrapolations of sea level critical tensions;
- in short, dive conservatively, remembering that tables and meters are not bends proof.

Procedures such as those above are prudent, theoretically sound, and safe diving protocols. Ultimately, they link to free phase and bubble mechanisms.

Validation is central to diving, and significant testing of nonstop and saturation diving schedules has transpired. In between, repetitive (more than one dive in a 12 hour period), multilevel (arbitrary depths throughout the course of a single dive), reverse profile (second repetitive dive deeper than first), and multiday (repetitive dives over days) diving cannot claim the same benefits, though some ongoing programs are breaking new ground. Application of (just) dissolved gas models in latter cases possibly has witnessed slightly higher decompression sickness (bends) incidence than in the former ones, as discussed in newsletters, workshops, and technical forums. Some hyperbaric specialists also suggest higher incidence of rash (skin bends) under repetitive loading. While statistics are not yet conclusive, they raise some concerns theoretically addressed by considering both dissolved and free phase gas buildup and elimination in broader based bubble models. Such models often focus on the amount of free phase precipitated by compression-decompression, and contain dissolved gas models as subset. In limiting the volume of free phase in time, they must also limit the growth rate.

Pulmonary and Circulatory Networks

The pulmonary and circulatory organs are connected gas transfer networks, as Figure 31 suggests. Lung blood absorbs oxygen from inspired air in the alveoli (lung air sacs), and releases carbon dioxide into the alveoli. The surface area for exchange is enormous, on the order of a few hundred square meters. Nearly constant values of alveolar partial pressures of oxygen and carbon dioxide are maintained by the respiratory centers, with ventilated alveolar volume near 4 *l* in adults. The partial pressure of inspired oxygen is usually higher than the partial pressure of tissue and blood oxygen, and the partial pressure of inspired carbon dioxide less, balancing metabolic requirements of the body.

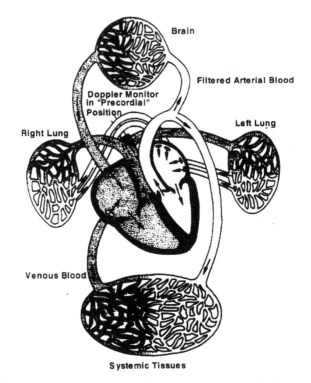

Brain

Filtered Arterial Blood

Doppler Monitor in "Precordial" Position

Left Lung

Right Lung

Venous Blood

Systemic Tissues

Figure 31. Pulmonary And Circulatory Gas Transfer Network

The heart, lungs, arterial circulation, and venous circulation are a gas transfer network, supplying oxygen and removing carbon dioxide from the body. Oxygen is consumed and carbon dioxide produced in cellular metabolic processes. Gas exchange between tissue and blood depends upon blood flow rates, and diffusivities of tissue and blood. If blood flow rates control the exchange process, transfer is perfusion limited. If diffusivities control the exchange process, transfer is diffusion limited. Certainly, both interplay strategically in the body.

Gas moves in direction of decreased concentration in any otherwise homogeneous medium with uniform solubility. If there exist regions of varying solubility, this is not necessarily true. For instance, in the body there are two tissue types, one predominantly aqueous (watery) and the other (lipid), varying in solubility by a factor of five for nitrogen. That is, nitrogen is five times more soluble in lipid tissue than aqueous tissue. If aqueous and lipid tissue are in nitrogen equilibrium, then a gaseous phases exists in equilibrium with both. Both solutions are said to have a nitrogen tension equal to the partial pressure of the nitrogen in the gaseous phase, with the concentration of the dissolved gas in each species equal to the product of the solubility times the tension according to Henry's law. If two nitrogen solutions, one lipid and the other aqueous, are placed in contact, nitrogen will diffuse towards the solution with decreased nitrogen tension. The driving force for the transfer of any gas is the pressure gradient, whatever the phases involved, liquid-to-liquid, gas-to-liquid, or gas-to-gas. Tensions and partial pressures have the same dimensions. The volume of gas that diffuses under any gradient is a function of the interface area, solubility of the media, and distance traversed. The rate at which a gas diffuses is inversely proportional to the square root of its atomic weight. Following equalization, dissolved volumes of gases depend upon their individual solubilities in the media.

Lipid and aqueous tissues in the body exhibit inert gas solubilities differing by factors of roughly five, in addition to different uptake and elimination rates. Near standard temperature and pressure (32 ^oF, and 1 *atm*), roughly 65% of dissolved nitrogen gas will reside in aqueous tissues, and the remaining 35% in lipid tissues at equilibration, with the total weight of dissolved nitrogen about 0.0035 *lb* for a 150 *lb* human.

The circulatory system, consisting of the heart, arteries, veins, and lymphatics, convects blood throughout the body. Arterial blood leaves the left heart via the aorta (2.5 *cm*), with successive branching of arteries until it reaches arterioles (30 μm), and then systemic capillaries (8 μm) in peripheral tissues. These capillaries join to form venules (20 μm), which in turn connect with the vena cava (3 *cm*), which enters the right heart. During return, venous blood velocities increase from 0.5 *cm/sec* to nearly 20 *cm/sec*. Blood leaves the right heart through the pulmonary arteries on its way to the lungs. Upon oxygenation in the lungs, blood returns to the left heart through the pulmonary veins, beginning renewed arterial circulation. Flow patterns in lowest (still representative) order follow streamlines, for initial and final states, i and f,

$$mv_f^2 + 2h_f + 2mgz_f = mv_i^2 + 2h_i + 2mgz_i = \gamma$$

with blood mass, m, velocity, v, enthalpy, h, position, z, and constant, γ, as the entrained blood routinely circulates. Obviously, as systemic vessels change size, branch, and recollect, blood cursing through them experiences speed changes according to mass flow conservation, that is, denoting mass flow rate, dm/dt,

$$\frac{dm}{dt} = \rho_i A_i v_i = \rho_f A_f v_f$$

with A the cross sectional area of the blood vessel and more simply where, $\rho_i = \rho_f$, for incompressible fluids, like blood.

Blood has distinct components to accomplish many functions. Plasma is the liquid part, carrying nutrients, dissolved gases (excepting oxygen), and some chemicals, and makes up some 55% of blood by weight. Red blood cells (erythrocytes) carry the other 45% by weight, and through the protein, hemoglobin, transport oxygen to the tissues. Enzymes in red blood cells also participate in a chemical reaction transforming carbon dioxide to a bicarbonate in blood plasma. The average adult carries about 5 *l* of blood, 30–35% in the arterial circulation (pulmonary veins, left heart, and systemic circulation), and 60–65% in the venous flow (veins and right heart). About 9.5 *ml* of nitrogen are transported in each liter of blood. Arterial and venous tensions of metabolic gases, such as oxygen and carbon dioxide differ, while blood and tissue tensions of water vapor and nitrogen are the same. Oxygen tissue tensions are below both arterial and venous tensions, while carbon dioxide tissue tensions exceed both. Arterial tensions equilibrate with alveolar (inspired air) partial pressures in less than a minute. Such an arrangement of tensions in the tissues and circulatory system provides the necessary pressure head between alveolar capillaries of the lungs and systemic capillaries pervading extracellular space.

Tissues and venous blood are typically unsaturated with respect to inspired air and arterial tensions, somewhere in the vicinity of 8–13% of ambient pressure. That is, summing up partial pressures of inspired gases in air, total venous and tissue tensions fall short in that percentage range. Carbon dioxide produced by metabolic processes is 25 times more soluble than oxygen consumed, and hence exerts a lower partial pressure by Henry's law. That tissue debt is called the *inherent unsaturation*, or *oxygen window*, in diving applications

Inherent Unsaturation

Inert gas transfer and coupled bubble growth are subtly influenced by metabolic oxygen consumption. Consumption of oxygen and production of carbon dioxide drops the tissue oxygen tension below its level in the lungs (alveoli), while carbon dioxide tension rises only slightly because carbon dioxide is 35 times more soluble than oxygen. Figure 32 compares the partial pressures (fsw) of oxygen, nitrogen, water vapor, and carbon dioxide in dry air, alveolar air, arterial blood, venous blood, and tissue (cells).

Arterial and venous blood, and tissue, are clearly unsaturated with respect to dry air at 1 *atm*. Water vapor content is constant, and carbon dioxide variations are slight, though sufficient to establish an outgradient between tissue and blood. Oxygen tensions in tissue and blood are considerably below lung oxygen partial pressure, establishing the necessary ingradient for oxygenation and metabolism. Experiments also suggest that the degree of unsaturation increases linearly with pressure for constant composition breathing mixture, and decreases linearly with mole fraction of inert gas in the inspired mix. A rough measure of the inherent unsaturation, Δ_u, is given as a function of ambient pressure, P, and mole fraction, f_{N_2}, of nitrogen in the air mixture, in fsw

$$\Delta_u = (1 - f_{N_2})P - 2.04\, f_{N_2} - 5.47.$$

Since tissues are unsaturated with respect to ambient pressure at equilibrium, one might exploit this *window* in bringing divers to the surface. By scheduling the ascent strategically, so that nitrogen (or any other inert breathing gas) supersaturation just takes up this unsaturation, the total tissue tension can be kept equal to ambient pressure, the zero supersaturation ascent.

Surface Tension

Discontinuities in types of materials and/or densities at surfaces and interfaces give rise to interfacial forces, called *surface tension*. Discontinuities in density produce cohesive gradients tending to diminish density at the surface region. At the interfaces between immiscible materials, cohesive forces produce surface tension, but adhesional forces between dissimilar materials tend to offset (decrease) the interfacial tension. Surface and interfacial tension are readily observed in fluids, but less readily in solids. In solids, very little stretching of the surface region can occur if the solids are rigid. Upon heating rigid solids to higher temperature, surface tension becomes a discernible effect.

Any two phases in equilibrium are separated by a surface of contact, the existence of which also produces surface tension. The thin contact region is a transition layer, sometimes called the *film* layer. Phases can be solid, liquid, or vapor, with surface tension in each case different. The actual position, or displacement, of the phase boundary may alter the area of the phases on either side, leading to pressure differences in the phases. The difference between phase pressures is known as the surface, or film, pressure. The phase equilibration condition requires the temperatures and chemical potentials (Gibbs free energy) of phases be equal, but certainly not the pressures.

A simple description of measurable surface tension, γ, is linked to the magnitude of cohesive forces in materials a and b, denoted, χ_a and χ_b, wanting to pull the surfaces together, and the adhesional forces, α_a and α_b, wanting to draw the surfaces apart. The net surface tension, γ, is the sum of cohesive forces minus adhesive forces, that is,

$$\gamma = \chi_a + \chi_b - \alpha_a - \alpha_b.$$

Thermodynamically, surface tension contributes a differential work term, $d\omega$, to system balance equations given in terms of surface contact area, dA,

$$d\omega = \gamma \, dA,$$

Surface tension pressure, τ, is surface tension force per unit area, that is, in terms of work function, ω,

$$\tau = -\left[\frac{\partial \omega}{\partial V}\right]_{S,T},$$

at constant entropy, S, and temperature, T. Interfacial tension in liquids is measured by the pressure difference across surfaces, again denoted a and b,

$$\tau = \gamma \left[\frac{1}{r_a} + \frac{1}{r_b}\right],$$

given radii of curvature, r_a and r_b. For thin films, such as bubbles, $r_a \approx r_b = r$, and we see,

$$\tau_{bub} = \frac{2\gamma}{r},$$

deduced by Young and Laplace almost two centuries past. For water, $\gamma = 50 \, dyne \, cm$, while for watery tissue, $\gamma = 18 \, dyne \, cm$.

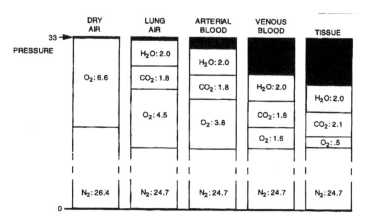

Figure 32. Inherent Unsaturation

Tissues and blood are typically undersaturated with respect to ambient pressure, that is, summed partial pressures of oxygen, nitrogen, water vapor, and carbon dioxide in tissue and blood (total tension) are always less than ambient pressure. Carbon dioxide produced in metabolic processes is 25 times more soluble than the oxygen consumed, and hence, by Henry's law, exerts a smaller partial pressure than the oxygen replaced. The picture above corresponds to sea level pressure, but experiments confirm that the unsaturation increases linearly with pressure for constant composition breathing mixture, and decreases linearly with mole fraction of inert breathing gas. Tensions below are listed in fsw.

Adsorption

The surface of all solids and liquids adsorb foreign molecules from their surroundings. These adsorbed molecules change most of the chemical and physical properties of the underlying substrate. Adhesion, catalysis, corrosion, fracture, lubrication, and wear are affected by the topmost molecular layers on a surface. Understanding these changes involves close study of films themselves, as described.

The forces of attraction that cause adsorption are relatively weak and are the long range interactions existing between all atoms and molecules.

Surfactants

Water, gasoline, glycerin, and salad oil are clearly liquids. Pancake syrup, paster, eggwhite, silly putty, paint, glue, and soap are also liquids, that is, they flow on the application of stress, but border on classification otherwise. In mechanical response, the latter class differs from each other as much as they differ from solids. And the response is variable in time. Syrup becomes sticky as it dries. Dishwashing soap often dries into light flakes. Silly putty flows on tilt, but shatters on sudden impact. Airplane glue is springy and rubbery.

Substances in the latter category are called structured fluids, owing their distinctive and unusual properties to large polyatomic composites, many times the size of a water molecule. Fluids containing polyatomic structures manifest a wide variety of mechanical response and self organization. Body tissues and fluids host an uncountable variety of organic and inorganic matter, with many biochemical substances falling into structured fluid category. Among the structured fluids, a class of self assemblies, called surfactants, are very interesting, possessing properties which can stabilize microbubbles in various stages of evolution by offsetting surface tension.

A surfactant is a structured fluid which is *ambiphillic*, incorporating parts that assume preferential orientations at water-oil (immisicible) interfaces. A surfactant molecule usually consists of a bulky ion at one end, and a counter ion at the other. Isolated molecules cannot usually exist in one media type, or the other, but instead orient themselves into *micelles*, configurations in which like parts clump together, that is head in one substance and tail in the other. Micelles typically possess diameters near 10^{-3} μm, and render the interfaces unlike anything measured in the components. Lipid-aqueous tissue interfaces potentially present favorable environments for surfactants.

Under certain conditions, a surfactant can reduce interfacial surface tension, allowing the interface to grow and wrap around itself. The result is a microbundle full of alternating surfaces and interfaces, spherical in structure to minimize thermodynamic energy constraints. Many substances may be bound up in the microbundle. If small gas nuclei, but typically much larger than a micelle, are in contact with the interfaces, or surfactants directly, a spherical gas micronucleus-microemulsion can develop, varying in size and surfactant content. The assembly is stable when the effective surface tension is zero, when surfactant skin pressure just balances mechanical (Laplace) surface tension. If the effective surface tension of the microbubble, γ, is not zero, the collection will grow or contract until stable, or disassemble. In the case of gas microemulsions, the surfactant is thought to coat the inside boundary layer mostly, with free gas in the interior. The actual picture is probably more complex, but such a picture can be drawn for computational simplicity. Surfactant stabilized micronuclei may theoretically destabilize under compression-decompression processes in diving, perhaps spawning bubble growth fueled by high gas tension in surrounding media. Microbubbles may remain at the interfaces, but probably migrate. Sources of initial gas nuclei, surfactant composition, and tissue sites await description.

Micronuclei

Bubbles, which are unstable, are thought to grow from micron size, gas nuclei which resist collapse due to elastic skins of surface activated molecules (surfactants), or possibly reduction in surface tension at tissue interfaces or crevices. If families of these micronuclei persist, they vary in size and surfactant content. Large pressures (somewhere near 10 *atm*) are necessary to crush them. Micronuclei are small enough to pass through the pulmonary filters, yet dense enough not to float to the surfaces of their environments, with which they are in both hydrostatic (pressure) and diffusion (gas flow) equilibrium. When nuclei are stabilized, and not activated to growth or contraction by external pressure changes, the skin (surfactant) tension offsets both the Laplacian (film) tension and any mechanical help from surrounding tissue. Then all pressures and gas tensions are equal. However, on decompression, the seed pockets are surrounded by dissolved gases at high tension and can subsequently grow (bubbles) as surrounding gas diffuses into them. The rate at which bubbles grow, or contract, depends directly on the difference between tissue tension and local ambient pressure, effectively the bubble pressure gradient, denoted G. At some point in time, a critical volume of bubbles, or separated gas, is established and bends symptoms become statistically more probable. On compression, the micronuclei are crunched down to smaller sizes across families, apparently stabilizing at new reduced size. Bubbles are also crunched by increasing pressure because of Boyle's law, and then additionally shrink if gas diffuses out of them. As bubbles get smaller and smaller, they probably restabilize as micronuclei.

Under compression-decompression, gas nuclei may grow as bubbles, depending on their effective bubble radius. Below a certain critical radius, r_c, listed in Table 10 below as a function of pressure according to a bubble model (varying permeability), as fitted to gel experiments, bubbles tend to collapse on themselves, while at larger equilibrium radius, they grow as gas diffuses into them. Stabilized nuclei evolve into unstable bubbles when their effective surface tension is greater than zero, or a sufficient diffusion gradient exists to drive gas into, or out of, the nucleus. At sea level, the model excitation radius is near .8 μm, smaller than living cells, having dimensions starting at a few microns.

Table 10. Micronuclei Excitation Radii

Pressure P (fsw)	Excitation radius r_s (μm)	Pressure P (fsw)	Excitation radius r_s (μm)
13	.89	153	.49
33	.80	173	.46
53	.72	193	.44
73	.66	213	.41
93	.61	233	.39
113	.57	253	.37
133	.53	273	.36

Micronuclei can be broadly classified as *homogeneous* or *heterogeneous*, depending upon their composition and that of the surrounding media. If the composition of both micronuclei and parent media are essentially the same, the nucleation process is termed homogeneous. If the composition of micronuclei and parent media differ, the nucleation process is termed heterogeneous. Spontaneous bubble formation in pure supersaturated liquids under explosive decompression is mainly homogeneous, while bubble formation on dust particles in supersaturated fluids is mostly heterogeneous. Homogeneous nucleation and bubble formation usually require large decompressions (many tens of atmospheres), while heterogeneous nucleation and bubble formation processes transpire with very small decompressions (tenths of atmospheres). Homogeneous nucleation in body tissue under nominal and controlled conditions of decompression appears much less likely than heterogeneous nucleation, considering pressure change and host of organic and inorganic body substances.

Nucleation theory is consistent with a number of diving observations. Divers can significantly increase tolerance against bubble formation, and therefore bends, by following three simple practices:

- make the first dive a deep, short (crush) dive, thereby constricting micronuclei down to smaller, safer size;
- make succeeding dives progressively more shallow, thus diving within crush limits of the first dive and minimizing excitation of smaller micronuclei;
- make frequent dives (like every other day), thus depleting the number of micronuclei available to form troublesome bubbles.

An underlying point can be made here. If nucleation sites are extinguished, reduced in number, or ill-disposed to excitation, bubble formation and risk are commensurately reduced. Regeneration times for classes of micronuclei are estimated to be near a week, underscoring physiological adaptation to recurring pressure environments. The mechanics of nucleation, stabilization, and bubble growth are fairly complex, with stabilization mechanisms only recently quantified. Source and generation mechanisms before stabilization are not well understood. Some candidates include cosmic radiation and charged particles, dissolved gases in fluids we drink, lymph draining tissues into veins, collisional coalescence, blood turbulence and vorticity, exercise, the stomach, and the thin air-blood endothelium in the lungs. Once formed, micronuclei must stabilize very rapidly with surfactant material. Passing through the pulmonary filters of the lungs, only sub-micron sizes might survive. If nuclei are persistent, it is not clear that they populate all tissue sites, nor possess the same size distributions. Some can argue that gel findings are not relevant because biological fluids are formed, and contained, in a sealed environment (the body), but the Strauss and Yount studies confirm the existence of preformed gas micronuclei in serum and egg albumin. Nuclei seem to pervade all manner of fluids.

Abandoning preformed nuclei, other methods of instantaneous bubble formation are certainly possible. Cavitation, produced by the rapid tearing, or moving apart, of tissue interfaces, is a candidate, as well as surface friction (tribonucleation). Crevices in tissues may form or trap gas phases, with later potential for release. Vorticity in blood flow patterns might cause small microbubbles. Stable, or unstable, the copious presence of microbubbles in the venous circulation would impact dissolved gas elimination adversely, also possibly impairing the lungs or the arterial network. The presence of bubbles in the arterial circulation might result in embolism. Bubble clogging of the pulmonary circulation is thought to relate to the chokes, a serious form of decompression sickness, while cerebral decompression sickness is believed due to emboli. Microbubbles in the venous circulation would render gas uptake and elimination asymmetric, with uptake faster than elimination. Displacing blood, microbubbles would reduce the effective area and volume for tissue-blood gas exchange.

Free Phases

Henry's law tells us that a gas will tend to separate from solution (pass from the dissolved state to the free state) if the tension of the gas in the dissolved state exceeds its partial pressure in the adjacent free state. And the opposite holds true if the gradient is reversed. Phase separation can be delayed if some remnant of a free phase does not already exist in the liquid, providing a pathway for the dissolved gas to *dump* over into the free state, rendering the dissolved gas *metastable* during the delay. The challenge in tracking phase separation is the presence and quantification of free phase precursors, or seeds, that facilitate gas transfer in a process called *nucleation*.

Nucleation

Metastable states are unstable thermodynamic states lying close to stable configurations, that is, separated by relatively small energy differences. A substance in a metastable state will eventually transition into a stable state. For instance, a supercooled vapor will eventually condense into a liquid, a supercooled liquid will eventually become solid, and a superheated liquid will eventually evaporate into a gas. Bubble formation can be a process in which a gas, or vapor, phase is initially formed from a metastable liquid environment, one that is usually supersaturated with dissolved gas.

Metastable phase transitions deposit an unstable phase onto a stable phase, with aggregates in the stable phase serving as *nuclei* for the transition. Liquid drops in a supercooled vapor, if sufficiently large, become centers of condensation of the vapor, for example. Nuclei will form in both phases because of statistical fluctuations, but the nuclei in the metastable phase will disappear in time, while those in the stable phase will remain. Such nuclei form statistically as a result of thermal fluctuations in the interior of the media, with a certain (small) number reaching *critical* radius for growth. If large enough, nuclei in the stable phase seed the continuing process of phase transitions from the metastable state. For each metastable state, there is a minimum size which nuclei in the stable phase must possess to afford more stability than the metastable state. This size is called the critical radius, r_c. Nuclei smaller than the critical radius will not support phase transitions from the metastable state, and will also disappear in time. In assigning a critical radius to nuclei, spherical aggregate symmetry is assumed, and is requisite to minimize surface energy.

Homogeneous nucleation processes occur in single component systems, while heterogeneous nucleation processes involve more than one component. To describe nucleation, a heterogeneous model, ascribed to Plesset, containing the homogeneous case as a subset, has been useful in applications. A solid hydrophobic sphere, of radius r_0, is surrounded by a concentric layer of vapor, out to a radius r. The instantaneous (Boltzmann) probability, dw, for the state depends on the difference in free energy, ΔG, associated with the vapor phase,

$$dw = exp\,(-\Delta G/kT)\,dG,$$

at temperature, T, for (Gibbs) free energy change, ΔG,

$$\Delta G = \frac{4}{3}\pi r^2 \, \gamma_{lv} + \frac{4}{3}\pi r_0^2 \, (\gamma_{vs} - \gamma_{ls}),$$

and γ_{lv}, γ_{vs}, and γ_{ls} surface tensions associated with the liquid-vapor, vapor-solid, and liquid-solid interfaces. The homogeneous case corresponds to $r_0 = 0$, that is, no solid and only liquid-vapor nucleation.

Tensions, pulling parallel to their respective surfaces, at equilibrium have zero net component,

$$\gamma_{lv} \cos \theta = \gamma_{vs} - \gamma_{ls},$$

with liquid-vapor contact angle, θ, measured through the liquid.   Wetted (hydrophillic) solids exhibit acute contact angle, occurring when,

$$\gamma_{vs} - \gamma_{ls} > 0,$$

so that the meniscus of the liquid phase is concave. In this case, the solid has greater adhesion for the liquid than the liquid has cohesion for itself, the free energy required to maintain the vapor phase is large (because the solid surface tension term is positive), and the probability of nucleation is decreased by the solid impurity. For a nonwetting (hydrophobic) solid, the situation is reversed, that is, the contact angle is obtuse,

$$\gamma_{vs} - \gamma_{ls} < 0,$$

the meniscus is convex, the solid has less adhesion for the liquid than the liquid has cohesion for itself, the free energy is reduced because the solid surface tension term is negative, and the probability of formation is increased. In the limiting case, $\cos \theta = -1$, the free energy is given by,

$$\Delta G = \frac{4}{3}\pi \gamma_{lv} \, (r^2 - r_0^2),$$

which becomes small for cavity radius, r, near impurity radius, r_0.

While theories of heterogeneous and homogeneous nucleation work well for a number of liquids, the application of the heterogeneous model to water with impurities is not able to reduce the tensile strength to observable values. The homogeneous theory of nucleation predicts a tensile strength of water near 1,400 *atm*, the heterogeneous theory, with a variety of solid impurities, drops the tensile strength down to 1,000 *atm*, and the measured value for water is approximately 270 *atm*.

In any solution, gas nuclei can be deactivated (crushed) by the application of large hydrostatic pressures. The process of *crushing* is also termed *denucleation*. When denucleated solutions are decompressed in supersaturated states, much higher degrees of supersaturation are requisite to induce bubble formation. In diving, denucleation has been suggested as a mechanism for acclimatization. If denucleation is size selective, that is, greater hydrostatic pressures crush smaller and smaller nuclei, and if number distributions of nuclei increase with decreasing radius (suggested by some experiments), than a conservative deep dive, followed by sufficient surface interval, should in principle afford a margin of safety, by effectively crushing many nuclei and reducing the numbers of nuclei potentially excited into growth under compression-decompression.

The mechanisms of nucleation in the body are obscure. Though nucleation most probably is the precursor to bubble growth, formation and persistence time scales, sites, and size distributions of nuclei remain open questions. Given the complexity and number of substances maintained in tissues and blood, heterogeneous nucleation would appear a probable mechanism.

Cavitation

Simply, *cavitation* is the process of vapor phase formation of a liquid when pressure is reduced. A liquid cavitates when vapor bubbles are formed and observed to grow as consequence of pressure reduction. When the phase transition results from pressure change in hydrodynamic flow, a two phase stream consisting of vapor and liquid results, called a cavitating flow. The addition of heat, or heat transfer in a fluid, may also produce cavitation nuclei in the process called boiling. From the physico-chemical perspective, cavitation by pressure reduction and cavitation by heat addition represent the same phenomena, vapor formation and bubble growth in the presence of seed nuclei. Depending on the rate and magnitude of pressure reduction, a bubble may grow slowly or rapidly. A bubble that grows very rapidly (explosively) contains the vapor phase of the liquid mostly, because the diffusion time is too short for any significant increase in entrained gas volume. The process is called vaporous cavitation, and depends on evaporation of liquid into the bubble. A bubble may also grow more slowly by diffusion of gas into the nucleus, and contain mostly a gas component. In this case, the liquid degasses in what is called gaseous cavitation, the mode observed in the application of ultrasound signals to the liquid. For vaporous cavitation to occur, pressure drops below vapor pressure are requisite. For gaseous cavitation to occur, pressure drops may be less than, or greater than, vapor pressure, depending on nuclei size and degree of liquid saturation. In supersaturated ocean surfaces, for instance, vaporous cavitation occurs very nearly vapor pressure, while gaseous cavitation occurs above vapor pressure.

In gaseous cavitation processes, the inception of growth in nuclei depends little on the duration of the pressure reduction, but the maximum size of the bubble produced does depend upon the time of pressure reduction. In most applications, the maximum size depends only slightly on the initial size of the seed nucleus. Under vaporous cavitation, the maximum size of the bubble produced is essentially independent of the dissolved gas content of the liquid. This obviously suggests different cavitation mechanisms for pressure (reduction) related bubble trauma in diving. Slowly developing bubble problems, such as limb bends many hours after exposure, might be linked to gaseous cavitation mechanisms, while rapid bubble problems, like central nervous system hits and embolism immediately after surfacing, might link to vaporous cavitation.

In a flowing fluid (or body moving through a stationary liquid), the cavitation number, κ, is an indication of the degree of cavitation, or the tendency to cavitate. Describing the similarity in the liquid-gas system, the cavitation number relates gas pressure, p, to absolute pressure, P, through,

$$\kappa = 2 \, \frac{P - p}{\rho u^2}$$

with ρ and u the fluid density and velocity. Cavitation and cavitating flows have long been of interest in ship-building and hydraulic machinery, underwater signal processing, propellor design, underwater detection, material damage, chemical processing, high pressure and temperature flows in nuclear reactors, volatility of rocket fuels, and bubble chambers for detection of high energy particles, to list a few. Cavitation processes in flowing blood and nearby tissue are also of considerable interest to decompression modelers and table designers.

Today we know that the inception of cavitation in liquids involves the growth of submicroscopic nuclei containing vapor, gas, or both, which are present within the liquid, in crevices, on suspended matter or impurities, or on bounding layers. The need for cavitating nuclei at vapor pressures is well established in the laboratory. There is some difficulty, however, in accounting for their presence and persistence. For a given difference between ambient and gas-vapor pressure, only one radius is stable. Changes in ambient, gas, or vapor pressures will cause the nuclei to either grow, or contract. But even if stable hydrostatically, bubbles and nuclei, because of constricting surface tension, will eventually collapse as gas and vapor diffuse out of the assembly. For instance, an air bubble of radius 10^{-3} *cm* will dissolve in saturated water in about 6 *sec*, and even faster if the water is undersaturated or the bubble is smaller. In saturated solutions, bubbles will grow by diffusion, and then tend to be quickly lost at free surfaces as buoyant forces raise them up. A 10^{-2} *cm* air bubble rises at the rate of 1.5 *cm/sec* in water. If nuclei are to persist in water, or for that matter, any liquid media, some mechanism must prevent their dissolution or buoyant exit.

A number of possibilities have been suggested to account for the presence of persistent, or stabilized, nuclei in undersaturated liquids, liquids that have been boiled, or denucleated. Crevices in the liquid, or surrounding boundary, may exert mechanical pressure on gas nuclei, holding them in place. Microscopic dust, or other impurities, on which gas and vapor are deposited, are stabilized already. Surface activated molecules, (such as hydrogen and hydroxyl ions in water), or surface activated skins formed from impurities may surround the nuclei and act as rigid spheres, offsetting constrictive surface tension, preventing diffusion of gas out of the nuclei and collapse. In all cases, the end result is a family, or group of families, of persistent nuclei. Time scales for stabilization and persistence of nuclei would obviously equate to the strength and persistence of stabilizing mechanism. Experimentally, trying to differentiate stabilization modes is very difficult, because (eventual) growth patterns of nuclei are the same in all cases. The ultimate crumbling of surrounding shells, release of crevice mechanical pressure, removal of dust and impurity nucleation centers, and deactivation of surface chemicals leads to the onset of cavitation and bubble growth.

Keyed Exercises

• *What is the (Doppler) frequency shift, Δf, of a boat horn, $f = 32.5$ hertz, moving toward a stationary snorkeler at speed of $v_s = 6$ knots?*

$$\Delta f = f \frac{v_s}{u - v_s}$$

$$u = 333 \ m/sec, \ v_s = 6 \times .514 \ m/sec = 3.08 \ m/sec$$

$$\Delta f = 32.5 \times \frac{3.08}{333 + 3.08} \ hertz = .0314 \ hertz$$

• *In the adiabatic limit, what is the sound speed, u, in an ideal gas at atmospheric pressure, $P = 1.009 \times 10^6 \ dynes/cm^2$?*

$$u^2 = \frac{Y}{\rho}, \ Y = 5/3P, \ \rho = .00024 \ g/cm^3$$

$$u = \left[\frac{5/3P}{\rho} \right]^{1/2} = \left[\frac{5/3 \times 1.009 \times 10^6}{.00024} \right]^{1/2} \ cm/sec = 837.2 \ m/sec$$

• *What is the approximate bubble diameter, d, for audible bubbles moving with speed, $u = 35 \ cm/sec$, in the pulmonary artery?*

$$d = 78 \ \mu m$$

• *Blood is mainly incompressible water of density, $\rho = 1 \ g/cm^3$. So, if blood moving at speed, $u = 1.2 \ cm/sec$, through an artery of cross sectional area, $A_i = .6 \ cm$, under pressure, $p_i = 1.012 \ atm$, encounters a vessel constriction of cross section, $A_f = .24 \ cm$, what is the blood speed at the constriction, assuming constant elevation and no external heat or work exchanged in flow?*

$$p_i = 1.012 \ atm = 1.012 \times 1.013 \times 10^6 \ dynes/cm^2 = 1.0252 \times 10^6 \ dynes/cm^2$$

$$\rho_i = \frac{m}{V_i} = \rho_f = \frac{m}{V_f} = \rho = 1.0 \ g/cm^3, \ v_i = u$$

$$\rho_i v_i A_i = \rho_f v_f A_f$$

$$v_f = \frac{\rho_i A_i}{\rho_f A_f} v_i = \frac{A_i}{A_f} v_f = \frac{.6}{.24} \times 1.2 \ cm/sec = 3.0 \ cm/sec$$

What is the mass flow rate, dm/dt?

$$\frac{dm}{dt} = \rho A_i v_i = \rho A_f v_f = 1.0 \times .6 \times 1.2 \ g/sec = 1.0 \times .24 \times 3 \ g/sec = .72 \ g/sec$$

If a rupture develops in the artery, allowing blood to exit at atmospheric pressure,
$p_f = 1.0$ *atm, what is the change in kinetic energy per unit mass,* $\Delta k = 1/2(v_f^2 - v_i^2)$,
at the rupture point?

$$\Delta k = \frac{1}{2}(v_f^2 - v_i^2) = \frac{(p_i - p_f)}{\rho}$$

$$\Delta k = \frac{.012 \times 1.013 \times 10^6}{1.0} \ ergs/g = 12.2 \times 10^3 \ ergs/g$$

- *What is the inherent unsaturation,* Δ_u, *for an equilibrated diver at 33 fsw using
  76/24 nitrox?*

$$\Delta_u = (1 - f_{N_2})P - 2.04 f_{N_2} - 5.47 \ fsw$$

$$f_{N_2} = .76, \quad P = P_0 + d = 33 + 33 \ fsw = 66 \ fsw$$

$$\Delta_u = .24 \times 66 - 2.04 \times .76 - 5.47 \ fsw = 8.82 \ fsw$$

- *Laboratory bubble seed counts in gels and (some) living tissue suggest the seed size
  (radius), r, distribution, n, is exponential, decreasing in number as the seed radius
  increases, so that (differentially),*

$$n_i = n_0 \ exp \ (-\beta r_i)$$

with n_0 *and* β *constants. For small sample counts (microscope),* $n_1 = 9865$, $r_1 = .7$ *microns and* $n_2 = 5743$, $r_2 = 1.4$ *microns, what are* n_0 *and* β *?*

$$n_i = n_0 \ exp \ (-\beta r_i), \quad \ln \ (n_1/n_2) = -\beta(r_1 - r_2)$$

$$\beta = \frac{1}{r_2 - r_1} \ln \ (n_1/n_2) = \frac{1}{.7} \ln \ (9865/5743) = .773$$

$$n_0 = n_i \ exp \ (\beta r_i) = n_1 \ exp \ (\beta r_1) = 9865 \ exp \ (.773 \times .7) = 16947$$

Assuming β *is determined (given), how is the distribution function, n, normalized to
the total seed count, N, across all sizes?*

$$n_0 \int_0^\infty exp \ (-\beta r) \ dr = \frac{n_0}{\beta} = N$$

$$n_0 = \beta N$$

- *What is the work function,* ω, *for thin film (Laplacian) bubbles of radius, r, at
  constant temperature and entropy)?*

$$\frac{\partial \omega}{\partial V} = -\tau = -\frac{2\gamma}{r}$$

$$V = \frac{4}{3}\pi r^3$$

$$\frac{\partial \omega}{\partial V} = \frac{\partial \omega}{\partial r}\frac{\partial r}{\partial V} = \frac{1}{4\pi r^2}\frac{\partial \omega}{\partial r}$$

$$\frac{\partial \omega}{\partial r} = -4\pi r^2 \frac{2\gamma}{r} = -8\pi\gamma r$$

$$\omega = \int -8\pi\gamma r \, dr = -4\pi\gamma r^2$$

- *What is the probability, dw, for purely homogeneous bubble nucleation in (watery) tissue, for any temperature, T, and radius, r?*

$$dw = exp\,(-\Delta G/kT), \quad \Delta G = \frac{4}{3}\pi\gamma r^2, \quad \gamma = 18 \, dyne/cm$$

What happens to the nucleation probability as seed radii shrink, that is, as $r \to 0$?

$$\lim_{r\to0} dw = \lim_{r\to0} exp\,(-4\pi\gamma r^2/3kT) \to exp(0) \to 1$$

How would this probability function be normalized over all bubble radii?

$$\Gamma = \int_0^\infty exp\,(-4\pi\gamma r^2/3kT) \, dr = \left[\frac{3kT}{16\gamma}\right]^{1/2}$$

$$dw = \Gamma^{-1} exp\,(-4\pi\gamma r^2/3kT) \, dr$$

What is the cumulative probability, Π, for nucleation in the range, $r_{min} \le r \le r_{max}$?

$$\Pi = \Gamma^{-1} \int_{r_{min}}^{r_{max}} exp\,(-4\pi\gamma r^2/3kT) \, dr$$

Assuming $(3kT/16\gamma)^{1/2} = 1 \, \mu m$, evaluate the probability function (integral), Π, in the range, $0.1 \le r \le 0.5 \, \mu m$, using any convenient technique (analytic, approximate, numerical integration)?

$$\Gamma = \left[\frac{3kT}{16\gamma}\right]^{1/2} = 1 \, \mu m$$

$$\Pi = \Gamma^{-1} \int_{0.1}^{0.5} exp\,(-\pi r^2/4\Gamma^2) dr = .3673$$

- *What is the cavitation index, κ, for blood flowing through the pulmonary arteries at a speed, $u = 5 \, cm/sec$, while saturated with metabolic and inert gases, $p = .95 \, atm$, at depth, $d = 45 \, fsw$?*

$$\kappa = 2\frac{P-p}{\rho u^2}, \quad \rho = 1.04 \, gm/cm^3$$

$$p = .95 \times 1.013 \times 10^6 \, dynes/cm^2 = .962 \times 10^6 \, dynes/cm^2$$

$$P = (1+45/33) \times 1.013 \times 10^6 \, dynes/cm^2 = 2.394 \times 10^6 \, dynes/cm^2$$

$$\kappa = 2 \times \frac{1.41 \times 10^6}{1.04 \times 25} = 73.3 \times 10^6$$

Part 3

GAS KINETICS AND PHASE TRANSFER

Gas Kinetics

Air is a mixture of inert and metabolic gases, composed of nitrogen and oxygen mainly, with variable amounts of carbon dioxide, water vapor, ozone, sulfur dioxide, and nitrogen dioxide, and fixed trace amounts of xenon, helium, krypton, argon, methane, nitrous oxide, hydrogen, and neon. By volume, air is 78.1% nitrogen, 20.9% oxygen, and 1% everything else. Over nominal pressure and temperature ranges encountered in the Earth's atmosphere, air can be treated as an *ideal*, or dilute, gas.

Ideal Gases

Ideal gas molecules occupy no space, do not interact, scatter elastically from each other, and cannot be distorted upon collision, in short, act as vanishingly small, perfectly elastic, hard spheres in constant random motion from collisions. Real gases, in the limit of very large confining volumes, all behave like ideal gases, as well as over select ranges of pressure, temperature, and density. Simple monatomic (one atom molecules) and diatomic (two atom molecules) gases and mixtures, such as air, at room temperatures and atmospheric pressures are considered ideal, and satisfy an equation-of-state (EOS) linking pressure P, volume, V, and and temperature, T, of the form,

$$PV = nRT$$

with n the number of moles of gas, and R the universal gas constant (8.317 *joule/gmole* $^o K$). Temperature is measured in absolute, or Kelvin ($^o K$), units. In conservative processes, n is constant and changes in the state variables, P, V, and T, are linked to each other by the $P - V - T$ relationship. If each variable is alternatively held fixed, we get three well known ideal gas law corollaries,

$$PV = \gamma_T \quad (Boyle's\ law),$$

$$\frac{P}{T} = \gamma_V \quad (Amonton's\ law),$$

$$\frac{V}{T} = \gamma_P \quad (Charles'\ law),$$

with $\gamma_T = nRT$, $\gamma_V = nR/V$, and $\gamma_P = nR/P$ all constant. The relationships connect any number of arbitrary changes of state for constant temperature, volume, or pressure, respectively. In a mixture of ideal gases, the total pressure is the sum of component gas partial pressures, intuitively obvious, but also known as Dalton's law. Denoting gas partial pressures, p, the total pressure, P, is given by,

$$P = \sum_{j=1}^{J} p_j,$$

with p_j the partial pressure of the jth gas species in a J component mixture.

Temperatures, which really measure average kinetic energy of gas molecules in the ensemble, are measured in Centigrade (^oC), Fahrenheit (^oF), Kelvin (^oK), and Rankine (^oR) degree units, related by,

$$^oF = \frac{9^o}{5} C + 32,$$

$$^oK = {}^o C + 273,$$

$$^oR = {}^o F + 460.$$

Real Gases

All gas molecules occupy space, exert short-ranged forces on each other, scatter inelastically at times, and possibly distort with collision, in short, act as nonideal gas molecules. Then equations-of-state need include such effects, particularly in appropriate pressure, temperature, and density regimes. The most general form of the equation-of-state can be cast in *virial* form, in terms of the molal specific volume, v,

$$v = \frac{V}{n}$$

for n the number of moles,

$$Pv = RT \left[1 + \frac{a}{v} + \frac{b}{v^2} + \frac{c}{v^3} + ... \right],$$

with a, b, c functions mostly of temperature, possibly specific volume. For ideal gases, $a = b = c = 0$, but in general these virial constants are nonzero. Certainly as the specific volume, v, or real volume, V, gets large, the virial expansion collapses to the ideal case. The virial expansion and coefficients can be fitted to sets of experimental data for gases. Such fits to even very complicated gas behavior all have one feature in common. The quantity, pv/T, always approaches the universal gas constant, R, as temperature, T, approaches absolute zero ($-273\ ^oC$ or $-460\ ^oF$).

Clausius suggested that the volume, V, available to a single gas molecule be reduced by the actual volume occupied by all other molecules in the assembly, as shown in Figure 33. Accordingly, a correction factor, b, enters the ideal gas law through the simple relationship,

$$P(v-b) = RT$$

and is called the Clausius equation of state. Van der Waals, in 1873, suggested that a second correction term, accounting for forces between molecules, a, also be added to the ideal equation of state,

$$(P+a/v^2)(v-b) = RT$$

giving the van der Waals relationship. Both a and b are functions of temperature, T, and not simple constants. Again, as $a,b \to 0$, the van der Waals and Clausius equations go over to the ideal gas limit.

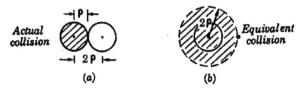

Figure 33. Volume Reduction For Ideal Gas Law

The center of a moving gas molecule is excluded from a spherical volume of radius, 2ρ, and this volume is called the excluded sphere by Clausius and van der Waals. Only the hemisphere facing the moving molecule is excluded, so the total volume, B, excluded by N other gas molecules, is $1/2$ the total exclusion volume of the molecules,

$$B = \frac{N}{2}\frac{4}{3}\pi(2\rho)^3 = \frac{16N}{3}\pi\rho^3$$

and we recast the ideal gas expression,

$$p(V-B) = nRT$$

The van der Waals equation can be put in virial form by first rewriting,

$$Pv = RT\left[1-\frac{b}{v}\right]^{-1} - \frac{a}{v}$$

and then using the binomial expansion,

$$\left[1-\frac{b}{v}\right]^{-1} \approx 1 + \frac{b}{v} + \frac{b^2}{v^2} +$$

so that,

$$Pv = RT + \frac{RTb-a}{v} + \frac{RTb^2}{v^2} +$$

The Beattie-Bridgman equation is a modified virial equation which fits the experimental data over a wide range of pressure, volume, and temperature,

$$Pv = \frac{RT(1-\delta/vT^3)}{v}(v+\beta) - \frac{\alpha}{v}$$

for α, β, and δ slowly varying (temperature) constants. The van der Waals gas law permits two degrees of freedom (a, b), while the Beattie-Bridgman equation is more flexible, admitting three degrees of freedom (α, β, δ), in fitting experimental data.

Collisional Phenomena

The properties of matter in bulk are predicted from kinetic, or dynamic, theory through application of the laws of mechanics to the individual molecules of the system, and from these laws, deriving expressions for the pressure of a gas, internal energy, and specific heat. Statistical mechanics, more broadly, ignores detailed considerations of molecules as individuals, and applies considerations of probability to the very large ensemble of molecules comprising matter. Both were developed on the assumption that the laws of mechanics, deduced from the behavior of matter in bulk, could be applied to molecules, atoms, and electrons. In the case of gases, these particles are in continuous collisional motion.

If we imagine that at a certain instance in time all the molecules of a gas, except one, are frozen in position, while the remaining single molecule continues to move among the others with ensemble average speed, $\bar{v}$, and that all molecules are perfectly elastic spheres, we can define a collision cross section, σ, as the area swept out by their total radial separation, 2ρ, with ρ the molecular radius (Figure 33),

$$\sigma = 4\pi\rho^2.$$

For gases, molecular radii are on the order of *angstroms* (10^{-10} *m*). In a time interval, dt, if there are N molecules in volume, V, the number, dN, with centers in the cylinder swept out by the molecule moving with velocity, $\bar{v}$, is,

$$dN = \sigma\frac{N}{V}\bar{v}dt,$$

also representing the number of collisions in that time interval. The collisional frequency, f, is the number of collisions per unit time interval,

$$f = \frac{dN}{dt} = \sigma\frac{N}{V}\bar{v}.$$

In ideal gases, collisional frequencies are on the order of 10^{10} sec^{-1}. The average distance between collisions, Λ, or the mean free path, equals distance covered, $\bar{v}dt$, divided by number of collisions, dN, that is,

$$\Lambda = \frac{V}{\sigma N}.$$

Typical values for Λ are near 10^{-7} *cm* for gases. Every collision removes a molecule from N, and the corresponding change, dN, in distance, dx, depends on N, and collision probability, χ,

$$dN = -\chi N dx,$$

with, in the simplest case of solid spheres,

$$\chi = \frac{1}{\Lambda}.$$

The standard survival equation follows upon integration of the above, with $N = N_0$ at $x = 0$,

$$N = N_0 \, exp \, (-x/\Lambda).$$

The viscosity, X, thermal conductivity, K, and diffusivity, D, in the kinetic picture depend on particle transport of momentum, energy, and mass by collisions. Considerations of the momentum, energy, and mass transfer across any imagined surface by molecular collisions yields,

$$X = \frac{1}{3}\frac{N}{V}m\bar{v}\Lambda,$$

$$K = \frac{1}{2}\frac{N}{V}\bar{v}k\Lambda,$$

$$D = \frac{1}{3}\bar{v}\Lambda,$$

with m the molecular mass, and k Boltzmann's constant. Obviously the density, ρ, is given by,

$$\rho = \frac{N}{V}m,$$

so that,

$$D = \frac{X}{\rho},$$

$$H = \frac{3}{2}\frac{X}{\rho}k.$$

Table 11 lists transport coefficients for a number of gases, that is, mean free path, molecular radius, viscosity, thermal conductivity, and diffusivity at room temperature.

Table 11. Kinetic Transport Coefficients.

gas	Λ (μm)	r (nm)	X (*dyne sec*/m^2)	K (*joule*/*cm sec* $^\circ K$)	D (cm^2/*sec*)
He	.186	.109	1.94	.144	.124
Ne	.132	.132	3.12	.046	.358
N_2	.063	.188	1.73	.023	.072
O_2	.068	.179	2.01	.024	.073
NH_3	.045	.222	.97	.021	.014
CO_2	.042	.232	1.45	.030	.009

Temperature

Temperature is a measure of hotness or coldness. But more particularly, temperature is a measure of the average kinetic energy of the molecular ensemble comprising the object, also called the internal energy. For an ideal gas, the mean molal kinetic energy, $\bar{\varepsilon}$, satisfies the Boltzmann relationship,

$$\bar{\varepsilon} = \frac{3}{2} kT,$$

with k Boltzmann's constant $(1.38 \times 10^{-23}$ $j/gmole$ $^{o}K)$, and T the absolute temperature. The first temperature measuring devices, employing displaced air volumes to define hotness of coldness according to the pronunciations of the instrument maker, were called thermometers in the 1600s. The liquid sealed in glass thermometers, based on thermal expansion and contraction, appeared in the latter half of the 1600s.

    Use of temperature as a measurement of hotness or coldness is based on two requirements, that is, a universal agreement on calibration and scale, and technology sufficient to produce reliable instruments giving identical readings under the same conditions. Wide adoption of the Fahrenheit scale, ^{o}F, was promoted by the trusty mercury (in glass) thermometers constructed in Danzig, by Fahrenheit, in the early 1700s. The scale was based on two fixed points, namely, the melting point of ice and the temperature of a healthy human body (later replaced by the boiling point of water). Celsius, at Uppsala, around the mid 1700s, introduced the Celsius (Centigrade) scale, ^{o}C, on which the degree was $1/100$ of the interval between the freezing and boiling points of water. Later, in the 1800s, Kelvin introduced the absolute scale, ^{o}K, based on the second law of thermodynamics and entropy, ultimately linked by statistical mechanics to an absolute zero, that is, a temperature at which random molecular motion ceases. By 1887, the international community adopted the constant volume hydrogen gas thermometer as defining measurements on the Kelvin scale.

    Kelvin (^{o}K), Centigrade (^{o}C), Rankine (^{o}R), and Fahrenheit (^{o}F) temperatures are linearly scaled, and are easily related,

$$^{o}F = \frac{9}{5} {}^{o}C + 32,$$

$$^{o}K = {}^{o} C + 273,$$

$$^{o}R = {}^{o} F + 460.$$

Kelvin and Rankine temperatures are employed in the gas laws.

First and Second Laws

The first law of thermodynamics is really a statement of conservation of energy in any system. Denoting the internal energy of the system, U, the net heat flow into the system, Q, and the work, W, done on the system, the first law requires that infinitesimal changes dQ, dU, and dW satisfy,

$$dU = dQ - dW.$$

The internal energy of an ideal gas is only dependent on temperature, and that is a good approximation in most other real gases near standard temperature and pressure. ($32\,^oF$, and 1 *atm*). Denoting the number of molecules of the gas, N, and the number of moles, n, with R the gas constant and k Boltzmann's constant, we have

$$dU = N\bar{e}dT = \frac{3}{2} NkdT = \frac{3}{2} nRdT,$$

as a measure of the internal energy change, dU, for temperature change, dT. Heat flow, dQ, into or out of the system occurs through conduction, convection, or radiation. Mechanical work, dW, performed on, or by, the system is associated with volume change, dV, under pressure, P,

$$dW = PdV,$$

so that,

$$dU = dQ - PdV,$$

in a mechanical system. We do not live in a reversible world, that is to say, processes usually proceed in only one direction. Collectively, the directionality ascribed to physical processes is termed *entropy*.

From experience, we know that some processes satisfying the first law (conservation of energy) never occur. For instance, a piece of rock resting on the floor will never cool itself down and jump up to the ceiling, thereby converting heat energy into potential energy. The second law defines a state *directional* variable, S, called the entropy, so that for any process, the heat transferred, dQ, is given by,

$$dQ = TdS$$

$$dS \geq 0.$$

The requirement that the entropy change, dS, associated with the process must be greater than or equal to zero imparts directionality to the process, or the process is forbidden. Put another way by Kelvin, there exist no thermodynamic processes, nor transformations, that extract heat from a reservoir and convert it entirely into work. Dissipative mechanisms, such as friction and viscosity, prevent a reduction in system entropy for any process. Processes for which the entropy change is zero,

$$dS = 0,$$

are termed reversible, or *isentropic*, represent an idealization of physical reality. Processes in which no heat is exchanged by the system are called *adiabatic*, that is,

$$dQ = 0.$$

Combining the first and second laws, and considering only mechanical work,

$$dW = PdV,$$

we see that,

$$dU = TdS - PdV$$

Simple energy considerations applied to the steady flow of a fluid (gas or liquid) in system able to exchange heat and do external work, such as a steam engine, refrigerator, turbine, compressor, and scuba regulator, provide a simple means to relate temperature, internal energy, kinetic and potential energy, and pressure changes to external work and heat. The simple, yet powerful, relationships detailed above can be applied to air and fluid flows in diving systems, such as regulators, compressors, tanks, hoses, and gauges to yield rough estimates of pressures, temperatures, heat, and work. Actual flow patterns can be extremely complicated, requiring numerical solution on high speed computers, especially high pressure flows.

Dissolved Phase Transfer

All gases dissolve in all liquids, but actual solubilities range over many orders of magnitude. Considering inert gases at room temperature, for illustration, the solubility of xenon in *n*-octane, a hydrocarbon liquid, is 470 times that of helium in water. Gas solubilities can vary much more for complex solutes and solvents. The solubility of the anesthetic gas halothane in olive oil is more than 10^6 times the solubility of common gases in liquid mercury. Inert gases such as helium and nitrogen are readily soluble in tissue and blood, and their solubility can fuel bubble growth with reduction in ambient pressure, a concern for decompressing divers.

Denoting the ambient partial pressure of a gas, p, and its solubility, S, in a liquid, the relative concentration of the dissolved gas component, c, is given by Henry's law,

$$c = Sp.$$

The corresponding *tension*, or dissolved gas partial pressure, is also p at equilibrium. By convention, partial pressures usually refer to the free gas phase, while tensions refer to the dissolved gas phase, though some folks use them interchangeably. When there exist differences, or *gradients*, between gas partial pressures and/or tensions across regions of varying concentration or solubility, gases will diffuse until partial pressures are equal, in short, move from regions of higher partial pressures to regions of lower partial pressures, regardless of the phases (free or dissolved) of the components. This movement is the crux of the decompression problem in divers and aviators, and modeling this movement is central to the formulation of decompression tables and dive computer algorithms.

Gas is driven across the tissue-blood interface by the gradient, but the rate at which bulk tissue transfers gas also depends on the blood flow rate and the degree of vascularity. Then both blood perfusion rate and gas diffusion rate contribute to the overall transfer process.

Perfusion Controlled Transport

Exchange of dissolved tissue and blood gas, controlled by blood flow rates across regions of varying concentration or solubility, is driven by the local tissue-blood gradient, that is, the difference between the arterial blood tension, p_a, and the instantaneous tissue tension, p, assuming that blood flow rates are considerably slower than gas diffusion rates across the regions. Such behavior is modeled in time, t, by simple classes of exponential response functions, bounded by p_a and the initial value of p, denoted p_i. These multitissue functions satisfy a differential *perfusion* rate equation,

$$\frac{\partial p}{\partial t} = -\lambda\ (p - p_a),$$

and take the form, tracking both dissolved gas buildup and elimination symmetrically,

$$p - p_a = (p_i - p_a)\ exp\ (-\lambda t),$$

$$\lambda = \frac{.6931}{\tau},$$

with perfusion constant, λ, defined by the tissue halftime, τ. Compartments with 2, 5, 10, 20, 40, 80, 120, 180, 240, 360, 480, and 720 minute halftimes, τ, are employed, and halftimes are independent of pressure.

   In a series of dives or multiple stages, p_i and p_a represent extremes for each stage, the initial tension and arterial tension at the beginning of the next stage. Stages are treated sequentially, with finishing tensions at one step representing initial tensions for the next step, and so on. Exposures are controlled through critical tensions, M, such that, throughout the dive,

$$p \leq M.$$

Diffusion Controlled Transport

Exchange of dissolved tissue and blood gas, controlled by diffusion across regions of varying concentration or solubility, is also driven by the local tissue-blood gradient, but solutions to the diffusion equation control transport. In simple planar geometry, the diffusion equation can be cast,

$$D\frac{\partial^2 p}{\partial x^2} = \frac{\partial p}{\partial t},$$

with D the diffusion coefficient. As in the perfusion case, solutions depend on initial values, and also on boundary conditions. Tissue is separated into intravascular and extravascular regions for application of boundary conditions, with the tissue tension, p, equal to the arterial tension, p_a, at the tissue-blood interface. Solving and applying initial and boundary conditions, and then averaging the solutions over the spatial region, of thickness, l, there obtains,

$$p - p_a = (p_i - p_a)\ \frac{8}{\pi^2}\ \sum_{n=1}^{\infty}\ \frac{1}{(2n-1)^2}\ exp\ (-\alpha_{2n-1}^2 Dt),$$

with,

$$\alpha_{2n-1} = \frac{(2n-1)\pi}{l}.$$

A decay constant, κ, fitted to exposure data, is related to the diffusion coefficient, D,

$$\kappa = \frac{\pi^2 D}{l^2} = 0.007928 \; min^{-1},$$

in the exponential expansion, and plays a similar role to λ in the perfusion controlled case. The diffusion expansion looks like a weighted sum of multitissue perfusion functions with decay constants, $(2n-1)^2 \; \kappa$. A diffusion equivalent halftime, ω, is simply defined,

$$\omega = \frac{.6931}{\kappa} = 87.4 \; min,$$

so that halftimes, ω_{2n-1}, in the weighted expansion, are given by,

$$\omega_{2n-1} = \frac{\omega}{(2n-1)^2}.$$

As before, p_i and p_a represent extremes for each stage. Critical gradients, G, control diving through the constraint,

$$p - p_a \leq G,$$

Free Phase Transfer

To satisfy thermodynamic laws, bubbles in blood and tissue assume spherical shapes in the absence of external or mechanical (distortion) pressures. Bubbles entrain free gases because of a thin film, exerting surface tension pressure on the gas, of magnitude, $2\gamma/r$, with γ the Laplacian surface tension and r the bubble radius. Hydrostatic pressure balance requires that the pressure inside the bubble, Π,

$$\Pi = \sum_{j=1}^{J} \pi_j,$$

with π_j bubble partial pressures of component (free) gases, exceed ambient pressure, P, by the surface tension pressure, $2\gamma/r$,

$$\Pi = P + \frac{2\gamma}{r},$$

as seen in Figure 34. At small radii, surface tension pressure is greatest, and at large radii, surface tension pressure is least.

Gases will also diffuse into or out of a bubble according to differences in gas partial pressures inside and outside the bubble, whether in free or dissolved phases outside the bubble. In the former case, the gradient is termed $free - free$, while in the latter case, the gradient is termed $free - dissolved$. Unless the surface tension, γ, is identically zero, there is always a gradient tending to force gas out of the bubble, thus making the bubble collapse on itself because of surface tension pressure. If surrounding external pressures on bubbles change in time, however, bubbles may grow or contract. The flow regime is depicted in Figure 35.

Bubbles grow or contract according to the strength of the free-free or free-dissolved gradient, and it is the latter case which concerns divers under decompression. The radial rate at which bubbles grow or contract is roughly given by,

$$\frac{\partial r}{\partial t} = \frac{DS}{r}(Q - \Pi),$$

with D and S tissue diffusivity and solubility, and total tissue tension, Q, the sum of component dissolved gas tensions,

$$Q = \sum_{j=1}^{J} p_j,$$

as before. A critical radius, r_c, separating growing from contracting bubbles is given by,

$$r_c = \frac{2\gamma}{Q - P}$$

and bubbles with radius $r > r_c$ will grow, while bubbles with radius $r < r_c$ will contract. Limiting bubble growth and impact upon nerves and circulation are issues when decompressing divers and aviators. The interplay between tissue tension and bubble growth is further complicated with ascent, since ambient pressure changes in time (depending on ascent rate). Figure 36 shows the effects of bubble growth in fast and slow tissue compartments for varying ascent rate.

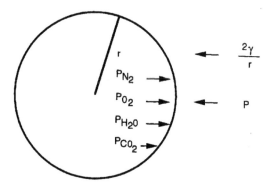

Figure 34. Bubble Pressure Balance

The total pressure, Π, within an air bubble equals the sum of ambient pressure, P, plus effective surface tension, $2\gamma/r$, according to,

$$\Pi = P + \frac{2\gamma}{r}$$

$$\Pi = P_{O_2} + P_{N_2} + P_{H_2O} + P_{CO_2} = \pi_{O_2} + \pi_{N_2} + \pi_{H_2O} + \pi_{CO_2}$$

so that the partial (free phase) pressures of O_2, N_2, H_2O, and CO_2 inside the bubble exceed ambient pressure by surface tension pressure. At small radii, surface tension effects are large, while at large radii effects of surface tension vanish. Effective surface tension is the difference between Laplacian (thin film) and skin (surfactant) tension. Stabilized bubble seeds or gas nuclei exhibit zero surface tension, so that gas pressures and tensions are equal. When nuclei are destabilized, any pressure gradients between free and dissolved gas phases will drive the system to different configurations, that is, expansion or contraction until a new equilibrium is established.

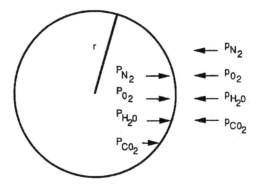

Figure 35. Bubble Gas Diffusion

An air bubble in hydrostatic equilibrium will grow or contract, depending on its size and any relative pressure gradients between free gas in the bubble and dissolved gas in tissue. Gradients are inward if tensions exceed bubble gas pressures, and outward if free phase pressures exceed tensions. A critical radius, r_c, separates growing from contracting bubbles for a given set of pressures. The critical radius depends on the total tissue tension, Q, ambient pressure, P, and effective surface tension, γ,

$$r_c = \frac{2\gamma}{Q - P}$$

$$Q = p_{O_2} + p_{N_2} + p_{H_2O} + p_{CO_2}$$

where growth occurs for $r > r_c$, and contraction for $r < r_c$. Some gas micronuclei in the body can be crushed and possibly eliminated by increasing pressure (compression), while others can be excited into growth by pressure changes (compression-decompression), as witnessed in vitro in the laboratory. Nuclei (stabilized over varying time scales) have been seen in virtually all aqueous substrates, including human blood, egg albumin, and water.

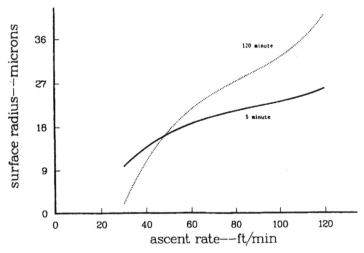

Figure 36. Bubble Growth With Varying Ascent Rate

Bubble growth on ascent depend on bubble size, surface tension, and the average difference between tissue tension and ambient pressure. For bubbles larger than a certain critical (cutoff) radius, faster ascents in the presence of elevated tensions in surrounding tissue sites tend to support growth, because average ambient pressure is lessened by fast ascents. Increasing ambient pressure always tends to restrict simple bubble growth, since internal bubble pressure is always greater than ambient by an amount, $2\gamma/r$, the surface tension pressure. In the calculation below, bubbles with initial radii of .35 microns, surrounded by tissues saturated at 120 fsw, and taking $2\gamma = 8.3$ fsw micron, are decompressed with different ascent rates. Unit solubility, concentration, and diffusivity are employed for simplicity. One notes that the growth rate in the 5 min compartment is less than in the 120 min compartment. Ostensibly, the faster compartment offgases more rapidly during ascent, presenting a lower average tension and weaker diffusion gradient for bubble growth. As also seen, ascent rates beyond 100 fsw/min theoretically spawn 60 to 100 fold increases in bubble radius upon surfacing.

Keyed Exercises

• *A tank initially at standard temperature and pressure, $P_i = 1$ atm, and, $T_i = 273\,^{\circ}K$, is heated to $313\,^{\circ}K$ by the Sun. What is the pressure, P, in the tank?*

$$P = \frac{T}{T_i}\,P_i = \frac{313}{273} \times 1\,atm = 1.146\,atm$$

- *The air in a dry suit at ambient sea level pressure, $P_0 = 33$ fsw, occupies volume, $V_0 = .3$ ft^3, at temperature, $T = 300\,^oK$. What is volume, V, occupied at depth, $P = 50$ fsw, and temperature, $T = 280\,^oK$?*

$$\frac{P_0 V_0}{T_0} = \frac{PV}{T}$$

$$V = V_0 \frac{P_0 T}{P T_0} = .3 \times \frac{33 \times 280}{50 \times 300}\ ft^3 = .185\ ft^3$$

- *What volume, V, does a gmole of an ideal gas occupy at standard temperature and pressure?*

$$p = 10.1\ newton/cm^2,\ \ T = 273\,^oK,\ \ R = 8.317\ j/gmole\,^oK$$

$$PV = nRT,\ \ V = \frac{nRT}{P}$$

$$V = \frac{8.317 \times 273}{.101}\ cm^3 = 22.48 \times 10^3\ cm^3 = 22.48\ l$$

- *Convert 37 ^oC to Fahrenheit (^oF), and then to Rankine (^oR) temperatures?*

$$^oF = \frac{9}{5}\,^oC + 32 = \frac{9}{5} \times 37 + 32 = 98.6$$

$$^oR =^o F + 460 = 98.6 + 460 = 558.6$$

- *Convert 80 ^oF to Centigrade (^oC), and then to Kelvin (^oK) temperatures?*

$$^oC = \frac{5}{9}\,(^oF - 32) = \frac{5}{9}\,(80 - 32) = 26.6$$

$$^oK =^o C + 273 = 26.6 + 273 = 299.6$$

- *A 10 qt plastic container is submerged to 100 ft in Lake Michigan. What is its volume, V?*

$$P_i = 33\ fsw,\ \ P = 33 + .975 \times 100\ fsw = 130.5\ fsw$$

$$P_i V_i = PV,\ \ V = V_i \frac{P_i}{P}$$

$$V = 10 \times \frac{33}{130.5}\ qt = 10 \times .253\ qt = 2.53\ qt$$

- *A weather balloon is partially inflated at 50 fsw to 20 ft^3, and allowed to drift to the ocean surface slowly. What is the volume, V_f, at 20 fsw?*

$$P_i = 33 + 50\ fsw = 83\ fsw,\ \ P_f = 33 + 20\ fsw = 53\ fsw,\ \ V_i = 20\ ft^3$$

$$P_i V_i = P_f V_f$$

$$V_f = V_i \frac{P_i}{P_f} = 20 \times \frac{83}{53}\ ft^3 = 31.3\ ft^3$$

- A skin diver with lung volume of 6 qt descends to a depth, $d = 85$ fsw. Assuming his lung tissues are 40% air space, what is his compressed lung volume, V?

$$V_i = .4 \times 6 \ qt = 2.4 \ qt, \quad V_{tis} = .6 \times 6 \ qt = 3.6 \ qt$$

$$P_i = 33 \ fsw, \quad P = 33 + d = 33 + 85 \ fsw = 118 \ fsw$$

$$P_i V_i = PV_f$$

$$V_f = V_i \frac{P_i}{P} = 2.4 \frac{33}{118} \ qt = .67 \ qt$$

$$V = V_f + V_{tis} = .67 + 3.6 \ qt = 4.27 \ qt$$

- A heliox gas mixture at pressure, $P_i = 225$ atm, occupying, $V_i = 1.2 \ ft^3$, and at temperature, $T_i = 293 \ ^\circ K$, is released to a larger tank with volume, $V = 4.5 \ ft^3$. Upon expansion, the mixture drops to a temperature $T = 283 \ ^\circ K$. What is the new pressure, P?

$$\frac{P_i \ V_i}{T_i} = \frac{P \ V}{T}$$

$$P = P_i \frac{V_i T}{V T_i} = 225 \times \frac{1.2 \times 283}{4.5 \times 293} \ atm = 51.6 \ atm$$

- If vapor is assumed an ideal gas in the Clausius-Clapeyron (phase) equation, and if the specific volume of the liquid and solid phase is very small, write an expression for the limiting form of the phase equation ?

$$\Delta v = \frac{RT}{P}, \quad \frac{dP}{dT} = \frac{l}{T \Delta v}$$

$$\frac{dP}{dT} = \frac{Pl}{RT^2}$$

Integrate the expression to give explicit dependence on temperature, T, for this case?

$$\frac{dP}{P} = \frac{l dT}{RT^2}$$

$$\ln P = -\frac{l}{RT} + \ln C$$

$$P = C \ exp \ (-l/RT), \quad C \text{ is integration constant}$$

- What is the mean molecular energy (molal), $\bar{\varepsilon}$, of an ideal gas at temperature, $T = 900 \ ^\circ K$?

$$\bar{\varepsilon} = \frac{3}{2}kT$$

$$\bar{\varepsilon} = \frac{3}{2} \times 1.38 \times 10^{-23} \times 900 \ j/gmole = 1.24 \times 10^{-20} \ j/gmole$$

- What is the molal specific heat, c_V, of an ideal gas at constant volume ?

$$dQ = dU + PdV, dV = 0, \quad dU = \frac{3}{2}nRdT$$

$$c_V = \frac{1}{n}\left[\frac{dQ}{dT}\right]_V = \frac{3}{2}R$$

- What is the temperature, T, of a kgmole van der Waals gas at pressure, $P = 500 \ newton/m^2$, and a specific volume, $v = 2 \ m^3/kgmole$, taking the virial coefficients, $a = 100 \ newton \ m/kgmole$, and $b = .03 \ m^3/kgmole$?

$$RT = \left[P + \frac{a}{v^2}\right](v - b)$$

$$T = \left[500 + \frac{100}{4}\right] \times (2 - .03) \times \frac{1}{8.31 \times 10^{-3}} = 124.5 \times 10^3 \ {}^o K$$

- A reef ecologist at depth, $d = 35 \ fsw$, on a dive computer registers a spectrum of nitrogen tensions, $p = (50, 48, 43, 41, 40, 42, 44) \ fsw$, in tissues, $\tau = (5, 10, 20, 40, 80, 120, 240) \ min$. What are the corresponding tissue gradients, $g = p - p_a$?

$$g = p - p_a, \quad P = 33 + 35 \ fsw = 68 \ fsw, \quad p_a = .79 \ P = 53.7 \ fsw$$

$$g = (-3.7, -5.7, -10.7, -12.7, -13.7, -11.7, -9.7) \ fsw$$

Since tissue gradients are inward (all negative), what is the implication for the present dive?

Present Dive Has Been Short And Shallow

What might higher tissue tensions in the two slowest compartments, relative to faster middle compartments, suggest?

Repetitive Diving Within 12 − 24 hr

- What is the total pressure, Π, inside a bubble lodged in an arteriole of diameter, $2r = 10 \ \mu m$, if ambient pressure, $P = 45 \ fsw$, and assuming a watery surface tension, $\gamma = 50 \ dyne/cm$?

$$P = \frac{45}{33} \times 10.1 \ newton/cm^2 = 13.77 \ newton/cm^2$$

$$\frac{2\gamma}{r} = \frac{100}{5 \times 10^{-6}} \ dyne/cm^2 = 2 \ newton/cm^2$$

$$\Pi = P + \frac{2\gamma}{r} = 13.77 + 2 \ newton/cm^2 = 15.77 \ newton/cm^2$$

- *For ambient pressure, P = 28 fsw, what is the watery critical bubble radius, r_c, at total tissue tension, Q = 20 newton/cm²?*

$$2\gamma = 1.0 \times 10^{-3} \ newton/cm^2$$

$$Q = 20 \ newton/cm^2, \quad P = \frac{28}{33} \times 10.1 \ newton/cm^2 = 8.56 \ newton/cm^2$$

$$r_c = \frac{2\gamma}{\Pi - P} = \frac{1.0 \times 10^{-3}}{20 - 8.56} \ cm = 1.14 \ \mu m$$

- *A bubble of radius 1.2 μm in tissue interstice at 165 fsw will grow to what radius if decompressed to sea level pressure (just Boyle's law expansion)?*

$$P_i r_i^3 = P_f r_f^3, \quad P_i = 198 \ fsw, \quad P_f = 33 \ fsw, \quad r_i = 1.2 \ \mu m$$

$$r_f = \left[\frac{P_i}{P_f}\right]^{1/3} r_i = \left[\frac{198}{33}\right]^{1/3} \times 1.2\mu m = 1.80 \times 1.2\mu m = 2.17 \ \mu m$$

- *After 6 halftimes, t = 6τ, what is the ratio, ω, of tissue saturation gradient, (p − pₐ), to initial tissue saturation gradient, (p − pᵢ)?*

$$\omega = \frac{p - p_a}{p_i - p_a} = exp\,(-\lambda t) = exp\,(-.693 \times 6) = .016$$

Decompression

Bubbles can form in tissue and blood when ambient pressure drops below tissue tensions, according to the rules of established phase mechanics. Trying to track free and dissolved gas buildup and elimination in tissue and blood, especially their interplay, is extremely complex, beyond the capabilities of even supercomputers. But safe computational prescriptions are necessary in the formulation of dive tables and digital meter algorithms. The simplest way to stage decompression, following extended exposures to high pressure with commensurate dissolved gas buildup, is to limit tissue tensions. Historically, Haldane first employed that approach, and it persists today.

Critical Tensions

To maximize the rate of uptake or elimination of dissolved gases, the *gradient*, simply the difference between p_i and p_a, is maximized by pulling the diver as close to the surface as possible. Exposures are limited by requiring that the perfusion-dominated tissue tensions, p, never exceed criticality, M, for instance, written for each tissue compartment in the US Navy approach employing 5, 10, 20, 40, 80, and 120 *minute* tissue halftimes, τ,

$$M = M_0 + \Delta M d,$$

with,

$$M_0 = 152.7\tau^{-1/4},$$

$$\Delta M = 3.25\tau^{-1/4},$$

as a function of depth, d, for ΔM the change per unit depth. Figure 37 plots the US Navy critical tensions.

Surfacing values, M_0, are principal concerns in nonstop diving, while values at depth, ΔMd, concern decompression diving. In both cases, the staging regimen tries to pull the diver as close to the surface as possible, in as short a time as possible. By contrast, free phase (bubble) elimination gradients, as seen, *increase* with depth, directly opposite to dissolved gas elimination gradients which *decrease* with depth. In actuality, decompression is a playoff between dissolved gas buildup and free phase growth, tempered by body ability to eliminate both. But dissolved gas models cannot handle both, so there are problems when extrapolating outside tested ranges.

In absolute pressure units, the corresponding critical gradient, G, is given by,

$$G = \frac{M}{.79} - P = 1.27\,M - P,$$

with P ambient pressure, and M critical nitrogen pressure. In bubble theories, supersaturation is limited by the critical gradient, G. In decompressed gel experiments, Strauss suggested that $G \approx 20\ fsw$ at ambient pressures less than a few atmospheres. Other studies suggest, $14 \leq G \leq 30\ fsw$, as a range of critical gradients (G-values).

In diffusion-dominated approaches, the tissue tension is often limited by a single, depth-dependent criterion, such as,

$$M = \frac{709\,P}{P + 404},$$

a continuous parameterization lying between fixed gradient and multitissue schemes. The corresponding critical gradient, G, is shown in Figure 38.

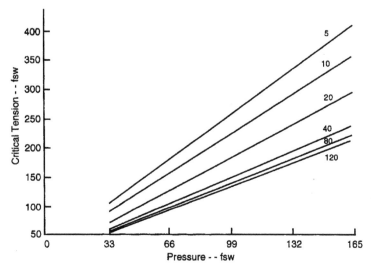

Figure 37. Perfusion Limited Nitrogen Critical Tensions

Critical tensions are linear functions of pressure in the Haldane scheme, obviously increasing with ambient pressure. Faster compartments permit larger amounts of dissolved nitrogen, slower compartments less. During any dive, compartment tensions must stay below the depicted lines in the Haldane approach. The critical tensions, M, below (Workman USN) can be reduced to an approximate form,

$$M = M_0 + \Delta Md = 152.7\tau^{-1/4} + 3.25d\tau^{-1/4}$$

for depth, d, and units of fsw. Extensions of the curves to altitude, $P \leq 33$ fsw, have been effected linearly and exponentially. In the linear case, the zero pressure intercepts are positive (Buhlmann), while in the exponential case, the intercepts are zero (Wienke). Any set of nonstop time limits (bounce dive NDLs) can be plugged into the model equations, and ensuing sets of tensions for compartments can be scanned for maximum surfacing tensions, M_0, across all depths and tissue halftimes, τ. Fits to decompression, or saturation, data can be employed to estimate increases in critical tension, ΔM, with depth, d.

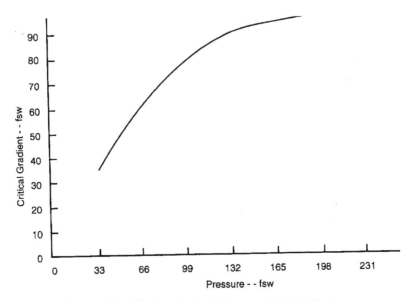

Figure 38. Diffusion Limited Nitrogen Critical Gradient

A single tissue is assumed in diffusion models, characterized by a diffusion coefficient, D. The difference between tissue tension, Q, and ambient pressure, P, is limited by a critical gradient, G, depicted below in absolute units of fsw,

$$G = Q - P = P \left[\frac{493 - P}{P + 404} \right]$$

In terms of nitrogen critical tensions, M, obviously,

$$Q = \frac{M}{.79}$$

Controlling Tissues

Blood rich, well perfused, aqueous tissues are usually thought to be *fast* (small τ), while blood poorer, scarcely-perfused, lipid tissues are thought to be *slow* (large τ), though the spectrum of halftimes is not correlated with actual perfusion rates in critical tissues. As reflected in relationship above, critical parameters are obviously larger for faster tissues. The range of variation with compartment and depth is not insignificant. Fast compartments control short deep exposures, while slow compartments control long shallow, decompression, and saturation exposures.

As is well known, bounce exposures are often limited by a depth-time law of the form,

$$d\, t_n^{1/2} \leq C,$$

with t_n the nonstop time limit, and $400 \leq C \leq 500$ *fsw min*$^{1/2}$. For $C = 465$ *fsw min*$^{1/2}$, Figure 39 depicts the depth-time relationship. One can obtain the corresponding tissue constant, λ, controlling the exposure at depth d, for nonstop time t_n, by differentiating the tissue equation with respect to depth, d, and setting the result, to zero. With $p_a = 0.79 \, (d + 33)$ at sea level, there results,

$$1 - exp \, (-\lambda t_n) \, (1 + 2 \, \lambda t_n) = 0.$$

Corresponding critical tensions, M, are then easily obtained from the tissue equation using d, λ, and t_n. In the above case, the transcendental equation is satisfied when,

$$\lambda t_n = 1.25,$$

thus providing a means to estimate controlling tissue halftime at depth for corresponding nonstop time limits.

Time Remaining

Time remaining before a stop or surfacing, time at a stop, or surface interval before flying can all be obtained by inverting the tissue equation. Taking the perfusion equation, and denoting the limiting critical tension at some desired stage (lower ambient pressure), M, the initial tension, p_i, and the instantaneous tension at that particular time, p, at stage, p_a, the limiting time, t, follows from,

$$t = \frac{1}{\lambda} \, \ln \left[\frac{p_i - p_a}{p - p_a} \right]$$

as the inversion of the tissue equation in time.

The nonstop time limit, t_n, follows by replacing the instantaneous tension, p, with the (limiting) critical tension, M, that is,

$$t_n = \frac{1}{\lambda} \, \ln \left[\frac{p_i - p_a}{M - p_a} \right]$$

while time remaining, t_r, at level, p_a, before ascension to new level with limiting critical tension, M, is given by,

$$t_r = \frac{1}{\lambda} \, \ln \left[\frac{p - p_a}{M - p_a} \right],$$

with p the instantaneous tension now the initial tension. These hold for each compartment, λ. Across all compartments, the smallest t_n limits time at the present level when ascent is permitted, while the largest t_r prescribes wait time at the present level when ascent is not permitted. Table 12 lists compartment time limits using the critical tensions, M_0, from Figure 37 (USN) for the six compartments, $\tau = 5, 10, 20, 40, 80$, and 120 *min*, that is, $M_0 = 104, 88, 72, 58, 52, 51 \, fsw$. Note the blank entries correspond to depths less than the critical tension, so tissue loading to that critical tension is not possible.

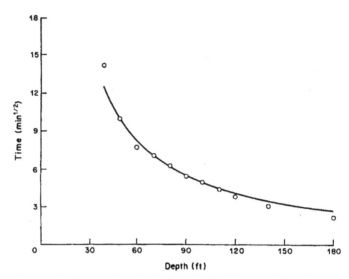

Figure 39. Depth-Time Relationship For Nonstop Time Limits

Diffusion models exhibit characteristic $t^{1/2}$ temporal behavior for inert gas uptake and elimination, serving as the basis for the Hempleman law limiting nonstop time and depth, as depicted below,

$$dt_n^{1/2} = 475 \ fsw \ min^{1/2}$$

with t_n the nonstop time limit, and d the depth. In diffusion models, the inert gas tissue penetration depth, as a function of time, plays a role analogous to tissue halftime in perfusion models.

Generally, the t_n are monotonically decreasing functions of depth, while t_r are monotonically increasing functions of depth, for fixed M_0.

Saturation Curve and Separated Phase

In elegant experiments, using both animals and humans, subjects were first saturated at various pressures, Q, then decompressed to lower absolute pressures, P, and closely checked for bends development. Various values of Q and P can be determined in a controlled *titration*, that is, by holding one variable fixed and changing the other very slightly over times spans of a day, or more. In analyzing this saturation data, it is possible to draw a linear relationship, in the hyperbaric regime, separating bends from no bends for ranges of P and Q. For instance, Figure 40 portrays the linear relationship for air, the saturation curve. The line takes the form, in fsw,

$$Q = \zeta P + \xi,$$

with an approximate spread over different studies, depending on statistics,

$$1.20 \le \zeta \le 1.40$$

$$7.5 \; fsw \le \xi \le 15.3 \; fsw,$$

and a range of ambient pressures, P,

$$33 \; fsw \le P \le 300 \; fsw.$$

Table 12. Compartment Time Limits At Depth.

τ (min)	5	10	20	40	80	120
M_0 (fsw)	104	88	72	58	52	51
d (fsw)						
40					198	269
50				95	123	173
60			100	65	91	129
70			51	50	73	103
80		56	37	41	61	87
90		30	30	34	52	75
100	31	22	25	30	46	66
110	16	18	22	26	41	59
120	12	15	19	24	37	53
130	10	13	17	21	34	48
140	9	12	16	20	31	44
150	8	11	14	18	29	41
160	7	10	13	17	27	38
170	6	9	12	16	25	35
180	6	8	11	15	23	33
190	5	8	11	14	22	31
200	5	7	10	13	21	30

In the hypobaric regime, $P < 33 \; fsw$, recent studies suggest that the air saturation curve passes through the origin as ambient pressure drops, behavior predicted within phase models and discussed further on. Wienke deduced a general form, in (fsw),

$$Q = \left[2.37 - exp \left(-\frac{11.1}{P} \right) \right] P$$

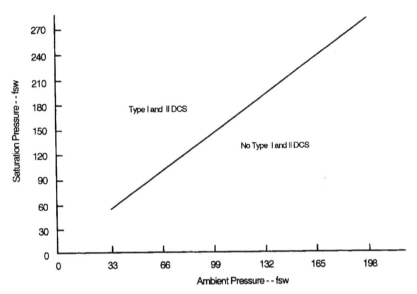

Figure 40. Air Saturation Curve

The classical saturation curve relates saturated tissue tension, Q, to permissible pressure, P, on decompression in a linear fashion, using absolute pressure units (fsw) for both Q and P,

$$Q = 1.37\,P + 11.1$$

holding in the hyperbaric region, $P \geq 33$ fsw, but questionable in the hypobaric region, $P \leq 33$ fsw, especially as P drops below 16 fsw. The above form was obtained by Hills, Hennessy and Hempleman, and Yount and Hoffman in applying the phase volume constraint to the saturation data. Wienke, in also applying a phase volume constraint within a bubble model, recovered the linear form for hyperbaric exposures, with an exponentially decreasing form (approaching zero supersaturation) in the hypobaric regime, generalizing the saturation curve,

$$Q = [2.37 - exp\,(-11.1/P)]\,P$$

Such curves are usually assigned as the critical tension in the slowest compartment in multitissue (Haldane) approaches.

using the permissible bubble (Doppler) excess as a phase limit point. For all exposures, $0 \leq P \leq \infty$, the supersaturation, Q, is bounded, with linear asymptotic behavior for large P, and zero intercept for small P. That is,

$$\lim_{P \to 0} Q \to 2.37\,P \to 0$$

$$\lim_{P \to \infty} Q \to \left[2.37 - 1 + \frac{1.11}{P}\right]\,P \to 1.37\,P + 11.1$$

Hennessy and Hempleman, and later Yount and Hoffman, established the linear titration curve for the data assuming that the same critical volume of released gas provokes mild attacks of decompression sickness. Such analyses offer explanations for changes in signs and symptoms which follow changes in the nature of the exposure to pressure. Findings press dissolved gas approaches. While the above titration expression is compatible with broad trends, it is clear that dissolved gas limiters, such as tensions, are often not the best critical flags. Indicators such as the volume fraction of separated gas are not only more natural, but seem to correlate more strongly with experiment. Computational algorithms, coupling phase equilibration or observed numbers of bubbles to critical volumes, offer more rational physical alternatives to the matrix of critical tensions. The critical volume hypothesis is an important development in decompression modeling, and certainly extends to breathing mixtures other than air.

Critical Phase Volumes

The rate at which gas inflates in tissue depends upon both the excess bubble number, Λ, and the supersaturation gradient, G. The critical volume hypothesis requires that the integral of the product of the two must always remain less than some limit point, αV, with α a proportionality constant. Accordingly this requires,

$$\int_0^\infty \Lambda G dt \leq \alpha V,$$

for bubble number excess, Λ, an approximately linear function of excitation seed radius (difference) on compression-decompression, ΔP,

$$\Lambda = N(r_i - r)$$

with N, β seed constants, r_i, r seed sizes, and V the limiting gas volume. Assuming that tissue gas gradients are constant during decompression, t_d, while decaying exponentially to zero afterwards, and taking limiting condition of the equal sign, yields for a bounce dive,

$$\Lambda G(t_d + \lambda^{-1}) = \alpha V.$$

With compression-decompression, ΔP, the excitation radius, r, follows from micronuclei growth experiments in gels and tissue,

$$\frac{1}{r} = \frac{1}{r_i} + \frac{\Delta P}{\zeta}$$

where ζ and r_i are structure functions at initial pressure, P_i, for final pressure, P_f, so that, $\Delta P = P_f - P_i$, and with, $130 \ \mu m \ fsw \leq \zeta \leq 180 \ \mu m \ fsw$. At sea level, consistent fits to exposure data suggest that, $r_i = .80 \ microns$. From the above, $r \leq r_i$, as, $P_f \geq P_i$, that is, smaller seeds grow on decompression. With all exposures, the integral must be evaluated iteratively over component decompression stages, maximizing each G while satisfying the constraint equation. In the latter case, t_d is the sum of individual stage times plus interstage ascent times, assuming the same interstage ascent speed, v. Employing the above iteratively, and one more constant, δ, defined by,

$$\delta = \frac{\gamma_c \alpha V}{\gamma \beta r_i N} = 7500 \; fsw \; min,$$

we have,

$$\left[1 - \frac{r}{r_i}\right] G(t_d + \lambda^{-1}) = \delta \frac{\gamma}{\gamma_c} = 522.3 \; fsw \; min,$$

from the Spencer bounce and Tektite saturation data. A set of critical phase volume gradients, G, appears in Table 13 below, and the gradient representation, G, is of the usual form,

$$G = G_0 + \Delta G d$$

at depth, d.

Table 13. Critical Phase Volume Gradients.

Halftime τ (min)	Threshold depth δ (fsw)	Surface gradient G_0 (fsw)	Gradient change ΔG
2	190	151	.518
5	135	95	.515
10	95	67	.511
20	65	49	.506
40	40	36	.468
80	30	27	.417
120	28	24	.379
240	16	23	.329
480	12	22	.312

For repetitive diving, the gradients, G, above are replaced with a reduced set, $\bar{G}$, with the property,

$$\bar{G} \leq G.$$

tending to reduce bottom time for repetitive activities and exposures. Because of this constraint, the approach is termed a reduced gradient bubble model. The terms, ΛG and $\Lambda \bar{G}$, differ by effective bubble elimination during the previous surface interval. To maintain the phase volume constraint during multidiving, the elimination rate must be downscaled by a set of bubble growth, regeneration, and excitation factors, cumulatively designated, ξ, such that,

$$\bar{G} = \xi G.$$

A conservative set of bounce gradients, G, can be employed for multiday and repetitive diving, provided they are reduced by ξ. Three bubble factors, η, reduce the diving gradients to maintain the phase volume constraint. The first bubble factor, η^{rg}, reduces G to account for creation of new stabilized micronuclei over time scales, ω^{-1}, of days,

$$\eta^{rg} = exp\,(-\omega t_{cum}),$$

$$7\ min \le \omega^{-1} \le 21\ days,$$

for t_{cum} the cumulative (multiday) dive time. The second bubble factor, η^{rd}, accounts for additional micronuclei excitation on reverse profile dives,

$$\eta^{rd} = \frac{(\Lambda)_{prev}}{(\Lambda)_{pres}} = \frac{(rd)_{prev}}{(rd)_{pres}},$$

for excitation radius, r, at depth, d, and the subscripts referencing the *previous* and *present* dives. Obviously, η^{rd} remains one until a deeper point than on the previous dive is reached. The third factor, η^{rp}, accounts for bubble growth over repetitive exposures on time scales, χ^{-1}, of hours,

$$\eta^{rp} = 1 - \left[1 - \frac{G^{bub}}{G_0\,exp\,(-\omega t_{cum})}\right] exp\,(-\chi t_{sur}),$$

$$10\ min \le \chi^{-1} \le 120\ minutes,$$

$$0.05 \le \frac{G^{bub}}{G_0} \le 0.90,$$

according to the tissue compartment, with t_{sur} the repetitive surface interval.

In terms of individual bubble factors, η, the multidiving fraction, ξ, is defined at the start of each segment, and deepest point of dive,

$$\xi = \eta^{rg}\,\eta^{rp}\,\eta^{rd}$$

with surface and cumulative surface intervals appropriate to the preceding dive segment. Since η are bounded by zero and one, ξ are similarly bounded by zero and one. Corresponding critical tensions, M, can be computed from the above,

$$M = \xi G + P,$$

with G listed in Table 13 above. Both G and ξ are lower bounded by the shallow saturation data,

$$G \ge G^{bd} = .303\,P + 11,$$

for P ambient pressure, and similarly,

$$\xi \ge \xi^{bd} = \frac{.12 + .18\,exp\,(-480\lambda_{bd})}{.12 + .18\,exp\,(-\tau\lambda_{bd})},$$

$$\lambda_{bd} = 0.0559\ min^{-1}.$$

A set of repetitive, multiday, and excitation factors, η^{rp}, η^{rg}, and η^{rd}, are drawn in Figures 5, 6, and 7, using conservative parameter values, $\chi^{-1} = 80\ min$ and $\omega^{-1} =$

7 *days*. Clearly, the repetitive factors, η^{rp}, relax to one after about 2 *hours*, while the multiday factors, η^{rg}, continue to decrease with increasing repetitive activity, though at very slow rate. Increases in χ^{-1} (bubble elimination halftime) and ω^{-1} (nuclei regeneration halftime) will tend to decrease η^{rp} and increase η^{rg}. Figure 41 plots η^{rp} as a function of surface interval in minutes for the 2, 10, 40, 120, and 720 minute tissue compartments, while Figure 42 depicts η^{rg} as a function of cumulative exposure in days for $\omega^{-1} = 7$, 14, and 21 *days*. The repetitive fractions, η^{rp}, restrict back-to-back repetitive activity considerably for short surface intervals. The multiday fractions get small as multiday activities increase continuously beyond 2 weeks. Excitation factors, η^{rd}, are collected in Figure 43 for exposures in the range 40–200 *fsw*. Deeper-than-previous excursions incur the greatest reductions in permissible gradients (smallest η^{rd}) as the depth of the exposure exceeds previous maximum depth. Figure 43 depicts η^{rd} for various combinations of depths, using 40, 80, 120, 160, and 200 *fsw* as the depth of the first dive.

In trying to retrofit the reduction parameters, η, to Haldane critical tensions and nonstop time limits, it is advantageous to use a slightly different picture for the multidiving fraction, ξ,

$$\xi = \gamma_{rg}\eta^{rg} + \gamma_{rp}\eta^{rp} + \gamma_{rd}\eta^{rd}$$

for γ a set of weighting factors normalized,

$$\gamma_{rg} + \gamma_{rp} + \gamma_{rd} = 1$$

and specific reduction factors, η^j, of a general Gaussian form ($j = rg, rp, ex$),

$$\eta^j = 1 - \alpha_j \, exp \left[-\frac{(t_{sur} - \beta_j)^2}{4\beta_j^2} \right]$$

with α_j and β_j weighting fractions and Doppler relaxation halftimes following repetitive, reverse profile, and multiday diving, and α_j functions of depth differences on reverse dives and depth in general. Likelihood regression analysis is used to fit parameters to data, with typical ranges,

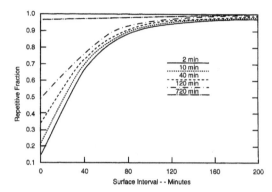

Figure 41. Repetitive Reduction Factors

Within phase volume constraints, bubble elimination periods are shortened over repetitive diving, compared to bounce diving. Therefore, a gradient reduction factor, η^{rp}, proportional to the difference between maximum and surface bubble inflation rate, is employed to maintain the separated phase volume below a limit point, deduced from bounce and saturation diving in the varying permeability (VPM) and reduced gradient bubble (RGBM) models. Repetitive fractions are plotted for various tissue compartments (2, 10, 40, 120, 720 min) for surface intervals up to 200 min. Faster compartments are impacted the most, but all fractions relax to one after a few hours or so.

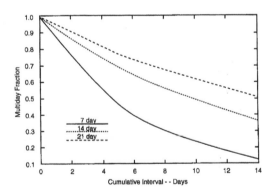

Figure 42. Regeneration Reduction Factors

Micronuclei are thought to regenerate over adaptation time scales of days, replenishing existing pools of gas seeds. Persistence and regeneration time scales need not be the same according to theromodynamics and statistical mechanics. A factor, η^{rg}, accounting for creation of new micronuclei reduces permissible gradients by the creation rate, thus maintaining the phase volume constraint over multiday diving. Multiday fractions are plotted for 7, 14, and 21 day regeneration times. Shorter regeneration times impart greater multiday penalties.

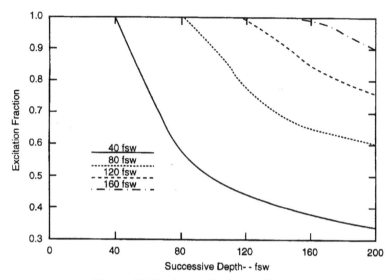

Figure 43. Excitation Reduction Factors

Reverse profile (deeper-than-previous) diving activities are thought to excite bubble seeds into growth according to the varying permeability and reduced gradient bubble models (VPM and RGBM). Scaling gradients by the ratio of bubble models excesses on the present dive to the bubble excess on the deepest point of earlier dives, η^{rd}, maintains the phase volume constraint for multidiving. Excitation fractions are plotted for a series of deeper exposures, following initial dives to 40, 80, 120, and 160 fsw. Shallow initial excursions, followed by deep dives, or yo-yo dives, incur the largest reductions in permissible gradients on reverse dives.

$$0.15 \leq \alpha_{rp} \leq 0.65$$

$$0.25 \leq \alpha_{rd} \leq 0.85$$

$$0.10 \leq \alpha_{rg} \leq 0.40$$

$$15 \; min \leq \beta_{rp} \leq 130 \; min$$

$$25 \; min \leq \beta_{rd} \leq 190 \; min$$

$$2 \; days \leq \beta_{rg} \leq 24 \; days$$

Ascent Staging

Clearly, from all of the foregoing, the dominant modes for staging diver ascents depend upon the preponderance of separated or dissolved phases in the tissues and blood, their coupling, and their relative time scales for elimination. This is (and will always be) the central consideration in staging hyperbaric or hypobaric excursions to lower ambient pressure environments. The dynamics of elimination are directly opposite, as depicted in Figure 44. To eliminate dissolved gases (the central tenet of Haldane decompression theory), the diver is brought as close as possible to the surface. To eliminate free phases (the coupled tenet of bubble decompression theory), the diver is maintained at depth to both crush bubbles and squeeze gas out by diffusion across the bubble film surface. Since both phases must be eliminated, the problem is a playoff in staging. In mathematical terms, staging is a minimax problem, and one that requires full blown dual phase models, exposure data, and some consensus of what is an acceptable level of DCI incidence.

Another transfer pathway that needs highlighting is seen in Figure 45. Many competing transfer pathways exist between tissues and blood (dissolved and free gas phases in both). The central problem of the table and meter designer is to stage ascents so that both free and dissolved phases are removed from tissues by the capillary system in optimal fashion. This is equally as difficult since we know little about the composition and susceptibility of tissue sites, blood perfusion rates, and geometries for modeling gas transfer. And even if we did, the complexity of the model and the computing power of our largest and fastest supercomputers would mitigate solutions. As seen graphically in Figure 4, the complexity of ascent rates, tissue tensions, and ambient pressures on bubble growth, especially with tensions and ambient pressures varying widely on ascent, is not a simply tracked quantity in diving exposures even when we know all the variables.

Attempts to track free phases within patently dissolved phase models may not optimize, but still can be mocked up for consistency with phase dynamics. One approach is to slow ascent rates and/or introduce safety stops strategically. As far as net gas exchange is concerned, most combinations of stops and rates can be equivalenced to almost any other set at given pressure, so there is always some leeway. Growth minimization and free phase elimination favor slow ascents. Figure 4 plots surfacing radius of an initially small bubble ($r = 0.36$ *microns*), held in both fast and slow tissue compartments, as a function of ascent rate. The results are typical for classes of bounce and repetitive diving, and underscore growth minimization with slow ascent rate due to increased ambient pressure on the average.

Based on suggestions at an American Academy of Underwater Sciences ascent workshop, recorded by Lang and Egstrom, discretionary safety stops for 2–4 *min* in the 10–20 *fsw* zone are recommended. Calculations reported by Wienke and others, and summarized in Tables 14 and 15, underscore the bases of the suggestions for a number of reasons. Relative changes in three computed trigger points, tissue tension, separated phase volume, and bubble radius, are listed for six compartments following a nominal bounce dive to 120 *fsw* for 12 *min*, with and without a safety stop at 15 *fsw* for 3 *min*. Stop procedures markedly restrict bubble and phase volume growth, while permitting insignificant levels of dissolved gas buildup in the slow tissues. The reduction in growth parameters far outstrips any dissolved gas buildup in slow compartments, and faster compartments naturally eliminate dissolved gases during the stop, important for deeper diving.

THE PLAYOFFS

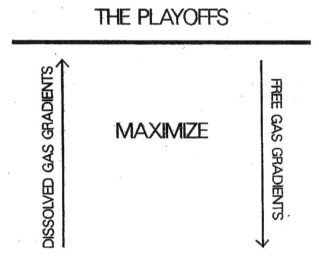

Figure 44. Free And Dissolved Gas Gradients

Staging diver ascents is a minimax problem. To eliminate dissolved gas, the diver is brought as close to the surface as possible. To eliminate free phases, the diver is kept at depth. Obviously, staging diver ascents with dual phase (free and dissolved gases) treatments is a playoff. Both must be eliminated, but timescales and pressures for both are different.

COMPETING GAS PATHWAYS

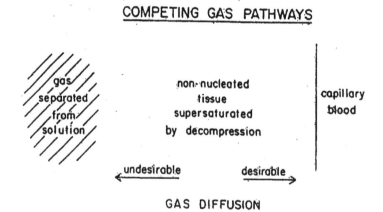

Figure 45. Dual Phase Gas Diffusion Pathways

The hope in staging diver ascents is to eliminate both free and dissolved gas phases as rapidly as possible through the capillary blood flow. Dumping dissolved phases into existing free phases (bubbles) increases the separated volume, reducing diver ascent choices.

Table 14. Relative Changes In Critical Parameters After Safety Stop

τ (*min*) halftimes	tissue tension relative change	critical volume relative change	bubble radius relative change
5	-21%	-34%	-68%
10	-11%	-24%	-39%
20	-6%	-11%	-24%
40	-2%	-8%	-18%
80	1%	3%	-2%
120	2%	4%	1%

Safety stop time can be added to bottom time for additional conservatism, but the effect of neglecting stop time is also small, as seen in Table 15. A stop at 15 *fsw* for 2 *min* is roughly equivalent to more than halving the standard ascent rate at depths in excess of 120 *fsw*. Procedures such as this, as well as reduced nonstop time limits, appear beneficial in multiday, multilevel, and repetitive diving. A safety stop near 15 *fsw* is easier than 10 *fsw* in adverse water conditions, such as surge and surface disturbances. Slower ascent rates afford additional advantages, but safety stops in the 2–4 *min* range are easier and more efficient.

Table 15. Comparative Surfacing Tissue Tensions

τ (*min*) Halftimes	Surfacing Tension (*fsw*) 120 *fsw*/15 *min*	Surfacing Tension (*fsw*) 120 *fsw*/12 *min* 15 *fsw*/3 *min*	Surfacing Tension (*fsw*) 120 *fsw*/15 *min* 15 *fsw*/3 *min*
5	101.5	77.0	79.7
10	87.5	73.0	78.1
20	66.9	59.0	64.0
40	49.9	45.7	49.2
80	39.0	36.9	38.9
120	34.9	33.5	34.8

At altitude the same procedures can be employed, with depths, ascent rates, and stops conservatively scaled by the altitude correction factors (ratio of sea level pressure to ambient pressure at altitude) when using tables for which critical tensions need extrapolation at reduced ambient pressure. Tables with critical tensions fitted to altitude data have their own rules, as do meters.

Generally, bubble growth and excitation are compounded at altitude because of reduced pressure. The modeling work of Wienke, Gernhardt and Lambertsen underscores this fact, indicating why critical tension models often fall short in hypobaric applications. Bubbles grow faster as they get bigger, and as pressure drops. With decreased pressure, bubbles will also expand by Boyle's law. Bigger bubbles are not as constricted by Laplacian film tension, while reduced pressure supports a faster rate of tissue gas diffusion into the bubble itself. Lanphier and Lehner performed extensive aerial decompression studies with goats, concluding that aerial decompression sickness strongly resembles underwater decompression sickness following saturation exposure. For ranging profiles followed by decompression to reduced ambient pressure, a high incidence of chokes was noted. Chokes is thought to result from microemboli interfering with pulmonary function. It is easy to speculate that rapid decompression to reduced pressure contributes to the buildup and growth of pulmonary emboli for the same reasons. Lanphier also concluded that slow tissue ($\tau \geq 80$ *min*) compartments do not correlate with chokes, suggesting that pulmonary microemboli are linked to fast compartments. Clearly, such an assertion also points out differences between types of decompression sickness, inferred critical tissue half-lives, and bubble formation time scales. Chokes and limb bends result from different critical insults, at different places, and over possibly different time scales.

The point to be made here in all cases is simple. Increased offgassing pressures reduce bubble growth rates dramatically in shallow zones, while impacting dissolved gas buildup in the slowest compartments minimally. Fast compartments also offload gas during safety stops, important for repetitive diving. Stops and slow ascent rates are always advisable, but particularly in multiexposures.

Consistent Critical Parameter Sets

For Haldane computational algorithms, the process of constructing closed sets of time limits, tissue halftimes, and limiting tensions becomes an important activity. We detail a method for this closure, applying the approach to some exposure relationships. The approach maximizes the tissue perfusion equation, subject to a depth-time law (theoretical, fitted, inferred, or otherwise) at the exposure time limit, coupling exposure limits, halftimes, depths, and maximum tensions in the process.

Dissolved gas models limit tissue supersaturation, assuming that gas exchange is controlled by perfusion or diffusion in blood-tissue media. A perfusion equation quantifies bulk gas transfer,

$$\frac{\partial(p - p_a)}{\partial t} = -\lambda(p - p_a),$$

with the exchange of inert gas driven by the local gradient, that is, the difference between arterial blood, p_a, and local tissue tension, p. Obviously the exchange process is very complicated, and models are only approximate. The solutions are well known, simple classes of exponential functions, bounded by arterial and initial tissue tensions, p_a and p_i,

$$(p - p_a) = (p_i - p_a) \, exp \, (-\lambda t),$$

with λ the decay rate, defined in terms of the halftime, τ,

$$\lambda = \frac{.693}{\tau}$$

with instantaneous tissue tension, p, in that compartment. Compartments with 2, 5, 10, 20, 40, 80, 120, 240, 360, 480, and 720 minute halftimes, τ, are employed in applications, and halftimes are assumed to be independent of pressure.

Next, algorithms limit degrees of dissolved gas buildup, p, hypothetical absolute compartment supersaturation, by *critical* values, M, such that,

$$p \leq M,$$

across all compartments at all times during exposure, and upon surfacing. Equivalently, critical ratios, R, and critical gradients, G are also employed, with,

$$R = \frac{M}{P},$$

$$G = M - P,$$

for ambient pressure, P. Critical parameters evolved from self consistent application of assumed tissue response functions to sets of exposure data, that is, trial and error bootstrapping of model equations to observed exposure time limits. Newer compilations ultimately extend older ones to extended data ranges.

In a diffusion framework, nonstop air limits, t_n, roughly satisfy a bulk transfer law,

$$dt_n^{1/2} = 465 \; fsw \; min^{1/2},$$

at depth, d (Hempleman *square root* law), generalized by writing,

$$dt^a = b,$$

for a and b some constants. Ranges subtended today in tables and meters include:

$$0.25 \leq a \leq 0.65,$$

$$250 \; fsw \; min^a \leq b \leq 500 \; fsw \; min^a,$$

A separated phase model for nonstop air diving suggests,

$$\delta \, d \, (t_n + 1/\lambda) = 8750 \; fsw \; min,$$

for number factor, δ, collectively representing bubble seeds excited by compression-decompressio that is, from surface pressure, P_0, to ambient pressure, P, and back to P_0,

$$\delta = \frac{P}{P_0} - 1.$$

The phase law generalizes obviously to,

$$\delta \, d \, (t + 1/\lambda)^a = \frac{d^2}{P_0 + d} \, (t + 1/\lambda)^a = b,$$

with,

$$P = P_0 + d.$$

The depth-time law and tissue equation present a minimax problem, here, maximization of the tissue equation at depth subject to the constraint of the depth-time law. The standard approach sets the depth derivative of the tissue equation (tension) to zero at the exposure time limit, under the primary constraint of the depth-time equation. First writing ambient gas partial pressure, p_a, as

$$p_a = p_0 + fd,$$

for surface partial pressure, p_0, mole fraction, f, and then differentiating tension, p, with respect to depth, d, we find in general,

$$\frac{\partial p}{\partial d} = f - f\ exp\ (-\lambda t) + (p_0 + fd - p_i)\lambda\ exp\ (-\lambda t)\frac{\partial t}{\partial d} = 0,$$

as the maximization condition. The time derivative with respect to depth, $\partial t/\partial d$, is evaluated from the assumed exposure law (theoretical, fitted, inferred), and then inserted above. The resulting expression couples halftime, τ, to exposure limit, t_n, and the value of the tissue tension at those values is the (maximized) critical tension, M_0.

Table and meter algorithms still rely heavily on (Haldane) dissolved gas treatments to schedule diving, with square root-like nonstop limits folded into a multitissue perfusion framework. So, as example, consider the bulk relationship, so that,

$$\frac{\partial t}{\partial d} = -\frac{t}{ad}.$$

Setting $p_i = p_0$, substituting the derivative, and maximizing at the nonstop limit, t_n, there results,

$$1 - exp\ (-\lambda t_n) - \frac{\lambda t_n}{a}\ exp\ (-\lambda t_n) = 0.$$

At nonstop time, $t = t_n$, the tissue tension is maximized, that is, $p = M_0$, so that,

$$M_0 = p_a + (p_i - p_a)\frac{a}{a + \lambda t_n}.$$

The maximization condition links λ and t_n together, while M_0 falls out of the tissue equation. The quantity λt_n is pivotal to the solution. Table 16 gives thumbnail solutions to,

$$exp\ (x) = 1 + \frac{x}{a},$$

for a, as function of dimensionless parameter, $x = \lambda t_n$.

Table 16. Maximization Parameters

a	$1/a$	x
.157	6.37	3.00
.323	3.09	2.00
.435	2.29	1.50
.455	2.20	1.40
.488	2.05	1.30
.500	2.00	1.25
.517	1.93	1.20
.549	1.82	1.10
.581	1.72	1.00
.771	1.29	0.50
.951	1.05	0.10
1.00	1.00	0.00

In the separated phase model, we have differentiating,

$$\frac{\partial t}{\partial d} = -\frac{2(t+1/\lambda)}{ad},$$

so that,

$$1 - exp\,(-\lambda t_n) - \frac{2(\lambda t_n + 1)}{a}\,exp\,(-\lambda t_n) = 0,$$

as the maximization constraint. Or, equivalently, one needs,

$$exp\,(y) = 1 + \frac{2(y+1)}{a},$$

with $y = \lambda t_n$. Then, the critical tension, M_0, is given by,

$$M_0 = p_a + (p_i - p_a)\,\frac{a}{a + 2(\lambda t_n + 1)}$$

The procedures for constructing a consistent set can be summarized as follows:

- first, from experiment, wet or dry tests, Doppler, or otherwise, a set of nonstop time limits, t_n, at depth, d, is obtained;
- next, the set is fitted to the two parameter power law given above, and the constants a and b determined;
- then, with a and b determined, the controlling halftime, τ, is obtained from t_n at d;
- finally, from τ, t_n, d, and a, the critical tension, M_0, is extracted, closing the whole set;
- compute and recalibrate parameters against a set of test profiles, data, or exposure information.

The set a, b, τ, d, t_n, x, y, and M_0 then close self consistently when derived according to the above set of equations and constraints.

Results for some air limits are summarized in Table 17, using a standard nonlinear least squares (NLS) approach in fitting t_n to the depth-time relationship, with usual L_2 error norm, the square root of the sum of the squares of the differences in the fit. The labels RGBM, DCIEM, ZHL, Spencer, and USN refer to nonstop time limits for popular Haldane models.

Table 17. Fits, Limits, Halftimes, And Critical Tensions.

	RGBM	DCIEM	ZHL	Spencer	USN
		Fit Parameters			
a	.94	.48	.46	.39	.41
$b(fsw\ min^a)$	6119	362	385	290	355
x	1.40	1.34	1.39	1.65	1.58
y	2.00	1.08	1.65	1.16	1.57
$L_2(fsw)$	12.8	57.7	62.3	85.5	56.5
		Nonstop Limits $t_n(min)$			
$d(fsw)$					
30	200	150	290	225	
40	110	90	125	135	200
50	70	70	75	75	100
60	50	50	54	50	60
70	35	35	38	40	50
80	26	25	26	30	40
90	20	20	20	25	30
100	16	15	20	20	25
110	13	12	17	15	20
120	11	10	15	10	15
130	9	8	11	5	10
		Halftimes $\tau(min)$/Critical Tensions $M_0(fsw)$			
$d(fsw)$					
30	69/46	98/44	122/45	134/45	178/45
40	38/53	53/49	68/51	60/52	88/52
50	24/60	33/55	42/57	37/58	52/57
60	17/67	22/61	28/63	23/64	33/64
70	12/74	17/67	20/69	16/71	23/69
80	9/79	12/73	15/73	11/77	16/76
90	7/87	10/87	12/82	8/84	12/83
100	6/94	8/85	9/88	7/90	10/89
110	5/101	6/91	8/84	6/96	8/95
120	4/108	5/96	6/100	4/103	6/101
130	3/114	4/102	5/106	3/109	5/107

The structure and range above is interesting. Surfacing critical tensions, M_0, and tissue halftimes, τ, are bounded,

$$44\ fsw \le M_0 \le 114\ fsw$$

$$3\ min \le \tau \le 178\ min$$

with the DCIEM, ZHL, Spencer, and USN (all Haldane models) exhibiting roughly similar parameter clustering, but with the RGBM (phase model) rather different from the rest. And all said with nonstop time limits, t_n, pretty much the same across all models. In diving practice, this is just another manifestation of differences between dissolved gas (Haldane) and phase (RGBM) models. As seen, deeper stops and overall shorter decompression times are the result.

Keyed Exercises

• *What is the exact USN critical tension, M, in the 80 min tissue compartment at a depth, d = 80 fsw?*

$$M_0 = 52 \ fsw, \quad \Delta M = 1.26$$

$$M = M_0 + \Delta Md$$

$$M = 52 + 1.26 \times 80 \ fsw = 152.8 \ fsw$$

What is the critical ratio, R, and critical gradient, G?

$$R = \frac{M}{P}, \quad P = 80 + 33 \ fsw = 113 \ fsw, \quad R = \frac{152.8}{113} = 1.35$$

$$G = M - P = 152.8 - 113 \ fsw = 39.8 \ fsw$$

• *What is the critical tension, M, at depth, d = 34 fsw, for the nitrogen tissue compartment, $\tau = 7.56$ min?*

$$M = 152.7\tau^{-1/4} + 3.25\tau^{-1/4}d$$

$$M = 152.7 \times .603 + 3.25 \times .603 \times 34 \ fsw = 158.7 \ fsw$$

• *What is the instantaneous nitrogen pressure, p, in the 15 min tissue compartment of a Maine scallop diver at 67 fsw for 38 min, assuming initial sea level equilibration?*

$$\tau = 15 \ min, \quad f_{N_2} = .79$$

$$p_i = 33 \times .79 \ fsw = 26.1 \ fsw$$

$$p_a = f_{N_2}(P_0 + d) = (33 + 67) \times .79 \ fsw = 79 \ fsw$$

$$\lambda = \frac{.693}{15} \ min^{-1} = .046 \ min^{-1}$$

$$p = p_a + (p_i - p_a) \ exp \ (-\lambda t)$$

$$p = 79 + (26.1 - 79) \times .174 \ fsw = 69.7 \ fsw$$

What is the tension in the 240 min compartment?

$$\lambda = \frac{.693}{240} \ min^{-1} = .0029 \ min^{-1}, \quad p = 79 + (26.1 - 79) \times .896 \ fsw = 31.6 \ fsw$$

• *What is the critical tension, M, at a nominal depth of 10 fsw for the 15 min compartment, and corresponding critical ratio, R?*

$$M = 152.7\tau^{-1/4} + 3.25\tau^{-1/4}d$$

$$M = 152.7 \times .51 + 3.25 \times .51 \times 10 \ fsw = 94.4 \ fsw$$

$$R = \frac{M}{P} = \frac{94.4}{43} = 2.19$$

• *How long does it take for the 80 min compartment to approach its critical surfacing tension, $M = M_0 = 52$ fsw, at depth of 140 fsw, assuming initial nitrogen tension of 45 fsw?*

$$p_i = 45 \ fsw, \quad p_a = f_{N_2}(33+d)$$

$$p_a = .79 \times (33 + 140) \ fsw = 136.6 \ fsw$$

$$\lambda = \frac{.693}{80} \ min^{-1} = .0087 \ min, \quad M = 52 \ fsw$$

$$t = \frac{1}{\lambda} \ \ln \left[\frac{p_i - p_a}{M - p_a} \right] = 114.9 \times \ln \left[\frac{91.6}{84.6} \right] \ min = 9.1 \ min$$

What is the nonstop limit, t_n, for the 80 min tissue at this depth?

$$t_n = 9.1 \ min$$

• *If the nonstop time limit at depth, $d = 90$ fsw, is, $t_n = 22$ min, what is the surfacing critical tension, M_0, assuming that the 5 min compartment controls the exposure (has largest computed tissue tension at this depth)?*

$$\lambda = \frac{.693}{5} \ min^{-1} = .1386 \ min^{-1}$$

$$p_i = .79 \times 33 \ fsw = 26.1 \ fsw$$

$$p_a = .79 \times (33 + 90) = 97.1 \ fsw$$

$$M_0 = p_a + (p_i - p_a) \ exp \ (-\lambda t_n)$$

$$M_0 = 97.1 - 78.2 \ exp \ (-.1386 \times 22) \ fsw = 94 \ fsw$$

• *An oil rig diver is saturated at a depth of 300 fsw in the North Sea on heliox. For critical helium gradient (absolute), $G = M - P = 40$ fsw, what is the minimum depth (ceiling), d, accessible to the platform diver?*

$$M = 333 \ fsw, \quad P = M - G = (333 - 40) \ fsw = 293 \ fsw$$

$$d = (P - 33) \ fsw = (293 - 33) \ fsw = 260 \ fsw$$

If the mixture is 80/20 heliox, what is the tissue tension of helium, p_{He}, at the bottom, $d = 300$ fsw?

$$p_{He} = f_{He}P = f_{He}(33+d) \ fsw, \quad f_{He} = .80$$

$$p_{He} = .80 \times (33 + 300) \ fsw = .80 \times 333 \ fsw = 266.4 \ fsw$$

- In a gel experiment compression-decompression, $\Delta P = 120\ fsw$, at an ambient pressure, $P = 13\ fsw$, what is the seed excitation radius, r,?

$$\frac{1}{r} = \frac{1}{r_i} + \frac{\Delta P}{\zeta}, \quad \zeta = 158\ \mu m\ fsw, \quad r_i = .89\ \mu m$$

$$r = \frac{158 r_i}{158 + \Delta P r_i}\ \mu m = .47\ \mu m$$

- What is the reduction factor, ξ, for a repetitive dive, after 40 min surface interval, to a depth of 80 fsw, if a first dive was to 40 fsw following 6 consecutive days of diving, using the multiday regeneration timescale of 21 days for the compartment, $\tau = 40\ min$?

$$\xi = \eta^{rg}\ \eta^{rp}\ \eta^{rd}$$

$$\omega^{-1} = 21\ days, \quad \eta^{rg} = .74\ (7\ days\ cumulative)$$

$$\eta^{rp} = .70\ (40\ min\ surface\ interval,\ \tau = 40\ min)$$

$$\eta^{rd} = .52\ (d_{prev} = 40\ fsw,\ d_{pres} = 80\ fsw)$$

$$\xi = .74 \times .70 \times .52 = .29$$

What is the bounding reduction factor, ξ^{bd}, for this compartment and exposure?

$$\tau = 40\ min, \quad \lambda_{bd} = 0.0559\ min^{-1}$$

$$\xi^{bd} = \frac{.12 + .18\ exp\ (-480\lambda_{bd})}{.12 + .18\ exp\ (-\tau\lambda_{bd})}$$

$$\xi^{bd} = \frac{.12 + .18 \times 10^{-12}}{.12 + .18 \times .12} = .83$$

At depth, $d = 80\ fsw$, what is the critical gradient, $\bar{G}$, same exposure and tissue compartment?

$$\bar{G} = \xi G, \quad \xi = \xi^{bd} = .83, \quad d = 80\ fsw$$

$$G = G_0 + \Delta G d, \quad G_0 = 36\ fsw, \quad \Delta G = .468$$

$$\bar{G} = \xi(G_0 + \Delta G d) = .83 \times (36 + .468 \times 80)\ fsw = 60.9\ fsw$$

- Mark the following statements TRUE or FALSE.

_T_	F	Surfacing critical tensions are concerns for nonstop diving.
T	_F_	To eliminate dissolved gases increased pressure is best.
_T_	F	The Hempleman relationship links NDLs and depths.
T	_F_	The USN and Buhlmann critical tensions pass thru zero at zero pressure.
T	_F_	Critical phase volumes and critical tensions are the same.
_T_	F	RGBM reduction factors can reduce critical tensions.

T	_F_	Deep stops reduce dissolved gas buildup.
_T_	F	The critical volume hypothesis extends to all breathing gases.
T	_F_	Bubble models focus only on free phase growth.
T	_F_	Decompression diver staging is uniform across all models.
T	_F_	The VPM and Buhlmann ZHL-16 models are bubble models.

• Write and solve the perfusion rate equation with linear ascent or descent rates, that is, with ambient partial pressure, p_a, changing in time, t, as vt, with v diver ascent or descent rate and p_a initial ambient partial pressure.

$$\frac{\partial p}{\partial t} + \lambda(p - p_a - vt) = 0$$

or, changing variable, $q = p - p_a$,

$$\frac{\partial q}{\partial t} + \lambda q = \lambda vt$$

which has general solution for C_i an integration constant to be determined from the initial condition, $q_i = p_i - p_a$ at t = 0, for integrating factor, exp (λt), folded over the source term, vt, while interchanging differentiation and integration over λ and t within the inhomogeneous source term,

$$q = C_i \, exp\,(-\lambda t) + \lambda v \, exp\,(-\lambda t) \frac{\partial}{\partial \lambda} \int exp\,(\lambda t) dt$$

with end result,

$$q = C_i \, exp\,(-\lambda t) + vt - \frac{v}{\lambda}$$

so that, at t = 0,

$$q_i = C_i - \frac{v}{\lambda} \quad or, \quad C_i = q_i + \frac{v}{\lambda}$$

yielding finally, after collecting terms,

$$p - p_a = \left[p_i - p_a + \frac{v}{\lambda} \right] exp\,(-\lambda t) + vt - \frac{v}{\lambda}$$

Consistent with increasing ambient pressure, p_a, at increasing depth, what are the rate, v, sign conventions for ascents and descents?

$$+v \quad for \ descents$$

$$-v \quad for \ ascents$$

Velocity, v, has the same partial pressures units as ambient pressure, p_a.

- *For fast tissue compartments and λt very large, what is the limiting form of the rate equation?*

$$\lim_{\lambda t \to \infty} (p - p_a) \to vt - \frac{v}{\lambda}$$

For slow tissue compartment and λt very small, what is the limiting form of the rate equation?

$$\lim_{\lambda t \to 0} (p - p_a) \to p_i - p_a + vt$$

- *Write and solve the rate equation for a diver experiencing an uncontrolled buoyant ascent, that is, assuming constant acceleration, a, proportional to the buoyant force, F, which changes the ascent rate, v, in time, t, quadratically, $1/2at^2$, using the methodology of the foregoing.*

$$\frac{\partial q}{\partial t} + \lambda q = -\frac{1}{2}\lambda at^2$$

with formally,

$$q = C_i \exp(-\lambda t) - \frac{1}{2}\lambda a \exp(-\lambda t)\frac{\partial^2}{\partial \lambda^2}\int \exp(\lambda t)dt$$

yielding in analogy to the linear case,

$$q = C_i \exp(-\lambda t) - \frac{1}{2}at^2 + \frac{at}{\lambda} - \frac{a}{\lambda^2}$$

and, with $q = q_i$ at $t = 0$,

$$q_i = C_i - \frac{a}{\lambda^2} \text{ or, } C_i = q_i + \frac{a}{\lambda^2}$$

As with velocity, v, acceleration, a, has the same units as ambient pressure, p_a.

Reduced Atmospheric Pressure

Decompression at reduced ambient pressure, $P < 33 \ fsw$, has been a study in itself, as reported by many researchers over the years. Decompression studies developed separately above and below sea level, referenced as aerial and underwater decompression, also by the adjectives, hypobaric and hyperbaric. Aerial decompression differs from routine underwater decompression because the blood and tissues are equilibrated (saturated) with nitrogen ambient pressure before ascent. Breathing pure oxygen before ascent helps to protect against decompression sickness by washing out nitrogen. Up to about 18,000 ft, such procedure offers a considerable degree of protection. Beyond that, silent bubbles may retard nitrogen elimination. Simple bubble mechanics suggest that bubble excitation and growth are enhanced as ambient pressure decreases, and so decompression problems are theoretically exacerbated by altitude. Nucleation theory also suggests that critical radii increase with decreasing pressure, offering larger, less stable gas seeds for possible excitation and growth into bubbles. Larger bubbles possess smaller constricting surface tensions, and will thus grow faster in conducive situations. Such facts have been verified in the laboratory, and follow from simple bubble theory. Certainly the same considerations confront the diver at altitude, and are compounded with increasing inert gas tension upon surfacing at reduced atmospheric pressure.

Critical Extrapolations

Lower ambient pressures at elevation, as depicted in Figure 46, and the lesser density of fresh water in smaller degree, affect gas uptake and elimination rates in tissues and blood, as well as bubble growth and contraction. If critical tensions are employed to limit exposures, an immediate question centers upon their extrapolation and testing at altitude. Looking at Figure 46, a linear extrapolation of the critical tensions seems obvious, indeed just such an extrapolation of the US Navy critical tensions was proposed and tested by Bell and Borgwardt. Buhlmann, employing a different set of halftimes and critical tensions, also extended the Haldane algorithm to altitudes near 10,000 ft. Along with reduced critical tensions at altitude, reduced nonstop time limits, compared to sea level, are a natural consequence.

Another approach reduces critical tensions exponentially with decreasing ambient pressure. Such an extrapolation turns the curves in Figure 46 down through the origin at zero ambient pressure. Intuitively, an exponential extrapolation of critical tensions through the origin is more conservative than the linear extrapolation, since corresponding critical tensions for given ambient pressure are smaller, also noted by others. If the extrapolation of critical tensions is allowed to follow the same exponential decrease of ambient pressure with altitude, then the ratio of the critical tension over ambient pressure, R, remains constant. Nonstop time limits in the exponential scheme are also smaller than corresponding time limits in the linear scheme. As seen in Table 18, atmospheric pressure falls off approximately 1 fsw for every 1,000 ft of elevation. Exponential extrapolations of critical tensions have been tested, and serve as the operational basis of altitude procedures suggested by many others. Correlations of altitude chokes data for goats with constant ratio, R, trigger points have also been established, along with similar suggestions for the nitrogen washout data in aviators.

Altitude Procedures and Equivalent Sea Level Depth (ESLD)

Tables and meters designed for sea level need be conservatively modified at altitude if possible, otherwise, not employed. Decomputer and table use are best left to manufacturer and designer discretions, but in any case, modification of critical tensions is central to any Haldane altitude algorithm. We will describe a general technique and, for discussion purposes, the US Navy dive tables (or derivative) will suffice.

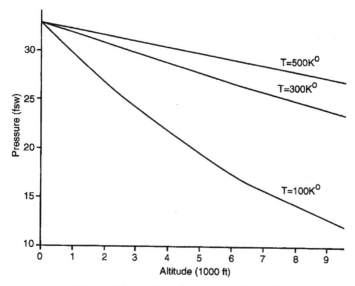

Figure 46. Ambient Pressure at Elevation

Ambient pressure, P, falls off exponentially with increasing altitude, approximately 1 fsw for each 1,000 ft of elevation. Such behavior affects not only diver physiology, but also gauges, instruments, buoyancy, and tables calibrated for sea level activity. Variation of atmospheric pressure with elevation is quantified with a phenomenological expression fitted to altitude pressure measurements,

$$P_h = 33 \; exp \; (-0.038h) = \frac{33}{\alpha}$$

with h measured in multiples of 1,000 ft, and pressure, P_h, given in fsw. The (theoretical) barometer equation factors temperature into the relationship,

$$P_h = 33 \; exp \; (-mg_0h/kT)$$

with m the mean molecular mass of constituent air molecules, g_0 the acceleration of gravity (sea level), k the Boltzmann constant, and T the temperature. The barometer equation assumes that air molecules satisfy Boltzmann statistics. The expression is plotted for temperatures of 100, 300, and 500 °K. The middle curve, depicting air pressure as a function of elevation at a temperature of 300 °K, also recovers the phenomenological fit extremely well, that is, to a percent or two. To good order, the atmosphere at lower elevations is an ideal gas at 300 °K.

Present diving schedules are based to large extent on the model discussed in the previous section, constraining activities so that *M* or *R* are never compromised. An approach to altitude diving that is roughly as conservative as the tested schemes of original researchers, holds the ratios, *R*, constant at altitude, forcing altitude exposures to be *similar* to sea level exposures. Such similarity will force M to decrease exponentially with increasing altitude, keeping R constant with commensurate exponential reduction in the ambient pressure, P. Constant R extrapolations of this sort should be confined to nominal diving activities, certainly not heavy repetitive, decompression, nor saturation exposures.

The sought ratio constancy, R, at altitude induces a necessary scaling of actual depth to *equivalent sea level depth* (ESLD) for table entry, while all times remain unchanged. Actual depths at altitude are multiplied by factors, α, called altitude correction factors, which are just the ratios of sea level atmospheric pressure to altitude atmospheric pressure, multiplied by the specific density of fresh water (0.975). Neglect of the specific density scaling is a conservative convenience, and one of minimal impact on these factors. Today, wrist altimeters facilitate rapid, precise estimation of α on site. They can be estimated from the *barometer* equation (shortly discussed) and are always greater than one. Table 18 lists correction factors at various altitudes, z, ranging to 10,000 ft. Up to about 7,000 ft elevation, $\alpha \approx 1 + 0.038\, h$, with h measured in multiples of 1,000 ft, that is, $z = 1,000\, h$. The higher one ascends to dive, the deeper is his relative exposure in terms of sea level equivalent depth. Figure 47 contrasts correction factors scaled by the specific density of fresh water for elevations up to 18,000 ft. Relative increases in correction factors hasten rapidly above 10,000 ft. As described in the Part 6 and seen in Table 18, P and α are reciprocally related, inverses actually. Again, time is measured directly, that is, correction factors are only applied to underwater depths, ascent rates, and stops.

Table 18. Altitude Correction Factors And US Navy Altitude Groups.

Altitude, or change $z\ (ft)$	Atmospheric pressure $P_h\ (fsw)$	Correction factor α	Penalty group on arrival at altitude	Permissible group for ascension to altitude
0	33.00	1.00		
1,000	31.9	1.04	A	L
2,000	30.8	1.07	B	K
3,000	29.7	1.11	B	J
4,000	28.5	1.16	C	I
5,000	27.5	1.20	D	H
6,000	26.5	1.24	E	G
7,000	25.4	1.29	E	F
8,000	24.5	1.34	F	E
9,000	23.6	1.39	G	D
10,000	22.7	1.45	H	C

The similarity rule for altitude table modification and applying correction factors to calculations is straightforward. Convert depths at altitude to sea level equivalent depths through multiplication by α. Convert all table sea level stops and ascent rates back to actual altitude through division by α. Ascent rates are always less than 60 fsw/min, while stops are always less than at sea level. Thus, a diver at 60 fsw at an elevation of 5,000 ft uses a depth correction of 72 fsw, taking $\alpha =$

1.2. Corresponding ascent rate is 50 *fsw/min*, and a stop at 10 *fsw* at sea level translates to 8 *fsw*. A capillary gauge at altitude performs these depth calculations automatically, and on the fly, as described below. Here the 3% density difference between salt and fresh water is neglected. Neglecting the 3% density correction is conservative, because the correction decreases equivalent depth by 3%. The effect on ascent rate or stop level is not on the conservative side, but is so small that it can be neglected in calculations anyway.

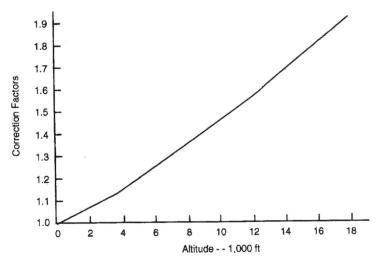

Figure 47. Altitude Correction Factors

Correction factors, β, are used to scale depths at altitude to sea level equivalence for use in standard tables. The factors are always greater than one, and are simply the ratios of sea level atmospheric pressures to atmospheric pressures at elevation, multiplied by the specific density, η, of fresh water,

$$\beta = \eta \left[\frac{33}{P_h} \right] = .975 \ exp \ (0.0381h) = .975 \alpha$$

with h measured in multiples of 1,000 ft elevation.

If a diver has equilibrated with ambient pressure at any elevation, than any reduction in ambient pressure will put the diver in a repetitive group, merely because tissue tensions exceed ambient pressure. If the original and new pressures are specified, it is possible to estimate tissue saturation and, hence, repetitive group for the excursion. Similar comments apply to pressure reductions following any diving activity, with sea level diving the usual bill of fare. These considerations are treated as follows.

At sea level, each repetitive group represents an increment of tissue pressure over ambient ($P_0 = 33 \ fsw$). For the US Navy tables, this increment is 2 *fsw* (absolute).

If we compute the difference between sea level pressure and altitude pressure, and then scale the difference by the ratio of sea level atmospheric pressure to that altitude atmospheric pressure (correction factor α), we can estimate the repetitive group in which a sea level diver finds himself following immediate ascent to altitude. These group specifications are listed in column 4 of Table 18, and represent penalty time for the excursion to altitude, Entries were computed using sea level as the baseline, but are also appropriate (conservative) for any excursion between differing elevations.

In similar fashion, excursions to higher altitude following diving are limited by tissue critical tensions, and minimal repetitive group designators can be attached to any planned excursion. For the 120 minute compartment, the surfacing critical tension (sea level) is 51 *fsw*. On the safer side, we take 44 *fsw* as the limiting tension, convert it to an absolute tension of 56 *fsw* (44/.79), and then inversely scale it to altitude by the ratio of sea level pressure to altitude pressure, that is, α. The resulting limiting tensions at altitude can then be converted to standard US Navy groups which are tabulated in column 5 of Table 18. Entries represent maximum permissible groups for immediate altitude excursions, and do not account for any travel time. Thus a diver would have to wait some length of time after a dive, until he dropped into the permissible group category, before ascending. The $D - Group$ rule for flying after diving is seen as a subcase for an altitude excursion to 9,000 *ft* (maximum cabin pressure). The question of altitude delay is an interesting one, a subject of recent discussions.

Altitude Delay

Time delays before altitude ascension, implicit to the permissible groups listed in the last column of Table 18, ultimately depend on the tissue compartment controlling the surface interval. In the US Navy tables, the 120 *minute* compartment controls surface intervals, and indeed Table 18 can be routinely applied to the US Navy Surface Interval Table to ascertain delay. With a 120 *minute* controlling compartment, corresponding time delays are compatible with a 12 hour rule for flying after diving. If a faster compartment is used to control surface intervals, a less conservative flying after diving rule would result, and similarly, if a slower compartment were employed, a more conservative rule would ensue.

Today, the 24 hour rule for flying after nominal diving is popular. Such a rule is more compatible with the 635 *minute* controlling compartment in Swiss tables (Buhlmann) than the 120 *minute* compartment in the US Navy tables (Workman). However, using a 635 *minute* compartment, we can still compute time delays for altitude excursions with the help of Table 18.

The calculation of permissible time for an altitude excursion following a dive, or flying after diving, amounts to determining the permissible altitude group from Table 18, the repetitive group following the dive, the standard (US Navy) surface interval to drop into the permissible altitude group, and multiplication of that surface interval by roughly 5.4. The factor of 5.4 results from replacement of the US Navy 120 *minute* compartment by the 635 *minute* compartment in the Surface Interval Table, so that intervals times are increased by roughly 635/120 plus rounding calculations at group boundaries. For given repetitive group and altitude excursion (change in elevation), Table 19 list minimum delay times for altitude excursions as a function of altitude and repetitive dive group. Entries are consistent with a 635 *minute* compartment controlling offgassing, and 44 *fsw* limiting dissolved gas buildup in that compartment.

Table 19. Altitude Delay Chart For The 24 Hour Rule.

Altitude change z (ft)	D	E	F	G	Group H	I	J	K	L
2,000	0:00	0:00	0:00	0:00	0:00	0:00	0:00	0:00	2:26
3,000	0:00	0:00	0:00	0:00	0:00	0:00	0:00	2:37	4:08
4,000	0:00	0:00	0:00	0:00	0:00	0:00	2:53	4:30	5:51
5,000	0:00	0:00	0:00	0:00	0:00	3:04	4:57	6:29	7:44
6,000	0:00	0:00	0:00	0:00	3:20	5:24	7:12	8:38	9:54
7,000	0:00	0:00	0:00	3:41	6:02	8:06	9:43	11:10	12:36
8,000	0:00	0:00	4:08	6:50	9:11	11:04	12:41	14:19	15:40
9,000	0:00	4:50	8:06	10:48	12:58	14:51	16:39	18:11	23:09
10,000	6:18	10:37	13.25	15:56	18.05	20:10	21:18	23:24	24:50

Note, in Table 19, that some 24 *hours* must elapse before the L-Group diver can ascend to an altitude of 10,000 ft, reflecting the current 24 hour delay recommended before flying after diving.

Equivalent Decompression Ratios

At altitude, the formal mathematical equivalence with diving at sea level can be established through the similarity method, by first noting that the ambient pressure, P, at depth, d, is less than at sea level,

$$P = P_h + d$$

with atmospheric pressure, P_h, at altitude, h, depicted in Figure 47 and given by (fsw),

$$P_h = 33 \, exp \, (-0.0381h) = \frac{33}{\alpha},$$

$$\alpha = exp \, (0.0381 \, h),$$

for h in multiples of 1,000 ft, and then requiring that dives at altitude be equivalent to dives at sea level as far as decompression ratios, R, are concerned. Extrapolations of critical tensions, below $P = 33 \, fsw$, must then fall off more rapidly than in the linear case, since surfacing ambient pressures decreases exponentially.

The similarity (exponential) extrapolation holds the ratio, $R = M/P$, constant at altitude. Denoting an *equivalent sea level depth* (ESLD), δ, at altitude, h, one has for an excursion to actual depth, d,

$$\frac{M(d)}{d + 33\beta^{-1}} = \frac{M(\delta)}{\delta + 33},$$

$$\beta = \eta \alpha$$

so that the equality is satisfied when,

$$\delta = \beta d$$

$$M(\delta) = \beta M(d).$$

As a limit point, the similarity extrapolation should be confined to elevations below 10,000 ft, and neither for decompression nor heavy repetitive diving. Again, the exponential factor, α, is the altitude correction factor and is plotted in Figure 47. Consequently at altitude, h, the previously defined fitted critical tensions, $M(d)$, are then written,

$$M_h(d) = \beta^{-1}M(\delta) = \beta^{-1}M_0 + \beta^{-1}\Delta M\delta = \beta^{-1}M_0 + \Delta Md$$

preserving the altitude similarity ratios as required above.

Extended Haldane Staging

Operational consistency of Haldane table and meter algorithms is also of interest here, and part of the reason is reflected in Table 20, which contrasts surfacing critical tensions, M_0, for a number of meter algorithms. Entries were estimated (computed) from quoted meter nonstop time limits, t_n, using the 5, 10, 20, 40, 80, and 120 *min* compartments for convenience of illustration, that is to say that arbitrary τ and M_0 can be fitted to any set of nonstop time limits. Ascent and descent rates of 60 fsw/min were also employed in calculations. The Workman, Buhlmann, and Spencer critical surfacing tensions are fixed, while the equivalent Wienke-Yount surfacing critical tensions vary, depending on repetitive exposure. Entries are also representative of critical tensions employed in related tables.

Table 20. Table and Meter Surfacing Critical Tensions (M_0).

Halftime τ (*min*)	Workman M_0 (*fsw*)	Spencer M_0 (*fsw*)	Buhlmann M_0 (*fsw*)	Wienke-Yount M_0 (*fsw*)
5	104	100	102	100–70
10	88	84	82	81–60
20	72	68	65	67–57
40	58	53	56	57–49
80	52	51	50	51–46
120	51	49	48	48–45

A glance at Table 20 underscores the operational consistency of classes of Haldane meter algorithms, with the Wienke-Yount approach effectively reducing critical tensions in multidiving applications as the simplest meter implementation of a dual phase model. The variation in M_0 within the same compartments is relatively small. Table 21 collates the corresponding nonstop time limits, t_n, for completeness.

Table 21. Table And Meter Nonstop Time Limits (t_n).

Depth d (fsw)	Workman t_n (min)	Spencer t_n (min)	Buhlmann t_n (min)	Wienke-Yount t_n (min)
30		225	290	250
40	200	135	125	130
50	100	75	75	73
60	60	50	54	52
70	50	40	38	39
80	40	30	26	27
90	30	25	22	22
100	25	20	20	18
110	20	15	17	15
120	15	10	15	12
130	10	5	11	9

Variation in the nonstop limits is greater than in the critical tensions, with the US Navy set the most liberal. Using the equivalent depth approach within the similarity method, the nonstop limits in Table 21 can be extrapolated to altitude with correction factors. Figure 48 plots the Wienke-Yount nonstop time limits at various altitudes directly, using a bubble model constraint on the separated phase volume. Correction factors, depicted in Figure 47, are routinely employed to scale (multiply) actual depths at altitude for direct table entry. Scaled depths for table entry at altitude are always greater than actual dive depths, as discussed earlier. If correction factors are applied to the Wienke-Yount critical tensions in Table 20, virtually the same set of nonstop limits at altitude result. This is no real surprise, since phase volume models recover Haldane predictions for short (nonstop) exposures.

Table 22 encapsulates calculations of altitude modifications using the above, gauge and meter corrections described in the following, and a set of modified US Navy Tables. The exercise pulls together a number of altitude considerations for operational diving.

Hypobaric and Hyperbaric Asymptotics

From discussions of the saturation curve, there are clearly differences in data fits across the full range of ambient pressures, $0 \leq P \leq \infty$, and more particularly, across the hypobaric, $P \leq 33$ fsw, and hyperbaric, $P \geq 33$ fsw, regimes. A physically consistent way to join the two regions can be effected within a dual phase model for gas transfer, as will be sketched shortly. Generally though, models for controlling and limiting hypobaric and hyperbaric exposures have long differed over ranges of applicability. Recent testing and comparison of altitude washout data question the hypobaric extension of the linear (hyperbaric) saturation curve, pointing instead to the correlation of altitude data (Conkin) with constant decompression ratios, R, in humans. Similar altitude correlations in sheep were noted by Lanphier and Lehner. Extensions of the saturation curve to altitude have been discussed by many, including Ingle, Bell and Borgwardt, Wienke, Cross, Smith, and Bassett in the not too distant past, with correlations and fits over small altitude excursions nicely established. However, in the limit of zero ambient pressure, P, these linear extrapolations are neither consistent with data nor with simple underlying physics (absolute law of entropy). Closure, then, of hypobaric and hyperbaric diving data is necessary, and must be effected with a more inclusive form of the saturation curve, one exhibiting proper behavior in both limits (pressure asymptotes).

Using the RGBM (or VPM) just such a saturation curve was obtained by Wienke in a coupled framework treating both free and dissolved gas buildup and elimination in tissues. Within the phase volume constraint in correlated bubble dynamics, a general saturation curve of the form,

$$M = [\zeta + 1 - exp\,(-\xi/P)]P$$

ensues for critical tensions, M, at ambient pressure, P, for ζ, ξ bubble number constants, and has the proper (zero entropy) limiting form. Obviously, in the hypobaric limit, as $P \to 0$, then $M \to 0$, while in the hyperbaric limit, as $P \to \infty$, then $M \to \zeta P + \xi$. Corresponding tissue ratios, $R = M/P$, are bounded for all pressures. In the hypobaric regime, as $P \to 0$, then $R \to \zeta + 1$, while in the hyperbaric limit, $P \to \infty$, then $R \to \zeta$. Thus a linear form of the saturation curve is recovered for hyperbaric exposures, while a nearly constant decompression ratio maintains for hypobaric exposures. Typical ranges for the bubble constants, ζ and ξ, when nested within other model requirements for extrapolations, are,

$$6.5\,fsw \le \xi \le 14.4\,fsw$$

$$1.25 \le \zeta \le 1.48$$

Just how the general form of the saturation curve listed above results can be seen in the following way. The integral form of the phase constraint couples permissible bubble excess, Λ, and gradient, G, in time,

$$\int_0^\infty \Lambda G dt \le \alpha V$$

as described previously, with V phase volume, and α a constant in time, t. The bubble excess, Λ, takes general form,

$$\Lambda = N\beta \int_0^r exp\,(-\beta r)dr \propto 1 - exp\,(-\beta r)$$

assuming all nuclei up to r are excited by the saturation exposure.

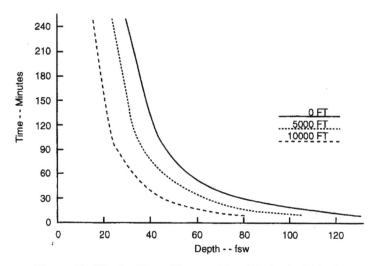

Figure 48. Wienke-Yount Nonstop Time Limits At Altitude

Nonstop time limits in any staging algorithm should decrease with elevation, on physical principles and existing hypobaric and hyperbaric exposure data. Reductions in critical tensions (linearily or exponentially), or near constancy of critical ratios, at altitude commensurately reduce bounce time limits. Using the phase volume limit, reductions in nonstop limits at elevation in the Wienke-Yount model (RGBM/VPM) follow directly. The Buhlmann critical tensions decrease linearily at elevation, thus shortening nonstop time limits. Within the similarity method, exponential reductions in the Workman and Spencer critical tensions at altitude effectively shorten those nonstop limits too.

with N the total number of bubbles, and β a scale length. For initial excitation radius, r_i, at pressure, P_i, the excitation radius, r, for compression to higher pressure, P, is given generally by,

$$\frac{1}{r} - \frac{1}{r_i} = \kappa(P - P_i)$$

with,

$$130 \ \mu m \ fsw \leq \frac{1}{\kappa} \leq 190 \mu m \ fsw$$

as a typical range in bubble excitation experiments in gels.

Clearly, from the above definitions, we see that,

$$\frac{1}{r} \propto P$$

Table 22. Altitude Worksheet

This Worksheet traces altitude corrections for an ocean diver journeying to higher elevation to make two dives. Embarkation altitude is 980 ft, and destination altitude is 4895 ft. The diver weighs 174 lbs, gear is an additional 46 lbs. On site, 2 hr are spent preparing for the dives. With capillary gauge, the first dive is 51 ft for 25 min, followed by 3 hr and 35 min on the surface, and the second dive to 27 ft for 65 min. After diving, the destination altitude is 10,755 ft.

Arrival

embarkation altitude = 980 ft
dive site altitude = 4895 ft
altitude correction factor = 1.2
arrival group = D

diver weight = 174 lbs
gear weight = 46 lbs
ΔB_{alt} = 1.5 lbs
ΔB_{sea} = - 5.5 lbs

Dive 1

group D (1:20) → group C
gauge depth/time = 51 fsw/25 min
correction/residual time = 6.5 fsw/15 min
actual depth/time = 57.5 fsw/40 min
sea level depth/time = 69 fsw/40 min
surfacing group = H

Ascent Rate And Surface Interval

ascent rate = 50 fsw/min
group H (3:35) → group C

Dive 2

gauge depth/time = 27 fsw/65 min
correction/residual time = 5.8 fsw/25 min
actual depth/time = 32.8 fsw/90 min
sea level depth/time = 39.4 fsw/90 min
surfacing group = I

Travel And Surface Interval

destination altitude = 10755 *ft*
permissible group = H
group I (0.34) → group H

On the dissolved gas side, we know that critical tensions scale with absolute pressure, P,

$$M \propto P$$

and on the free side, critical tensions depend upon the bubble excess,

$$M \propto \Lambda$$

Putting these qualitative expressions in mathematical terms, we can equate directly, for ζ and ξ proportionality constants, to the bilinear form,

$$M = \zeta P + \Lambda P = [\zeta + 1 - exp\,(-\xi/P)]\,P$$

and ζ and ξ subsuming all other previously defined parameters. The limiting forms drop from the following identities,

$$\lim_{P \to \infty} exp\,(-\xi/P) \to 1 - \xi/P$$

$$\lim_{P \to 0} exp\,(-\xi/P) \to 0$$

Figures 49, 50, and 51 depict the full behavior of M, R, and G, as function of P, with phase expression for M, and fitted values, ξ and ζ, that is,

$$M = [\zeta + 1 - exp\,(-\xi/P)]\,P$$

$$G = M - P = [\zeta - exp\,(-\xi/P)]\,P$$

$$R = \frac{M}{P} = [\zeta + 1 - exp\,(-\xi/P)]$$

with values, $\zeta = 1.31$ and $\xi = 11.3\ fsw$.
    In the hypobaric regime,

$$\lim_{P \to 0} M \to \lim_{P \to 0} (\zeta + 1)P \to 0$$

$$\lim_{P \to 0} G \to \lim_{P \to 0} \zeta P \to 0$$

$$\lim_{P \to 0} R \to \lim_{P \to 0} (\zeta + 1) \to (\zeta + 1)$$

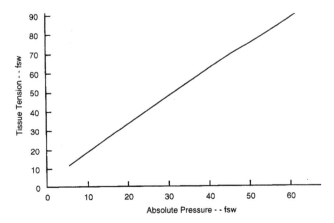

Figure 49. Phase Model Saturation Curve For Tissue Tensions

Within phase models, the critical tissue tensions, M, all satisfy the relationship,

$$M = [2.31 - exp\,(-11.3/P)]$$

for absolute pressure, P (fsw). At large P, the curve approaches a straight line (hyperbaric regime), while at small P, the curve falls off rapidly, passing through the origin (hypobaric regime).

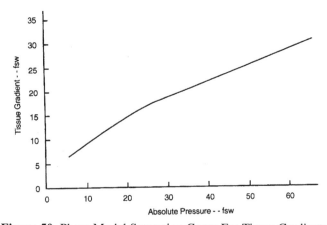

Figure 50. Phase Model Saturation Curve For Tissue Gradients

In analogy with tissue tensions, M, tissue gradients, G, exhibit similar asymptotic behavior,

$$G = [1.31 - exp\,(-11.3/P)]$$

approximating a straight line for large P, and curving through the origin as P approaches zero.

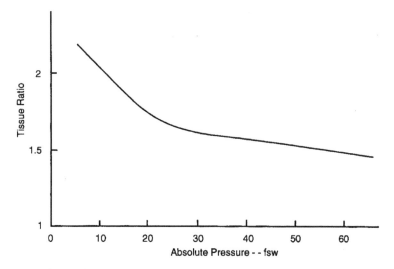

Figure 51. Phase Model Saturation Curve For Tissue Ratios

Tissue ratios, R, approach a constant value for both large and small P,

$$R = 2.31 - exp\,(-11.3/P)$$

that is, 2.31 for small P, and 1.31 for large P.

In the hyperbaric regime,

$$\lim_{P\to\infty} M \to \xi + \zeta P$$

$$\lim_{P\to\infty} G \to \xi + (\zeta - 1)P$$

$$\lim_{P\to\infty} R \to \zeta$$

The classical hyperbaric *straightline* tension and hypobaric *constant* ratio are thus recovered in a generalized phase representation.

Barometer Equation

The barometer equation is a simple application of Maxwell-Boltzmann statistics to an ensemble of colliding gas molecules in the presence of a gravitational field, to very good order, the situation posed by atmospheric gases surrounding the Earth. The equation was employed by Perrin in 1909 to estimate Avogadro's number, N_0, by counting gas molecules at various elevations.

In a mixture of N gases (ideal or noninteracting), the total pressure, P, at elevation, h, is the sum of component partial pressures, P_n, (Dalton's law),

$$P = \sum_{n=1}^{N} P_n$$

with each component Maxwellian distributed over elevation, h,

$$P_n = P_{n0} \, exp \, (-m_n g h / kT)$$

for molecular mass, m, acceleration of gravity, g, at elevation, h, temperature, T, and P_{0n} the partial pressure at sea level. The set are also known as the law of atmospheres. Using the above over all known atmospheric components, and the simple relationship,

$$k = \frac{R}{N_0}$$

linking Boltzmann's constant, k, to the universal gas constant, R, and Avogadro's number, N_0. Perrin estimated N_0 within 10%.

The atmosphere of the Earth is mostly nitrogen, and oxygen, in roughly 79/21 proportions. Neglecting the small variation in gravity, g, over elevations up to 15,000 ft, the total atmospheric pressure can be approximated,

$$P = 26.07 \, exp \, (-m_{N_2} g_0 h / kT) + 6.93 \, exp \, (-m_{O_2} g_0 h / kT)$$

for surface gravity, $g_0 = 9.8 \, m/sec^2$. Furthermore, the molecular masses of nitrogen and oxygen (diatomic) differ only by 4 amu, so that reasonably,

$$m_{O_2} \approx m_{N_2} = 28.16 \, amu = 4.708 \times 10^{-26} \, kg$$

yielding,

$$P = 33 \, exp \, (-0.0033 h / T)$$

For a moderate isothermal atmosphere, $T = 300 \,^{\circ}K$,

$$P = 33 \, exp \, (-0.038 h)$$

with h specifically in multiples of 1,000 ft elevation. For small values of h,

$$P \approx 33(1 - 0.038 h)$$

or put another way, atmospheric pressure drops roughly 3% for each 1,000 ft of elevation. In diving parlance, this is the Cross correction, the factor yielding equivalent sea level depths for table entry at altitude.

Keyed Exercises

• *What is ambient pressure, P_h, at an elevation of 6,500 ft?*

$$P_h = P_0 \, exp \, (-0.038 h), \quad P_0 = 33 \, fsw, \quad h = 6.5$$
$$P_{6.5} = 33 \, exp \, (-0.038 \times 6.5) \, fsw = 33 \times .78 \, fsw = 25.7 \, fsw$$

What is the altitude scaling factor, α, for depth, and what is the equivalent sea level depth, δ, for actual depth, $d = 78 \, ft$?

$$\alpha = exp \, (0.038 h) = exp \, (0.038 \times 6.5) = 1.28$$
$$\delta = \eta \alpha d = .975 \times 1.28 \times 78 \, fsw = 97.5 \, fsw$$

- *If a decompression stop is required at 20 fsw according to the USN Tables, what is the actual depth, d, of the stop at 6,500 ft elevation?*

$$\alpha = exp \, (0.038) = exp \, (0.038 \times 6.5) = 1.28$$

$$\delta = 20 \; fsw, \;\; d = \frac{\delta}{\eta \alpha} = \frac{20}{.975 \times 1.28} \; ft = 16 \; ft$$

- *Construct a set of critical surfacing ratios, R_7, at 7,000 ft elevation using the standard USN set, R_0, at sea level, and altitude similarity (downscaling) through the correction factor, α?*

$$\alpha = exp \, (0.0381h), \;\; h = 7$$

$$R_h = \frac{R_0}{\alpha} = R_0 \, exp \, (-0.0381h)$$

$$R_0 = (3.15, 2.67, 2.18, 1.76, 1.58, 1.55)$$

$$R_7 = R_0 \, exp \, (-0.0381 \times 7) = .77 \, R_0$$

$$R_7 = (2.43, 2.05, 1.67, 1.35, 1.20, 1.19)$$

- *At an altitude, $z = 10,000$ ft, what is the approximate nonstop limit, t_n, for an exposure at 60 fsw?*

$$t_n \approx 17 \; min$$

- *Using the similarity method, what is the nonstop time limit?*

$$\alpha = exp \, (0.038h), \;\; h = 10$$

$$\alpha = exp \, (.38) = 1.462, \;\; d = 1.462 \times 60 \; fsw = 87.7 \; fsw$$

$$t_n \approx 25 \; min$$

- *Using the fitted critical tensions for the, $\tau = 20$ min, compartment what is the specific time limit, t_n, at a depth, $d = 65$ fsw, at an elevation of 6,500 ft?*

$$\tau = 20 \; min, \;\; d = 65 \; fsw, \;\; h = 6.5, \;\; \alpha = exp \, (0.038 \times 6.5) = 1.28, \;\; \eta = .975$$

$$\beta = \eta \alpha = .975 \times 1.28 = 1.25, \;\; \delta = \beta d = 1.25 \times 65 \; fsw = 81.3 \; fsw$$

$$M_{6.5}(0) = \beta M_0 = .80 \times 152.7 \times .47 \; fsw = 57.4 \; fsw$$

$$p_i = .79 P_h = .79 \alpha_{-1} P_0 = .79 \times .78 \times 33 \; fsw = 20.33 \; fsw$$

$$p_a = .79(P_h + d) = .79 \times (.78 \times 33 + 65) \; fsw = 70.77 \; fsw$$

$$\lambda = \frac{.693}{20} \; min^{-1} = .0347 \; min^{-1}, \;\; p_i = 20.3 \; fsw, \;\; p_a = 70.8 \; fsw$$

$$t_n = \frac{1}{\lambda} \ln \left[\frac{p_i - p_a}{M_{6.5}(0) - p_a} \right] = 28.9 \times \ln \left[\frac{20.3 - 70.8}{57.4 - 70.8} \right] \ min = 38.3 \ min$$

What is the corresponding compartment limit, t_n, at depth, $d = 40 \ fsw$?

$$p_i = 20.33 \ fsw, \quad p_a = .79(P_h + d) = .79 \times (.78 \times 33 + 40) \ fsw = 51.9 \ fsw$$

$$M_{6.5}(0) = 57.4 \ fsw$$

$$M_{6.5}(0) > p_a \quad (maximum \ tension \ less \ than \ critical \ value)$$

$$t_n \to \infty \quad (for \ this \ compartment)$$

- *If descent rate, $s = 10 \ fsw/min$, is included, accounting for descent time, t_d, in the foregoing time limit estimation for the 20 min tissue at 6,500 ft elevation, what is the new nonstop time limit, t_n, for the same exposure depth, $d = 65 \ fsw$?*

$$p_i = 20.3 \ fsw, \quad p_a = 20.3 \ fsw, \quad \lambda = 0.0347 \ min^{-1}, \quad s = 10 \ fsw/min$$

$$t_d = \frac{d}{s} = \frac{65}{10} \ min = 6.5 \ min, \quad v = f_n s = .79 \times 10 \ fsw/min = 7.9 \ fsw/min$$

$$p_d = p_a + \left[p_i - p_a + \frac{v}{\lambda} \right] exp \ (-\lambda t_d) + v t_d - \frac{v}{\lambda}$$

$$p_d = 20.3 - \frac{7.9}{.0347} exp \ (-0.0347 \times 6.5) - \frac{7.9}{.0347} + 51.4 \ fsw = 25.6 \ fsw$$

$$t_n = \frac{1}{\lambda} \ln \left[\frac{p_d - p_a}{M_{6.5}(0) - p_a} \right] = 28.9 \times \ln \left[\frac{25.6 - 70.8}{57.4 - 70.8} \right] \ min = 35.1 \ min$$

Mixtures

Mixed breathing gases, across a spectrum of underwater activities, have been utilized successfully, mostly mixtures of nitrogen, helium, and oxygen, differing from pure air, and lately those with higher oxygen content than air (*enriched*), which can be employed efficiently in shallow diving. Non-enriched mixtures of nitrogen/oxygen (nitrox), helium/oxygen (heliox), and helium/nitrogen/oxygen (trimix), of course, have long been employed commercially in deep and saturation diving. Recently, mixtures of hydrogen/oxygen (hydrox) have also been tested. A closer look at these inert gases in a range of diving applications is illuminating, particularly gas properties, advantages and disadvantages, and interplay.

Biological Reactivities

Low pressure oxygen toxicity can occur if a gas mixture with 60% oxygen is breathed at 1 *atm* for 12 *hours* or more. Pulmonary damage, irritation, and coughing are manifestations (pulmonary toxicity). High pressure oxygen toxicity can occur when breathing pure oxygen at pressures greater than 1 *atm* for periods of minutes to hours, the lower the oxygen pressure the longer the time for symptoms to develop, and vice versa, as seen in Table 23 below. Twitching, convulsions, and dizziness are the symptoms (nervous system toxicity). On the other hand, if oxygen pressures fall below .16 *atm*, unconsciousness may result. Low levels of oxygen inhibit tissue cell metabolic function (hypoxia). Confusion and difficulty in maintaining coordination are milder symptoms. Severe hypoxia requires medical attention. Quantification of oxygen dose is taken up shortly.

Table 23. Oxygen Depth-Time Limits (t_x).

Oxygen depth d (*fsw*)	Air depth d (*fsw*)	Time limit t_x (*min*)
10	50	240
15	75	150
20	100	110
25	125	75
30	150	45
35	175	25
40	200	10

Clearly a constraint in mixed gas diving is the oxygen partial pressure. Inspired partial pressures of oxygen must remain below 1.6 *atm* (52.8 *fsw*) to prevent central nervous system (CNS) toxicity, and above .16 *atm* (5.3 *fsw*) to prevent hypoxia. This window, so to speak, is confining, some 1.44 *atm* (47.5 *fsw*). Denoting the mole fraction of oxygen, f_{O_2}, the upper and lower limits of this window, d_{max} and d_{min}, can be written (*fsw*),

$$\eta d_{max} = \frac{52.8}{f_{O_2}} - P_h,$$

$$\eta d_{min} = \frac{5.3}{f_{O_2}} - P_h,$$

$$\eta d_{max} - \eta d_{min} = \frac{47.5}{f_{O_2}},$$

with η the specific density (with respect to sea water) and with working depths, d, limited by d_{max} and d_{min},

$$d_{min} \le d \le d_{max}.$$

For fresh water, $\eta = 0.975$, and for sea water, $\eta = 1.000$. Certainly up to about 7,000 *ft* elevation, the lower limit, d_{min}, is no real constraint, with the surface accessible as the limit.

Another factor inhibiting performance underwater is inert gas narcosis, particularly at increasing ambient pressure. Although the common gases nitrogen and helium associated with diving are physiologically inert under normal atmospheric conditions, they both exhibit anesthetic properties as their partial pressures increase. The mechanism is not completely understood, but impaired carbon dioxide diffusion in the lungs, increased oxygen tension, fear, and related chemical reactions have all been implicated in the past. With 80/20 mixtures, symptom onset for nitrogen is near 100 *fsw*, and very much deeper for helium, in the 1,000 fsw range. Symptoms range from light headedness to unconsciousness at the extreme.

Nitrogen is limited as an inert gas for diving. Increased pressures of nitrogen beyond 200 fsw lead to excessive euphoria, and reduced mental and physical functional ability, while beyond 600 fsw loss of consciousness results. Individual tolerances vary widely, often depending on activity. Symptoms can be marked at the beginning of a deep dive, gradually decreasing with time. Flow resistance and the onset of turbulence in the airways of the body increase with higher breathing gas pressure, considerably reducing ventilation with nitrogen-rich breathing mixtures during deep diving. Oxygen is also limited at depth for the usual toxicity reasons. Dives beyond 300 fsw requiring bottom times of hours need employ lighter, more weakly reacting, and less narcotic gases than nitrogen, and all coupled to reduced oxygen partial pressures.

Comparative Properties

A number of inert gas replacements have been tested, such as hydrogen, neon, argon, and helium, with only helium and hydrogen performing satisfactorily on all counts. Because it is the lightest, hydrogen has elimination speed advantages over helium, but, because of the high explosive risk in mixing hydrogen, helium has emerged as the best all-around inert gas for deep and saturation diving. Helium can be breathed for months without tissue damage. Argon is highly soluble and heavier than nitrogen, and thus a very poor choice. Neon is not much lighter than nitrogen, but is only slightly more soluble than helium. Of the five, helium is the least and argon the most narcotic inert gas under pressure.

Saturation and desaturation speeds of inert gases are inversely proportional to the square root of their atomic masses. Hydrogen will saturate and desaturate approximately 3.7 times faster than nitrogen, and helium will saturate and desaturate some 2.7 times faster than nitrogen. Differences between neon, argon, and nitrogen are not significant for diving. Comparative properties for hydrogen, helium, neon, nitrogen, argon, and oxygen are listed in Table 24. Solubilities, S, are quoted in atm^{-1}, weights, A, in *atomic mass units* (amu), and relative narcotic potencies, v, are dimensionless (referenced to nitrogen in observed effect). The least potent gases have the highest index, v.

The size of bubbles formed with various inert gases depends upon the amount of gas dissolved, and hence the solubilities. Higher gas solubilities promote bigger bubbles. Thus, helium is preferable to hydrogen as a light gas, while nitrogen is preferable to argon as a heavy gas. Neon solubility roughly equals nitrogen solubility. Narcotic potency correlates with lipid (fatty tissue) solubility, with the least narcotic gases the least soluble. Different uptake and elimination speeds suggest optimal means for reducing decompression time using helium and nitrogen mixtures. Following deep dives beyond 300 fsw breathing helium, switching to nitrogen is without risk, while helium elimination is accelerated because the helium tissue-blood gradient is increased when breathing an air mixture. By gradually increasing the oxygen content after substituting nitrogen for helium, the nitrogen uptake can also be kept low. Workable combinations of gas switching depend upon the exposure and the tissue compartment controlling the ascent.

Table 24. Inert Gas and Oxygen Molecular Weights, Solubilities, and Narcotic Potency.

	H_2	He	Ne	N_2	Ar	O_2
A (amu)	2.02	4.00	20.18	28.02	39.44	32.00
S (atm^{-1})						
blood	.0149	.0087	.0093	.0122	.0260	.0241
oil	.0502	.0150	.0199	.0670	.1480	.1220
v	1.83	4.26	3.58	1.00	0.43	

Mixed gas diving dates back to the mid 1940s, but proof of principle diving experiments were carried out in the late 50s. In 1945, Zetterstrom dove to 500 fsw using hydrox and nitrox as a travel mix, but died of hypoxia and DCI when a tender hoisted him to the surface too soon. In 1959, Keller and Buhlmann devised a heliox schedule to 730 fsw with only 45 min of decompression. Then, in 1962, Keller and Small bounced to 1,000 fsw, but lost consciousness on the way up due to platform support errors. Small and another support diver, Whittaker, died as a result. In 1965, Workman published decompression tables for nitrox and heliox, with the nitrox version evolving into USN Tables. At Duke University Medical Center, the 3 man team of Atlantis III made a record chamber dive to 2250 fsw on heliox, and Bennett found that 10% nitrogen added to the heliox eliminated high pressure nervous syndrome (HPNS). In deep saturation diving, *normoxic* breathing mixtures of gases are often commonly employed to address oxygen concerns. A normoxic breathing mixture, helium or nitrogen, reduces the oxygen percentage so that the partial pressure of oxygen at the working depth is the same as at sea level, the obvious concerns, again, hypoxia and toxicity. Critical tensions can be employed in helium saturation diving in much the same fashion as nitrogen diving. A critical tension, recall, is the maximum permissible value of inert gas tension (M-value) for a hypothetical tissue compartment with specified halftime. An approach to helium exchange in tissue compartments employs the usual nitrogen set with halftimes reduced by 2.7, that is, the helium halftimes are extracted from the nitrogen halftimes following division by 2.7, and the same critical tension is assumed for both gas compartments. Researchers have tested schedules based on just such an approach. Tissue tensions scale as the relative proportion of inert gas in any mixture. More so than in air diving, computational methods for mixed gas diving and decompression are often proprietary information in the commercial sector.

Helium (normal 80/20 mixture) nonstop time limits are shorter than nitrogen, but follow a $t^{1/2}$ law similar to nitrogen, that is, depth times the square root of the nonstop time limit is approximately constant. Using standard techniques of extracting critical tensions from the nonstop time limits, fast compartment critical tensions can be assigned for applications. Modern bubble models, such as the varying permeability model, have also been used strategically in helium diving.

Today, the three helium and nitrogen mixtures (nitrox, heliox, trimix) are employed for deep and saturation diving, with a tendency towards usage of enriched oxygen mixtures in shallow (recreational) diving. The use of enriched oxygen mixtures by recreational divers is the subject of controversy, aptly a concern over diver safety. Breathing mixture purity, accurate assessment of component gas ratios, oxygen toxicity, and appropriate decompression procedures are valid concerns for the mixed gas diver. Care, in the use of breathing mixtures, is to be underscored. Too little, or too much, oxygen can be disastrous. The fourth hydrogen mixture (hydrox) is much less commonplace.

Nitrox

Mixtures of oxygen and nitrogen with less oxygen than 21% (pure air) offer protection from oxygen toxicity in moderately deep and saturation diving. Moderately deep here means no more than a few hundred feet. Hypoxia is a concern with mixtures containing as much as 15% oxygen in this range. Saturation diving on oxygen-scarce nitrox mixtures is a carefully planned exposure. The narcotic effects of nitrogen in the $100 \, fsw$ to $200 \, fsw$ depth range mitigate against nitrox for deep diving.

Diving on enriched nitrox mixtures need be carefully planned exposures, but for opposite reason, that is, oxygen toxicity. Mixtures of 30% more of oxygen significantly reduce partial pressures of nitrogen to the point of downloading tissue tensions compared to air diving. If standard air decompression procedures are used, enriched nitrox affords a safety margin. However, because of elevated oxygen partial pressures, a maximum permissible depth (floor) needs be assigned to any enriched oxygen mixture. With $1.6 \, atm$ ($52.8 \, fsw$) as oxygen partial pressure limit, the floor for any mixture is easily computed. Enriched nitrox with 32% oxygen is floored at a depth of $130 \, fsw$ for diving, also called the oxygen limit point. Higher enrichments raise that floor proportionately.

Decompression requirements on enriched nitrox are less stringent than air, simply because the nitrogen content is reduced below 79%. Many equivalent means to schedule enriched nitrox diving exist, based on the standard Haldane critical tension approach. Air critical tensions can be employed with exponential buildup and elimination equations tracking the (reduced) nitrogen tissue gas exchange, or equivalent air depths (always less than the actual depths on enriched nitrox) can be used with air tables. The latter procedure ultimately relates inspired nitrogen pressure on a nitrox mixture to that of air at shallower depth (equivalent air depth). For instance, a 74/26 nitrox mixture at a depth of $140 \, fsw$ has an equivalent air depth of $130 \, fsw$ for table entry. Closed breathing circuit divers have employed the equivalent air depth approach for many years.

Heliox

The narcotic effects of nitrogen in the several hundred feet range prompted researchers to find a less reactive breathing gas for deeper diving. Tests, correlating narcotic effects and lipid solubility, affirm helium as the least narcotic of breathing gases, some 4 times less narcotic than nitrogen according to Bennett, and as summarized in Table 24. Deep saturation and extended habitat diving, conducted at depths of 1,000 *ft* or more on helium/oxygen mixtures by the US Navy, ultimately ushered in the era of heliox diving. For very deep and saturation diving above 700 *fsw* or so, heliox remains a popular, though expensive, breathing mixture.

Helium uptake and elimination can also be tracked with the standard Haldane exponential expressions employed for nitrogen, but with a notable exception. Corresponding helium halftimes are some 2.7 times faster than nitrogen for the same hypothetical tissue compartment. Thus, at saturation, a 180 *minute* helium compartment behaves like a 480 *minute* nitrogen compartment. All the computational machinery in place for nitrogen diving can be ported over to helium nicely, with the 2.7 scaling of halftimes expedient in fitting most helium data.

When diving on heliox, particularly for deep and long exposures, it is advantageous to switch to nitrox on ascent to optimize decompression time, as discussed earlier. The higher the helium saturation in the slow tissue compartments, the later the change to a nitrogen breathing environment. Progressive increases of nitrogen partial pressure enhance helium washout, but also minimize nitrogen absorption in those same compartments. Similarly, progressive increases in oxygen partial pressures aid washout of all inert gases, while also addressing concerns of hypoxia.

An amusing problem in helium breathing environments is the high-pitched voice change, often requiring electronic voice encoding to facilitate diver communication. Helium is also very penetrating, often damaging vacuum tubes, gauges, and electronic components not usually affected by nitrogen. Though helium remains a choice for deep diving, some nitrogen facilitates decompression, ameliorates the voice problem, and helps to keep the diver warm. Pure helium, however, can be an asphyxiant.

Trimix

Diving much below 1400 *fsw* on heliox is not only impractical, but also marginally hazardous. High pressure nervous syndrome (HPNS) is a major problem on descent in very deep diving, and is quite complex. The addition of nitrogen to helium breathing mixtures (trimix), is beneficial in ameliorating HPNS. Trimix is a useful breathing mixture at depths ranging from 500 *fsw* to 2,000 *fsw*, with nitrogen percentages usually below 10% in operational diving, because of narcotic effect.

Decompression concerns on trimix can be addressed with traditional techniques. Uptake and elimination of both helium and nitrogen can be limited by critical tensions. Using a basic set of nitrogen halftimes and critical tensions, and a corresponding set of helium halftimes approximately 3 times faster for the same nitrogen compartment, total inert gas uptake and elimination can be assumed to be the sum of fractional nitrogen and helium in the trimix breathing medium, using the usual exponential expressions for each inert gas component. Such approaches to trimix decompression were tested by researchers years ago, and many others after them.

Hydrox

Since hydrogen is the lightest of gases, it is reasonably expected to offer the lowest breathing resistance in a smooth flow system, promoting rapid transfer of oxygen and carbon dioxide within the lungs at depth. Considering solubility and diffusivity, nitrogen uptake and elimination rates in blood and tissue should be more rapid than nitrogen, and even helium. In actuality, the performance of hydrogen falls between nitrogen and helium as an inert breathing gas for diving.

Despite any potential advantages of hydrogen/oxygen breathing mixtures, users have been discouraged from experimenting with hydrox because of the explosive and flammable nature of most mixtures. Work in the early 1950s by the Bureau of Mines, however, established that oxygen percentages below the 3%–4% level provide a safety margin against explosive and flammability risks. A 97/3 mixture of hydrogen and oxygen could be utilized at depths as shallow as 200 fsw, where oxygen partial pressure equals sea level partial pressure. Experiments with mice also indicate that the narcotic potency of hydrogen is less than nitrogen, but greater than helium. Unlike helium, hydrogen is also relatively plentiful, and inexpensive.

Haldane Decompression Procedures

In the case of mixtures of gases (nitrogen, helium, hydrogen), the Haldane decompression procedures can be generalized in a straightforward manner, using a set of nitrogen critical tensions, M, and halftimes, τ, as the bases. Denoting gas species, $j = N_2, He, H_2$, atomic masses, A_j, and partial pressures, p_j, each component satisfies a Haldane tissue equation, with rate modified coefficient, λ_j, given by,

$$p_j - p_{aj} = (p_{ij} - p_{aj}) \, exp \, (-\lambda_j t),$$

for p_{aj} and p_{ij} ambient and initial partial pressures of the jth species, and with decay constant, λ_j, related by Graham's law to the nitrogen coefficient, $\lambda_{N_2} = \lambda$, by,

$$\lambda_j = \left[\frac{A_{N_2}}{A_j} \right]^{1/2} \lambda.$$

Thus, for instance, one has,

$$\lambda_{He} = 2.7 \, \lambda,$$

$$\lambda_{H_2} = 3.7 \, \lambda.$$

In a mixture, the total tension, Π, is the sum of all J partial tensions, p_j,

$$\Pi = \sum_{j=1}^{J} [\, p_{aj} + (p_{ij} - p_{aj}) \, exp \, (-\lambda_j t) \,]$$

and the decompression requirement is simply,

$$\Pi = \sum_{j=1}^{J} p_j \le M,$$

for all exposures. Denoting ambient partial pressures, p_{aj}, as a fraction, f_j, of total pressure, P, that is,

$$p_{aj} = f_j P,$$

it follows that,

$$f_{O_2} + \sum_{j=1}^{J} f_j = 1$$

neglecting any carbon dioxide or water vapor in the mixture, of course. For 75/25 (enriched) nitrox, $f_{N_2} = 0.75$, for 90/10 heliox, $f_{He} = 0.90$, for 75/10/15 trimix, $f_{He} = 0.75$, $f_{N_2} = 0.10$, while for 95/5 hydrox, $f_{H_2} = 0.95$. For pure air obviously $f_{N_2} = 0.79$, as the common case. Clearly the treatment of breathing mixtures assumes a single critical tension, M, for each compartment, τ, in this case, extracted from the nitrogen data.

With enriched nitrox ($f_{N_2} < 0.79$), it is clear that the nitrogen decompression requirements are reduced when using the same set of M, that is, the air set of M are assumed to apply equally to both air and other nitrogen mixtures. The procedure has been applied to heliox, trimix, and hydrox mixtures in similar vein. One important constraint in any mixture is the oxygen content. Partial pressures of oxygen must be kept below 52.8 fsw (1.6 atm) to prevent toxicity, and above 5.3 fsw (.16 atm) to prevent hypoxia. Balancing diver mobility within this window at increasing depth is a delicate procedure at times.

Equivalent Air Depth (EAD)

In extending air tables to other breathing mixtures, an extrapolation based on critical tensions is crux of the *equivalent air depth* (EAD) method. The equivalent air depth method for table use derives from the imposed equality of mixture and inert gas partial pressures, and is very similar to the altitude equivalent depth method, but is not the same. For instance, with nitrox mixtures, the usual case, the equivalent air depth, δ, is related to the effective depth, d, by requiring equality of nitrogen partial pressures for air and nitrogen mixture with mole fraction f_{N_2},

$$\delta = \frac{f_{N_2}}{.79} (P_h + d) - P_h.$$

At altitude, the effective depth, d, is the equivalent sea level depth (ESLD) described earlier. At sea level, the actual depth and effective depth are the same.

With enriched mixtures ($f_{N_2} < 0.79$), it is clear that the equivalent air depth, δ, is less than the effective depth, d, so that nitrogen decompression requirements are reduced when using δ to enter any set of air tables. Obviously, the same set of M are assumed to apply equally to both air and other mixture in the approach. At sea level, the above reduces to the form,

$$\delta = \frac{f_{N_2}}{.79}(33+d) - 33,$$

with d the actual depth, and has been utilized extensively in ocean diving.

Equivalent Mixture Depth (EMD)

The same procedure can be applied to arbitrary heliox, trimix, and hydrox mixtures in theory, basically an extrapolation from a reference (standard) table with the same gas components (helium, nitrogen, or hydrogen with oxygen). Denoting the gas molar fractions in the standard (table) mixture, f_{sk}, with $k = N_2$, He, H_2, O_2, and molar fractions in the arbitrary mixture, f_k, we have for a balanced K component mixture,

$$\delta = \frac{(1-f_{O_2})}{(1-f_{sO_2})}(P_h+d) - P_h.$$

This is the *equivalent mixture depth* (EMD) method. At altitude, the ESLD is first determined, then converted to an EAD or EMD (conservative order).

Oxygen Rebreathing

As early as 1880, Fleuss developed and tested the first closed circuit, oxygen rebreathing system. At that time, of course, oxygen toxicity was not completely understood, though the effects of breathing pure oxygen were coupled to excitability and fever. In ensuing years, the apparatus was refined considerably, and was used by underwater combatants in World War II. During the 1950s, recreational divers used oxygen rebreathers. However, by the late 1950s, recreational divers switched to the popular open circuit device developed by Cousteau and Gagnan, thereby trading oxygen toxicity and caustic carbon dioxide concerns for decompression sickness and nitrogen narcosis. Today, rebreathers are witnessing a rebirth among technical divers. US Navy Underwater Demolition (UDT) and Sea, Air, Land (SEAL) Teams always employed rebreathers for tactical operations.

In closed circuit systems, exhaled gas is kept in the apparatus, scrubbed of carbon dioxide by chemical absorbents, and then returned to the diver. No gas is released into the water (no bubbles). Gas consumption is related only to the physiological consumption of oxygen. Only a small amount of oxygen is required for extended exposures. Oxygen is taken directly from a breathing bag, and exhaled gas passes separately through an alkaline, absorbent material, where it is scrubbed of carbon dioxide. A typical reduction process involves water vapor, sodium and potassium hydroxide, and carbon dioxide in the reaction chain, just mass balance without dissociation notation,

$$CO_2 + H_2 + O \rightarrow H_2 + CO_3,$$

$$2H_2 + CO_3 + 2NaOH + 2KOH \rightarrow Na_2 + CO_3 + K_2 + CO_3 + 4H_2 + O,$$

$$Na_2 + CO_3 + K_2 + CO_3 + 2Ca(OH)_2 \rightarrow 2CaCO_3 + 2NaOH + 2KOH.$$

Rebreathers today last about $3hr$, using approximately 6 m^3 of oxygen and 4 *lbs* of absorbent. Because of oxygen toxicity, depth is a limitation for oxygen rebreathing. Depth limitation for pure oxygen rebreathing is near 20 *fsw*. Today, closed circuit mixed gas rebreathers blend inert gases with oxygen (lowering oxygen partial pressure) to extend depth limitations. Two cylinders, one oxygen and the other inert gas (or a premixed cylinder), are employed, and the mixture is scrubbed of carbon dioxide before return to the breathing bag.

Closed circuit oxygen scuba takes advantage of gas conservation, but is limited in dive depth and duration by oxygen toxicity effects. Open circuit scuba offers greater depth flexibility, but is limited in depth and duration by the inefficiency of gas utilization. To bridge this gap, semiclosed circuit mixed gas rebreathers were developed. The semiclosed circuit rebreather operates much like the closed circuit rebreather, but requires a continuous, or frequent, purge to prevent toxic inert gas buildup. Two cylinders of oxygen and inert gas (or one premixed), are charged with safe levels of both, usually corresponding to safe oxygen partial pressure at the maximum operating depth. Gas flow from the high pressure cylinders the breathing circuit is controlled by a regulator and nozzle, admitting a continuous and constant mass flow of gas determined by oxygen consumption requirements. The diver inhales the mixture from the breathing bag and exhales it into the exhalation bag. Pressure in the exhalation bag forces the gas mixture through the carbon dioxide scrubber, and from the scrubber back into the breathing bag for diver consumption. When gas pressure in the breathing circuit reaches a preset limit, a relief valve opens in the exhalation bag, purging excess gas into the water.

Oxygen rebreathing at high partial pressures can lead to central nervous system (or pulmonary) oxygen poisoning. It is thought that high pressure oxygen increases the production of oxygen free radicals disrupting cell function. The US Navy conducted research into safe depths and durations for oxygen diving, and concluded that there is very little risk of central nervous system oxygen toxicity when partial pressures of oxygen are maintained below 1.6 *atm*. Additionally, risk only increases slightly when oxygen partial pressures are maintained below 1.8 *atm*.

Best Diving Mixture

Having discussed equivalent depths, a next question focuses on the best diving mixtures to minimize decompression requirements, inert gas narcosis, and oxygen toxicity (discussed in the next section). The procedure is straightforward across commercial, military, and technical diving sectors, and goes like this, neglecting water vapor, carbon dioxide, and all other trace gases, for ambient surface pressure, P_h, and depth, d, measured in fsw, and gas partial pressures, p_{O_2}, p_{N_2}, and p_{He}, given in *atm*:

- determine oxygen fraction, f_{O_2}, by specifying the maximum partial pressure, p_{O_2}, supported by the bottom depth and duration of the dive,

$$f_{O_2} = \frac{33 p_{O_2}}{\eta d + P_h}$$

with p_{O_2} in the 1.2–1.6 *atm* range;

- determine nitrogen fraction, f_{N_2}, by specifying maximum partial pressure, p_{N_2}, below narcosis threshold,

$$f_{N_2} = \frac{33 p_{N_2}}{\eta d + P_h}$$

with p_{N_2} somewhere in the 3.0–5.5 *atm* range;

- determine helium fraction, f_{He}, by subtracting oxygen and nitrogen fraction from one,

$$f_{He} = 1 - f_{O_2} - f_{N_2}$$

and is the expensive part of the dive mixture.

The same procedure is applied to gas switches on the way up (ascent), permitting decompression and oxygen management across the whole profile, top to bottom and then bottom to top. As such, it is an essential ingredient for decompression and extended range dive planning on mixed gases. And it applies to open circuit scuba and closed circuit (constant p_{O_2}) rebreathers.

Gas Mixing

There are a number of ways of mixing gases together for diving. Helium and oxygen can be added to air or other nitrox mixtures to effect the best diving mixture, detailed above. Or oxygen can be injected into continuous flow nitrox and helium mixtures. Nitrogen can be removed from a flowing stream of nitrox by membranes or molecular sieves. Same for helium.

Mixing processes are usually turbulent by nature, because of both high pressure in the cylinder, and high pressure and velocity flow regimes. Temperatures may also rise with rising tank pressure. However, and probably contrary to mixing folktales, within seconds or so, mixed gas components redistribute themselves uniformly over the cylinder. Layering is not a problem separating mixture components. All gases are pretty much ideal for simple mix quantification.

Upon equilibrium, the proportions of mix, f_{O_2}, f_{N_2}, f_{He}, are still ratios of component partial pressures divided by the total tank pressure. Simply,

$$p_i = f_i \Pi$$

for partial pressures, p_i, $(i = O_2,\ He,\ N_2,\ etc.)$, and tank pressure, Π, just the sum of partial mixture pressures,

$$\Pi = \sum_{i=1}^{I} p_i$$

for I the number of mixture components (2 or 3 these days). Of course, in filling tanks to best diving mix, the f_i are given, and it's up to the filler to adjust his mixing procedures to yield appropriate partial pressures, p_i, for given (or sought) Π.

The easiest way to blend gas mixtures is called partial pressure mixing. Helium, oxygen, or air at precomputed partial pressure can be injected into pure oxygen, air, nitrox, heliox, or trimix at some (given) tank pressure to produce the desired final mixture and pressure. Continuous flow blending inserts high purity oxygen into any base mixture, such as air, heliox, trimix, etc. As the blend exits, it can easily be analyzed for oxygen proportion. Pressure swing absorption is a removal mixing process, usually employed to produce nitrox from air. Molecular sieves are used to remove nitrogen from the flow gas. High purity oxygen is left, and can be blended back with air. Membranes may also be employed to remove nitrogen directly from the flow gas, which then exits as nitrox.

Perhaps the above is too cavalier in prose as far as gas mixing. Pure oxygen is, of course, explosive, in fact, mixtures above 40% oxygen need be handled with extreme care for the same reason. Combustion simulations with high pressure oxygen flows, through orifice constrictions, and in the presence of combustible materials found in mixing environments, compressors, and regulators support increasing explosion risk with increasing oxygen mix proportion. Cleaning of components involved in high pressure oxygen transfer is also suggested, and mixing of clean and unclean components is contraindicated. Obviously, and equally important, is verification of mixture fractions, f_i, by helium and oxygen analyzers. For nitrox, heliox, and helitrox, of course, just oxygen analysis pinpoints mixture fraction of inert gas (helium or nitrogen). For trimix, both helium and oxygen analysis is requisite.

Isobaric Countertransport

Isobaric countertransport simply denotes isobaric diffusion of two gases in opposite directions. Perhaps a better descriptor is countercurrent diffusion. Historically, both terms have been used, with the former mostly employed in the decompression arena. Countertransport processes are a concern in mixed gas diving, when differing gas solubilities and diffusion coefficients provide a means for multiple inert gases to move in opposite directions under facilitating gradients. While ambient pressure remains constant, such counterdiffusion currents can temporarily induce high tissue gas supersaturation levels, and greater susceptibility to bubble formation and DCI. In general, problems can be avoided when diving by employing light to heavy (breathing) gas mixture switches, and by using more slowly diffusing gases than the breathing mixture inside enclosure suits (drysuits). Such procedure promotes *isobaric desaturation*, as termed in the lore. The opposite, switching from heavy to light gas mixtures and using more rapidly diffusing gases than the breathing mixture inside exposure suits, promotes *isobaric saturation* and enhanced susceptibility to bubble formation. More simply, the former procedure reduces gas loading, while the latter increases gas loading. The effects of gas switching can be dramatic, as is well known. For instance, a dive to 130 *fsw* for 120 *min* on 80/20 heliox with a switch to 80/20 nitrox at 60 *fws* requires 15 *min* of decompression time, while 210 *min* is required without the switch (Keller and Buhlmann in famous mixed gas tests in 1965). Yet, skin leisions and vestibular dysfunctionality have developed in divers breathing nitrogen while immersed in helium (test chambers and exposure suits).

And nitrogen-to-helium breathing mixture switches are seldom recommended for diving. A closer look at the isobaric countertransport phenomenon is interesting.

In the perfusion case, for a mixture of J gases, the total tissue tension, Π, at time, t, for ambient partial pressure, p_{aj}, and initial partial pressure, p_{ij}, with j denoting the gas species, can be written,

$$\Pi = \sum_{j=1}^{J} [\, p_{aj} + (p_{ij} - p_{aj}) \, exp\,(-\lambda_j t)\,]$$

for, as usual,

$$\lambda_j = \frac{.693}{\tau_j}$$

and τ_j the tissue halftime. In the diffusion case, we similarly find

$$\Pi = \sum_{j=1}^{J} \left[p_{aj} + (p_{ij} - p_{aj}) \frac{8}{\pi^2} \sum_{n=1}^{\infty} \frac{1}{(2n-1)^2} exp\,(-\alpha_{2n-1}^2 D_j t) \right]$$

with,

$$\alpha_{2n-1} = \frac{(2n-1)\pi}{l}$$

for l a characteristic tissue scale parameter, and D_j the tissue diffusivity. These two expressions accommodate a multiplicity of initial conditions, gas switches, and provide a platform to discuss isobaric counterprocesses.

The form of the perfusion and diffusion total tensions, Π, is very similar. In fact, if we assume that the first term in the diffusion case dominates, we can write in general,

$$\Pi = \sum_{j=1}^{J} [p_{aj} + (p_{ij} - p_{aj}) \, exp\,(-\kappa_j t)]$$

with, in the perfusion limit,

$$\kappa_j = \lambda_j$$

and, in the diffusion limit, taking just the first term $(n = 1)$,

$$\kappa_j = \alpha_1^2 D_j = \frac{\pi^2 D_j}{l^2}$$

Simplifying matters by taking the case for two gases, $J = 2$, we have,

$$\Pi = (p_{a1} + p_{a2}) + (p_{i1} - p_{a1}) \, exp\,(-\kappa_1 t) + (p_{i2} - p_{a2}) \, exp\,(-\kappa_2 t)$$

for total tension, Π, as a function of individual gas initial tensions, time, and ambient partial pressures.

A local maxima or minima occurs in the total tension, Π, whenever,

$$\frac{\partial \Pi}{\partial t} = -\kappa_1 (p_{i1} - p_{a1}) \, exp\,(-\kappa_1 t) - \kappa_2 (p_{i2} - p_{a2}) \, exp\,(-\kappa_2 t) = 0$$

for constant ambient partial pressures, p_a. Or, equivalently written,

$$\frac{(p_{i1} - p_{a1})}{(p_{a2} - p_{i2})} = -\frac{\kappa_2}{\kappa_1} exp\left[(\kappa_1 - \kappa_2)t\right]$$

The equation is satisfied at a time, t_m, such that,

$$t_m = \frac{1}{(\kappa_1 - \kappa_2)} \ln\left[\frac{\kappa_2(p_{i2} - p_{a2})}{\kappa_1(p_{i1} - p_{a1})}\right]$$

and represents a local maxima in total tension, Π, if (after some algebra),

$$\left[\frac{\partial^2 \Pi}{\partial t^2}\right]_{t=t_m} < 0$$

or, a local minima, if,

$$\left[\frac{\partial^2 \Pi}{\partial t^2}\right]_{t=t_m} > 0$$

Some interesting features of isobaric counterdiffusion are imbedded in the above relationships, such as flow directionality, time scales, effects of switching, light versus heavy gases, and isobaric supersaturation or desaturation.

With positive time, $t_m > 0$, only two conditions are permissible:

$$\frac{\kappa_1(p_{i1} - p_{a1})}{\kappa_2(p_{a2} - p_{i2})} > 1, \ \kappa_1 > \kappa_2$$

or,

$$\frac{\kappa_1(p_{i1} - p_{a1})}{\kappa_2(p_{a2} - p_{i2})} < 1, \ \kappa_1 < \kappa_2$$

and the argument of the log function must be greater than zero always. The above relationships are complex functions of diffusivities, initial tensions, and ambient tensions before and after gas switching. The former case, $\kappa_1 > \kappa_2$, represents light-to-heavy gas switching (helium-to-nitrogen, for instance, where $\kappa_{He} = 2.7\kappa_{N_2}$), facilitating rapid desaturation of the lighter gas before heavier gas buildup. The latter case, $\kappa_1 < \kappa_2$, enhances supersaturation, as the lighter gas builds up rapidly before the heavier gas is eliminated.

Figure 52 tracks gas supersaturation following nitrogen-to-helium switching due to the isobaric counterdiffusion of both gases. For helium-to-nitrogen switching (usual case for technical and commercial divers), a state of gas desaturation would ensue due to isobaric counterdiffusion.

Oxygen Dose and Toxicity

Decompression sickness could be avoided by breathing just pure oxygen. And the usage of higher concentrations of oxygen in breathing mixtures not only facilitates metabolic function, but also aids in the washout of inert gases such as nitrogen and helium. Despite the beneficial effects of breathing oxygen at higher concentrations, oxygen proves to be toxic in excessive amounts, and over cumulative time intervals. Too little oxygen is equally detrimental to the diver. As discussed, limits to oxygen partial pressures in breathing mixtures range, 0.16 *atm* to 1.6 *atm*, roughly, but symptoms of hypoxia and hyperoxia are dose dependent. Or, in other words, symptom occurrences depend on oxygen partial pressures and exposure times, just like inert gas decompression sickness. The mixed gas diver needs to pay attention not only to helium and nitrogen in staged decompression, but also cumulative oxygen exposure over the dive, and possible underexposure on oxygen depleted breathing mixtures.

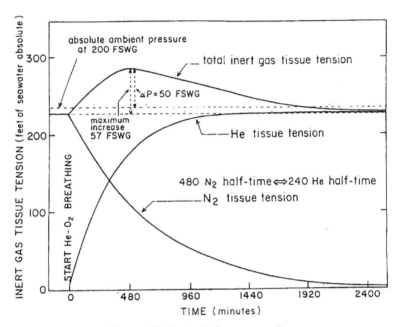

Figure 52. Isobaric Supersaturation

Switching from a heavy to a light breathing mixture results in higher degrees of tissue supersaturation than when breathing one or other gas, as depicted below for a nitrogen-to-helium switch with 480 min N_2 tissue compartment and 240 min He compartment at depth, d = 200 fsw. At zero time, the 80/20 nitrox mixture is switched to 80/20 heliox, assuming equilibration (saturation) on nitrox at that depth. Nitrogen outgasses some 2.85 times slower than helium ingasses, producing a local maxima in the total gas tension at 480 min. Subtracting the inherent unsaturation, the isobaric increase over saturated helium partial pressure is some 50 fsw, not insignificant. If the switch is helium-to-nitrogen a similar state of desaturation would occur.

The neurotoxic actions of high pressure oxygen are thought to relate directly to biochemical oxidation of enzymes, either those linked to membrane permeability or metabolic pathways. The list below is not exhaustive, but includes the following mechanisms:

- the inability of blood to remove carbon dioxide from tissue when hemoglobin is oxygen saturated;
- inhibition of enzymes and coenzymes by lipid peroxides;
- increased concentration of chemical free radicals which attack cells;
- oxidation of membranes and structural deterioration reducing electrical permeability for neuron activation:
- direct oxygen attack on smooth muscle fibres;
- oxygen induced vasoconstriction in arterioles;
- elevation of brain temperature due to lack of replacement of oxygen by carbon dioxide in hemoglobin;
- and, simple chemical kinetic redistribution of cellular carbon dioxide and oxygen with high surrounding oxygen tensions.

Fortunately for the diver, there are ways to avoid complications of hyperoxia. Careful attention to dose (depth-time) limitations for oxygen exposures is needed.

Despite the multiplicity and complexity of the above, limits for safe oxygen exposure are reasonably defined. Table 25 below lists NOAA CNS oxygen exposure time limits, t_x, for corresponding oxygen partial pressures, p_{O_2}. Below 0.5 *atm*, oxygen toxicity (CNS or pulmonary) is not really a problem. Variability in oxygen exposure limits is large, beyond variability in DCS limits for mixed gas exposures. While the 0.5 *atm* lower exposure limit is fairly well accepted, the upper exposure limits in Table 25 are neither hard and fast nor model predictable. Oxygen M-values and tissue compartments have never been specified, quantified, nor tested. In principle, such a construction is possible from existing oxygen data.

Table 25. Oxygen Dose-Time Limits

Oxygen partial pressure p_{O_2} (*atm*)	Oxygen time limit t_x (*min*)	Oxygen tolerance (OTU) Υ (*min*)
1.6	45	87
1.5	120	213
1.4	150	244
1.3	180	266
1.2	210	278
1.1	240	279
1.0	300	300
0.9	360	299
0.8	450	295
0.7	570	266
0.6	720	189

The data in Table 25 is easily fitted to a dose time curve, using least squares, yielding,

$$t_x = exp \left[\frac{3.0 - p_{O_2}}{.36} \right] = 4160 \, exp \, (-2.77 p_{O_2})$$

or, equivalently,

$$p_{O_2} = 3.0 - .36 \, ln \, (t_x)$$

in the same units, that is p_{O_2} and t_x in *atm* and *min* respectively. The last column tabulates a pulmonary exposure dose, Υ, for divers, called the oxygen tolerance unit (OTU), developed by Lambertsen and coworkers at the University of Pennsylvania. Formally, the oxygen tolerance, Υ, is given by,

$$\Upsilon = \left[\frac{p_{O_2} - 0.5}{0.5} \right]^{0.83} t$$

and can be cumulatively applied to diving exposures according to the following prescriptions:

- maintain single dive OTUs below 1440 *min* on the liberal side, or allow for 690 *min* of that as possible full DCI recompression treatment on the conservative side, that is, 750 *min*;
- maintain repetitive total dive OTUs below 300 *min*.

The expression is applied to each and all segments of a dive, and summed accordingly for total OTUs, and then benchmarked against the 750 *min* or 300 *min* rough rule. The 750 *min* and 300 *min* OTU rules are not cast in stone in the diving community, and 10% to 25% variations are common, in both conservative and liberal directions. Figure 53 depicts the depth-time relationships for oxygen dose. Formally, for multiple exposures (multilevel, deco, repetitive), the cumulative OTU, Υ, is the sum of segment doses, Υ_n, with segment times, t_n, and partial oxygen pressures, p_{nO_2}, at each nth segment,

$$\Upsilon = \sum_{n=1}^{N} \Upsilon_n = \sum_{n=1}^{N} \left[\frac{p_{nO_2} - 0.5}{0.5} \right]^{0.83} t_n$$

for N segments.

For exceptional and multiple exposures, the USN and University of Pennslyvania suggest the CNS limits summarized in Table 26, where for multiple exposures, N, and segment times, t_{x_n},

$$T_x = \sum_{n=1}^{N} t_{x_n}$$

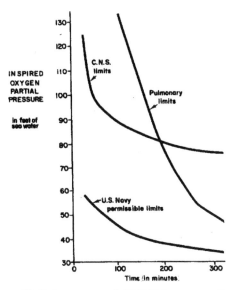

Figure 53. Pulmonary and CNS Tolerance to Oxygen

Oxygen is toxic in excessive amounts. Symptoms become apparent if exposures exceed certain limits, pictorialized below. Partial pressures, p_{O_2}, are in units of fsw, and times, t_x, are in units of min. The marginally safe limits resemble bounce dive curves for DCI, but are more variable between individuals and successive exposures.

Table 26 also summarizes the depth-time relationships for oxygen.

Table 26. Oxygen Exceptional Exposure Time Limits

oxygen partial pressure p_{O_2} (atm)	single exposure t_x (min)	multiple exposures T_x (min)
2.0	30	
1.9	45	
1.8	60	
1.7	75	
1.6	120	15
1.5	150	180
1.4	180	180
1.3	240	210
1.2	270	240
1.1	300	270
0.9	360	360
0.8	450	450
0.7	570	570
0.6	720	720

Note the severe reduction in multiple oxygen exposure time at 1.6 *atm* in Table 26. For this reason, technical divers generally restrict mixed gas diving exposures to $p_{O_2} \leq 1.6$ *atm* throughout any sequence of dives.

A similar toxicity unit, Φ, initially introduced by Lambertsen and called the unit pulmonary toxicity dose (UPTD) is closely related to the OTU, Υ, and is given by,

$$\Phi = \left[\frac{p_{O_2} - 0.5}{0.5} \right]^{1.2} t$$

and weights oxygen partial pressures more than time in dose estimates. Both are employed in the diving community as useful oxygen depth-time limiters.

For the diver, all the foregoing translates into straightforward oxygen management protocols for both CNS and pulmonary toxicity. They are similar to inert gas management, but individual susceptibilities to oxygen seem to vary more widely, though reported statistics are more scattered. Consider CNS oxygen management first, using the CNS clock as it is popularly termed, and then pulmonary oxygen management, using the OTU as described.

- CNS Toxicity Management
  The various oxygen time limits, t_x, tabulated in the Tables above, obviously bound exposures, t, at oxygen partial pressure, p_{O_2}. Converting the exposure time to a fraction of the limit, Ξ_n, we can define a CNS oxygen clock, Ξ, that is over N exposure levels,

$$\Xi = \sum_{n=1}^{N} \Xi_n$$

where,

$$\Xi_n = \frac{t_n}{t_{xn}}$$

for exposure time, t_n, at level, n, with oxygen time limit, t_{xn}. Tabulating Ξ is most easily done by a computer. The prescription might be, depending on degree of conservatism,

$$0.7 \leq \Xi \leq 1.3$$

and where $\Xi = 1$ is the nominal choice. The fit equation for p_{O_2} and t_x suffices to range estimates of Ξ across all depths.

For repetitive dives, a surface interval penalty, similar to the nitrogen penalty in the USN Tables, can be levied for oxygen. A 90 *min* halftime is employed today, that is, the decay constant for residual oxygen CNS management, λ_{O_2}, is,

$$\lambda_{O_2} = \frac{0.693}{90} = 0.0077 \ min^{-1}$$

For surface interval, t, initial CNS clock, Ξ_i, and for 90 *min* folding time, the penalty (or residual) CNS clock, Ξ, is simply,

$$\Xi = \Xi_i \ exp \ (-0.0077t)$$

The residual value is added to the planned repetitive dive additively, just like nitrogen penalty bottom time.

- Pulmonary Toxicity Management
Pulmonary oxygen toxicity, Υ, follows a similar management scheme. As described, the total exposure, Υ, is the sum of interval exposures, Υ_n,

$$\Upsilon = \sum_{n=1}^{N} \Upsilon_n = \sum_{n=1}^{N} \left[\frac{p_{nO_2} - 0.5}{0.5} \right]^{0.83} t_n$$

and is limited,

$$300 \ min \leq \Upsilon \leq 750 \ min$$

depending on desired degree of conservatism, and multiplicity of repetitive dives. Variations of 15% to 25% in the exposure limits are common.

There are many ways to measure oxygen, with devices called oxygen analyzers. They are employed in chemical plants and refineries, hyperbaric chambers, intensive care units, and nurseries. The paramagnetic analyzer is very accurate, and relies on oxygen molecular response to a magnetic field in displacing inert gases from collection chambers. Thermal conductivity analyzers differentiate oxygen and nitrogen conduction properties in tracking temperatures in thermistors, with difference in temperatures proportional to the oxygen concentration. Magnetic wind analyzers combine properties of paramagnetic and thermal analyzers. Polarographic analyzers measure oxygen concentration by resistance changes across permeable oxygen membranes. Galvanic cell analyzers are microfuel cells, consuming oxygen on touch and generating a small current proportional to the amount of oxygen consumed. In all cases, analyzer response is linear in oxygen concentration.

Although it is tempting to avoid problems of oxygen toxicity by maintaining oxygen partial pressures, p_{O_2}, far below toxic limits, this is not beneficial to inert gas elimination (free or dissolved state). Higher levels of inspired oxygen, thus correspondingly lower levels of inert gases, are advantageous in minimizing inert gas buildup and maximizing inert gas washout. Coupled to narcotic potency of helium and nitrogen, and molecular diffusion rates, balancing and optimizing breathing mixtures with decompression requirements is truly a complex and careful technical diving exercise.

Keyed Exercises

- *At elevation, $z = 3,800$ m, what are the working depths, d_{max} and d_{min}, for a 74/26 nitrox mixture, assuming 1.6 atm and .16 atm as the upper and lower oxygen partial pressure limits?*

$$f_{N_2} = .74$$

$$h = 3800 \times \frac{3.28}{1000} = 12.46, \ P_{12.46} = 33 \times exp\ (-.038 \ \times 12.46) \ fsw = 20.55 \ fsw$$

$$\eta d_{max} = \frac{52.8}{f_{O_2}} - P_h \ fsw, \quad \eta d_{min} = \frac{5.3}{f_{O_2}} - P_h \ fsw$$

$$\eta d_{max} = \frac{52.8}{.26} - 20.55 \ fsw = 182.5 \ fsw$$

$$d_{max} = \frac{182.5}{\eta} \ ft = 187.2 \ ft$$

$$\eta d_{min} = \frac{5.3}{.26} - 20.55 \ fsw = -.2 \ fsw \ (means \ surface \ is \ OK)$$

$$d_{min} = -\frac{.2}{\eta} \ ft = -.21 \ ft$$

- What is the equivalent air depth, δ, at ocean depth, $d = 98 \ fsw$, for enriched 74/26 nitrox?

$$f_{N_2} = .74$$

$$\delta = \frac{f_{N_2}}{.79}(33 + d) - 33 = \left[\frac{.74}{.79}\right] \times (33 + 98) - 33 \ fsw = 89.7 \ fsw$$

What is the equivalent depth, δ, for the same mixture and fresh water depth, $d = 98 \ fsw$, at an elevation of 10,000 ft?

$$P_h = 33 \ exp \ (-0.038h) = 33 \ exp \ (-0.038 \times 10) \ fsw = 22.6 \ fsw, \quad h = 10$$

$$\delta = \frac{f_{N_2}}{.79}(P_h + d) - P_h = \left[\frac{.74}{.79}\right] \times (22.6 + 98) - 22.6 \ fsw = 90.3 \ fsw$$

- What is the nitrogen fraction, f_{N_2}, for an equivalent air depth, $\delta = 110 \ fsw$, at ocean depth, $d = 125 \ fsw$?

$$f_{N_2} = \frac{.79(\delta + 33)}{(d + 33)} = \frac{.79 \times 143}{158} = .72$$

What is the corresponding oxygen floor, d_{max}?

$$f_{O_2} = .28, \quad P_0 = 33 \ fsw$$

$$d_{max} = \frac{52.8}{f_{O_2}} - P_0 \ fsw = \frac{52.8}{.28} - 33 = 156 \ fsw$$

- What is the relative concentration, c, of neon dissolved in oil at a partial pressure $p = 9.8 \ atm$?

$$c = Sp = .009 \times 9.8 = .0882$$

- *What is the ratio, ζ, of relative solubilities of neon in water and oil?*

$$\zeta = \frac{S_{water}}{S_{oil}} = \frac{.009}{.021} = .43$$

How many more times, ξ, is nitrogen soluble in oil versus water?

$$\xi = \frac{S_{oil}}{S_{water}} = \frac{.067}{.012} = 5.6$$

- *According to Graham, what roughly is the ratio, ψ, of molecular diffusion speeds of hydrogen to oxygen?*

$$\psi = \left[\frac{A_{O_2}}{A_{H_2}}\right]^{1/2} = \left[\frac{32}{2}\right]^{1/2} = 4$$

- *A commercial diving operation is constructing a set of helium proprietary tables using the popular DCIEM nitrogen tables as a basis before testing. If the spectrum of tissues, τ, in the DCIEM nitrogen tables is (2.5, 5, 10, 20, 40, 80, 160, 320 min), what are the corresponding set for the helium tables, assuming the same critical tensions, M, as the nitrogen tables?*

$$\tau_{He} = \left[\frac{A_{He}}{A_{N_2}}\right]^{1/2} \tau_{N_2} = \left[\frac{4}{28}\right]^{1/2} \tau_{N_2} = .38 \times \tau_{N_2}$$

$$\tau_{He} = (.94,\ 1.89,\ 3.78,\ 7.56,\ 15.12,\ 30.24,\ 60.48,\ 120.96)\ min$$

- *What is the ratio, ζ, of narcotic potency of helium to argon?*

$$\zeta = \frac{v_{He}}{v_{Ar}} = \frac{4.26}{.43} = 9.9$$

Which is the least potent?

$$Least\ Potent\ Gas = Helium$$

- *What is the surface oxygen partial pressure, p_0, for a normoxic breathing mixture at 450 fsw?*

$$p = .21\ atm\ (normoxic),\ \ P_0 = 33\ fsw,\ \ P = 450 + 33\ fsw = 483\ fsw$$

$$p_0 = \frac{P_0}{P}\,p = \frac{33}{483} \times .2\ atm = .0137\ atm$$

What can you say about such a mixture at the surface?

$$p_0 \leq .16\ atm$$

$$Mixture\ Is\ Hypoxic\ (Very\ Hypoxic)$$

- *Assuming surface equilibration on air, what is the total tissue tension, Π, in the, $\tau = 20$ min, compartment after 10 min at depth, $d = 90$ fsw, of a salvage diver breathing 60/25/15 trimix ($f_{He} = .60$, $f_{N_2} = .25$, $f_{O_2} = .15$)?*

$$\Pi = p_{He} + p_{N_2}, \quad d = 90\ fsw, \quad \tau_{N_2} = 20\ min, \quad \tau_{He} = \frac{20}{2.65} = 7.55\ min$$

$$\lambda_{N_2} = \frac{.693}{\tau_{N_2}} = \frac{.693}{20}\ min^{-1} = .0347\ min^{-1}$$

$$\lambda_{He} = \frac{.693}{\tau_{He}} = \frac{.693}{7.55}\ min^{-1} = .0918\ min^{-1}$$

$$p_{aN_2} = f_{N_2}p_a = f_{N_2}(33+d)\ fsw, \quad p_{iN_2} = .79P_0$$

$$p_{aHe} = f_{He}p_a = f_{He}(33+d)\ fsw, \quad p_{iHe} = 0.0\ fsw$$

$$p_{N_2} = p_{aN_2} + (p_{iN_2} - p_{aN_2})\ exp\ (-\lambda_{N_2}t)$$

$$p_{He} = p_{aHe} + (p_{iHe} - p_{aHe})\ exp\ (-\lambda_{He}t)$$

$$p_{iN_2} = .79 \times 33\ fsw = 26.01\ fsw, \quad p_{aN_2} = f_{N_2}p_a = .25 \times 123 = 30.7\ fsw$$

$$p_{N_2} = 30.7 + (26.1 - 30.7)\ exp\ (-.0347 \times 10)\ fsw = 27.4\ fsw$$

$$p_{iHe} = 0.0\ fsw, \quad p_{aHe} = f_{He}p_a = .60 \times 123\ fsw = 73.8\ fsw$$

$$p_{He} = 73.8 - 73.8\ exp\ (-.0918 \times 10)\ fsw = 44.3\ fsw$$

$$\Pi = 27.4 + 44.3\ fsw = 71.7\ fsw$$

What is the critical surfacing tension, M_0, for the 20 min compartment?

$$M_0 = 72\ fsw$$

Can this diver ascend to the surface on his trimix?

Probably — But Slowly

- *What is the critical tension, M, at depth, $d = 34$ fsw, in the helium tissue compartment, $\tau = 15$ min, using the air fit to critical tensions?*

$$\tau = 2.65\tau_{He} = 2.65 \times 15\ min = 39.8\ min, \quad d = 34\ fsw$$

$$M = 152.7\tau^{-1/4} + 3.25\tau^{-1/4}d$$

$$M = 152.7 \times 39.8^{-1/4} + 3.25 \times 39.8^{-1/4} \times 34\ fsw = 104.7\ fsw$$

- *What is the optimal diving mixture for a decompression dive to 300 fsw holding maximum oxygen partial pressure, $p_{O_2} = 1.2$ atm, and maximum nitrogen partial pressure, $p_{N_2} = 3.2$ atm in a fresh water lake at 2,300 ft in the mountains?*

$$\alpha = 0.038, \quad p_{N_2} = 3.2 \ atm, \quad p_{O_2} = 1.2 \ atm$$

$$\eta = 0.975, \quad h = 2.3, \quad d = 300 \ fsw, \quad P_h = 33 \ exp \ (-0.038 \times 2.3) \ fsw = 30.2 \ fsw$$

$$f_{O_2} = \frac{33 p_{O_2}}{\eta d + P_h} = \frac{33 \times 1.2}{.975 \times 300 + 30.2} = .123$$

$$f_{N_2} = \frac{33 P_{N_2}}{\eta d + P_h} = \frac{33 \times 1.2}{.975 \times 300 + 30.2} == .328$$

$$f_{He} = 1 - f_{O_2} - f_{N_2} = 1 - .123 - .328 = .549$$

- If an oil rig diver on 80/20 heliox saturated at $P_i = 6 \ atm$, switches to 80/20 nitrox at $P_a = 4 \ atm$ on ascent, how long after the switch, t_m, does isobaric counterdiffusion produce a minima in total gas tension, Π, in the $\tau_{N_2} = 54 \ min$ compartment?

$$\tau_{N_2} = 54 \ min, \quad \lambda_{N_2} = \frac{.693}{54} \ min^{-1} = .0128 \ min^{-1}$$

$$\tau_{He} = \frac{\tau_{N_2}}{2.7} = \frac{54}{2.7} \ min = 20 \ min, \quad \lambda_{He} = \frac{.693}{20} \ min^{-1} = .0347 \ min^{-1}$$

$$p_{iHe} = f_{He} P_i = .8 \times 6 \ atm = 4.8 \ atm, \quad p_{aHe} = f_{He} P_a = .8 \times 4 \ atm = 3.2 \ atm$$

$$p_{iN_2} = 0 \ atm, \quad p_{aN_2} = f_{N_2} P_a = .8 \times 4 \ atm = 3.2 \ atm$$

$$t_m = \frac{1}{\lambda_{He} - \lambda_{N_2}} \ ln \left[\frac{\lambda_{He}(p_{iHe} - p_{aHe})}{\lambda_{N_2}(p_{aN_2} - p_{iN_2})} \right]$$

$$t_m = \frac{1}{(.0347 - .0128)} \times ln \left[\frac{.0347 \times (4.8 - 3.2)}{.0128 \times (3.2 - 0)} \right] \ min = 13.9 \ min$$

If the gas switch is 80/20 nitrox to 80/20 heliox, how long after the switch (all else the same), t_m, does isobaric counterdiffusion produce a maxima in total gas tension, Π, in the same compartment?

$$p_{iN_2} = 4.8 \ atm, \quad p_{aN_2} = 3.2 \ atm, \quad p_{iHe} = 0 \ atm, \quad p_{aHe} = 3.2 \ atm$$

$$t_m = \frac{1}{\lambda_{N_2} - \lambda_{He}} \ ln \left[\frac{\lambda_{N_2}(p_{iN_2} - p_{aN_2})}{\lambda_{He}(p_{aHe} - p_{iHe})} \right]$$

$$t_m = \frac{1}{(.0128 - .0347)} \times ln \left[\frac{.0128 \times (4.8 - 3.2)}{.0347 \times (3.2 - 0)} \right] \ min = 77.1 \ min$$

- If a fish collector on a heliox rebreather with $p_{O_2} = 1.2 \ atm$ drops to 150 fsw for 20 min, and then spends an additional 45 min on ascent before exiting the water, what does his CNS clock, Ξ, register?

$$p_{O_2} = 1.2 \ atm, \quad t_x = 210 \ min, \quad t = 20 + 45 \ min = 65 \ min$$

$$\Xi = \frac{t}{t_x} = \frac{65}{210} = 0.31$$

After 3 hr on the surface, what is his CNS clock reading?

$$\Xi_i = 0.31, \quad t = 3 \ hr = 180 \ min$$

$$\Xi = \Xi_i \ exp \ (-0.0077t) = 0.31 \ exp \ (-0.0077 \times 180) = 0.31 \times 0.25 = 0.08$$

- *What is the equivalent mixture depth, δ, at ocean depth, $d = 220$ fsw, on 84/16 heliox, using 80/20 heliox tables as the standard?*

$$f_{sk} = f_{80/20} = .80, \quad f_k = f_{84/16} = .84, \quad d = 220 \ fsw, \quad P_h = P_0 = 33 \ fsw$$

$$\delta = \frac{f_k}{f_{sk}}(P_h + d) - P_h$$

$$\delta = \frac{.84}{.80}(33 + 220) - 33 \ fsw = 232 \ fsw$$

- *A tech diver on 12/40 trimix (12% oxygen 40% helium) at 280 fsw for 40 min registers what oxygen toxicity, Υ, as an ascent just begins?*

$$f_{O_2} = 0.12, \quad P_{sur} = 33 \ fsw, \quad d = 280 \ fsw$$

$$p_{O_2} = f_{O_2}\frac{d + P_{sur}}{33} = 0.12 \times \frac{280 + 33}{33} \ atm = 1.14 \ atm$$

$$\Upsilon = \left[\frac{p_{O_2} - 0.5}{0.5}\right]^{0.83} t = \left[\frac{0.64}{0.5}\right]^{0.83} \times 40 \ min = 49.1 \ min$$

What is the corresponding toxic limit, t_x, on this mixture at this depth?

$$t_x = 4160 \ exp\,(-2.77 p_{O_2}), \quad p_{O_2} = 1.14 \ atm$$

$$t_x = 4160 \times exp\,(-2.77 \times 1.14) \ min = 176.8 \ min$$

- *Mark the following statements TRUE or FALSE.*

T	*F*	*Isobaric counterdiffusion refers to gases moving in the same direction.*
T	F	*Pure oxygen is explosive.*
T	F	*EAD references exposures to $f_n = 0.79$.*
T	*F*	*EMD only applies to nitrox mixture.*
T	F	*HPNS is a concern on very deep diving.*
T	F	*Nitrox mixtures having higher oxygen concentrations than air.*
T	*F*	*Nitrox NDLs are shorter than air NDLs at same depth.*
T	F	*Heliox 80/20 NDLs are shorter than nitrox 80/20 NDLs.*
T	*F*	*The onset of full body oxygen toxicity is faster than CNS toxicity.*
T	*F*	*Hydrox is a good deep gas diving mixture.*
T	*F*	*Helium uptake and elimination is slower than nitrogen.*
T	F	*In a mixture, total gas tension is the sum of all gas components.*
T	*F*	*Haldane decompression procedures make deep stops.*
T	F	*Twitching, convulsions, and dizziness are manifestations of CNS.*
T	*F*	*Lower gas solubilities promote bigger bubbles.*
T	F	*Oxygen RBs recirculate and scrub oxygen in the breathing loop.*
T	F	*Best diving mixtures fix maximum oxygen and nitrogen partial pressures.*
T	F	*Oxygen dose and toxicity depend on exposure time and depth.*

- *Match the entries in the first column with the best single entry in the second column.*

(d) Paramagnetic analyzer	(a) Developed first rebreather
(j) Oxygen toxicity	(b) Found way to eliminate HPNS
(h) Isobaric countertransport	(c) Varies inversely with gas atomic mass
(a) Fleuss	(d) Oxygen response to magnetic field
(f) Rebreathers	(e) Inert gas breathing mixtures
(e) Hydrox, trimix, heliox	(f) Scrub carbon dioxide
(c) Saturation and desaturation speed	(g) Proportional to gas solubility
(g) Narcotic potency	(h) Helium and nitrogen moving in opposite directions
(b) Bennett	(i) Oxygen neurotoxicity
(i) Enzyme oxidation	(j) Full body and central nervous system
(l) CNS clock	(k) Oxygen concentration by electrical resistance change
(m) Pulmonary toxicity	(l) Sum of fractional oxygen exposure times
(k) Polarographic analyzer	(m) Limited by exposures of 300-750 min

Part 4

COMPUTING AND DIVING ALGORITHMS

Computing Advances

Computing technology has made incredible progress in the past 65 years. In 1945, there were no stored program computers. Today, a few thousand dollars will purchase a desktop personal computer with more performance, more memory, and more disk storage than a million dollar computer in 1965. This rapid rate of improvement has come from advances in technology used to build the computer and from innovation in computer design. Performance increase is sketched in Figure 54, in terms of a nominal 1965 minicomputer. Performance growth rates for supercomputers, minicomputers, and mainframes are near 20% per year, while performance growth rate for microcomputers is closer to 35% per year. Supercomputers are the most expensive, ranging from one to tens of millions of dollars, and microprocessors are the least expensive, ranging from a few to tens of thousands of dollars. Supercomputers and mainframes are usually employed in high end, general purpose, compute intensive applications. Minicomputers and microprocessors address the same functionality, but often in more diverse roles and applications. The latter class of computers is usually more portable, because they are generally smaller in size. They are on your desktop.

The label *supercomputer* usually refers to the fastest, biggest, and most powerful computer in existence at any time. In the 1940s, supercomputers were employed in the design of nuclear weapons (as still today). In the 1950s, supercomputers were first used in weather forecasting, while in the 1960s, computational fluid dynamics problems in the aerospace industry were solved on supercomputers. In the 1970s, 1980s, and 1990s seismological data processing, oil reservoir simulation, structural analysis of buildings and vehicles, quantum field theory, circuit layout, econometric modeling, materials and drug design, brain tomography and imaging, molecular dynamics, global climate and ocean circulation modeling, and semiconductor fabrication joined the supercomputing revolution. Very few areas in science and engineering have not been impacted by supercomputers. Diving is still on the fringes of supercomputing, but applications are growing, particularly in the areas of dive profile analysis, statistics, data management, and biomodeling. Smaller and less powerful computers are now employed for monitoring, controlling, directing, and analyzing dives, divers, equipment, and environments. Wrist computers perform rudimentary decompression calculations and stage ascents with Haldane models in the past, but with bubble models today.

Operational supercomputers today process data and perform calculations at rates of 10^9 floating point operations per second (*gigaflops*), that is, 10^9 adds, subtracts, multiplies, or divides per second. At the edge today, and in the marketplace, are shared memory processors (SMPs) providing users with 10^{12} floating point operations per second (*teraflops*), impressively opening yet another age in computational science. These machines are massively parallel processors (MPPs), involving thousands of computing nodes processing trillions of data points. To support these raw computing speeds, networks transmitting data at gigabits/sec, and fast storage exchanging terabytes of information over simulation times are also requisite. Ultrafast, high resolution, graphics servers, able to process voluminous amounts of information, offer an expeditious means to assess output data. Differences in raw processing speeds between various components in a high performance computing environment can degrade overall throughput, conditions termed *latencies*, or simply, manifest time delays in processing data. Latencies are parasitic to sustained computing performance. Latencies develop at the nodes connecting various computer, storage, network, terminal, and graphics devices, simply because of impedance mismatch in data handling capabilities.

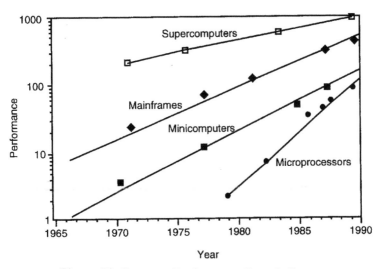

Figure 54. Computer Performance Growth Curves

Computer technology leapfrogs every few years, as seen below. The vertical axis denotes relative performance on a logarithmic scale, and the horizontal axis is the year. Classes of computers are loosely defined in terms of cost and raw power, with supercomputers the most powerful and expensive, and microprocessors the least powerful and expensive.

Obviously, computers work on processing information, doing calculations, and fetching and storing data in steps. A set of operations, performed in sequential fashion by one processor, is termed *serial*. A set of operations performed in any fashion, by any number of processors, is roughly termed *parallel*. Serial computing architectures, once the standard, are now being replaced by parallel computing architectures, with anywhere from tens to thousands of central processing units (CPUs). Processors themselves can be *scalar*, or *vector*, that is, operating on a single entity, or group of entities (numbers).

The architectural feature associated with supercomputers in the 1970s was vector processing. Vector processing allowed large groups of numbers, or vectors, to be processed in parallel, resulting in performance speedups by factors of ten or more (compared to generational improvements on the order of 2 or 3). In the early 1980s, parallel supercomputing was introduced, allowing multiple processors to work concurrently on a single problem. By the end of the century, significantly greater computing parallelism (combining tens of thousands of processing units perhaps), and architectures that integrate modalities, such as numeric and symbolic processing, may be possible. As in the past, software developments on future state of the art supercomputers will probably trail hardware advances, perhaps with increasing distance due to increasingly more complex superparallel systems.

Networks are the backbone of modern computer systems. Supercomputers without high speed communications links and network interfaces are degraded in application processing speed, limited by the slowest component in the computing platform. Gigaflop computers need gigabit/sec network transmission speeds to expedite the flow of information.

Data, voice, image, and full motion video can be digitally encoded, and sent across a variety of physical media, including wire, fiber optics, microwaves, and satellites. The assumption is that all information transmitted will be digital. The greater the number of systems, people, and processes that need to transmit information to one another, the greater the speeds and bandwidths required. Like water in a pipe, to get more information through a network, one can increase the rate of flow (*speed*), and/or increase the amount that can flow through cross sectional area (*bandwidth*). Applications under development today presage the needs to transfer data very quickly tomorrow. To perform as a utility, that is, usefully communicate anything, anytime, anywhere, a network must possess four attributes:

- connectivity—ability to move information regardless of the diversity of the media;
- interoperability—ability of diverse intelligent devices to communicate with one another;
- manageability—ability to be monitored, and to change with applications and devices;
- distributed applications and connective services—ability to provide easy access to tools, data, and resources across different computing platforms, or organizations.

Commercial telecommunications links (modem connections to the Internet) are extremely slow, in the vicinity of 10 kilobits/sec to 56 kilobits/sec. Even dedicated communications lines are low speed, that is, T1 and T3 links (1.4 megabits/sec and 43 megabits/sec respectively), and cannot feed supercomputers with information fast enough to support economical processing. The 4 terabytes from a seismic map of an oil field in the Gulf (8 square miles) would take about 3–4 days to transmit from one site to another for processing. The 1 million dive profiles projected in DAN Project Dive Exploration stacks up to hundreds of gigabytes, depending on resolution.

Advances in massively parallel, large memory computers, and high speed networks have created computing platforms, depicted in Figure 55, which allow researchers to execute supercodes that generate enormous data files. The supercomputing environment depicted in Figure 55 can be found in large Universities, National and Regional Laboratories, dedicated Commercial Computing Centers, and various Governmental Agencies. The one in Figure 55 depicts the superplatform at the Los Alamos National Laboratory. These facilities are available to the commercial user, and computing costs range from $100–$300 per hour on vector supercomputers (YMP, T90, J90) to $1–$4 per node per hour on massively parallel supercomputers (CM5, T3D, SP Cluster, Origin 2000).

Supercodes generate enormous amounts of data, and a typical large application will generate from tens of gigabytes up to several terabytes of data. Such requirements are one to two orders of magnitude greater than the comfortable capacities of present generation storage devices. New high performance data systems (HPDS) are online to meet the very large data storage and handling. Systems consist of fast, large capacity storage devices that are directly connected to a high speed network, and managed by software distributed across workstations. Disk devices are used to meet high speed and fast access requirements, while tape devices are employed to meet high speed and high capacity requirements. Storage devices usually have a dedicated workstation for storage and device management, and to oversee data transfer. Put simply, computer systems use a hierarchy to manage information storage:

- primary storage—fast, solid state memory contained in the processor;
- direct access storage—magnetic or optical disks, connected to the processor, providing fast access;
- sequential access storage—magnetic tape cassettes or microfilm, providing large capacity.

Transfer rates in fast HPDS systems are presently near 800 megabits/sec. Moving down the hierarchy, access time goes up, storage capacity increases, and costs decrease. Today, of all computing components, the cost of storage is decreasing the most rapidly. A few hundred dollars will buy gigabyte hard drives for your PC. Renting storage commercially is also cheap ($20 gigabyte/month).

In supercomputing today, there has been a paradigm shift towards shared memory processors (SMPs), many fast CPUs (64 or more) sharing common memory within an SMP, and communicating with other SMPs across very fast interconnects (switches) using message passing. Since 1999, the technology for their platform development has seen enormous advance, as depicted in Figure 56. Such advancement is ushering in the era of many tens of teraflops raw computing power.

Grand Challenge Applications

Grand Challenge problems are computational problems requiring the fastest computers, networks, and storage devices in existence, and problems whose solutions will have tremendous impact on the economic well being of the United States. Vortices in combustion engines, porous flow in oil bearing substrates, fluid turbulence, three dimensional seismic imaging, ductile and brittle fracture of materials under stress, materials by computer design, global convection of tectonic plates, geomagnetic field generation, ocean and atmospheric circulation, high impact deformation and flow, air and groundwater pollution, global climate modeling, elastic-plastic flow, brain tomography, HIV correlations, bubble generation and cavitating flow, and many others are just such problems. Statistical modeling coupled to maximum likelihood for millions of trials, as employed to estimate DCI incidence in DAN Project Dive Exploration, borders and pushes the Grand Challenge computational problem category, particularly as the number of model fit parameters increases beyond 5.

The scale of computational effort for nominal Grand Challenge problems can be gleaned from Table 27, listing floating point operations, computer memory, and data storage requirements. As a reference point, the 6 million volumes in the Library Of Congress represent 24 terabytes of information. The simulations listed in Table 27 run for hours on the CM5, the Thinking Machines Corporation massively parallel supercomputer. The CM5 is an old (1990s) 1024 node (Sparc processors) MPP supercomputer, with 32 gigabytes of fast memory, access to 450 gigabytes of disk storage, and a peak operational speed of 128 gigaflops. On the present (pedaflops) generation supercomputers, simulation times drop to seconds.

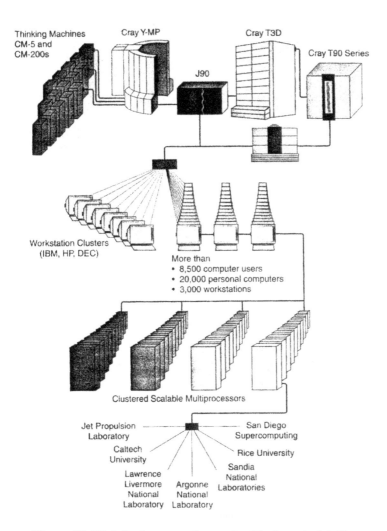

Figure 55. High Performance Computing Platform At LANL

Superplatforms, such as the one depicted below at the Los Alamos National Laboratory, cluster ultra fast supercomputers, high resolution graphics servers, workstations, terminals, archival storage, and high speed networks in user friendly environments.

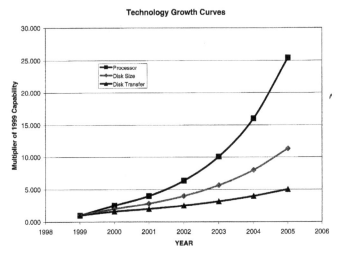

Figure 56. Processor And Disk Technology Growth Curves

Processor and disk technology curves drawn below suggest that technology advances double every few years. Limiting factors are microchip packing density and the speed of light for signal transmission.

Table 27. Grand Challenge Computing Requirements.

Problem	Description	Operations (*number*)	Memory (*terabytes*)	Storage (*terabytes*)
probabilistic decompression	DCI maximum likelihood	10^{14}	.030	.450
porous media	3D immisicible flow	10^{18}	1	4
ductile material	3D molecular dynamics	10^{18}	.30	3
	3D material hydro	10^{18}	1	20
plasma physics	numerical tokamak	10^{18}	1	100
global ocean	century circulation	10^{17}	4	20
brain topology	3D rendering	10^{15}	.015	.001
quantum dynamics	lattice QCD	10^{18}	.008	.008

Scientific advance rests on the interplay between theory and experiment. Computation closes the loop between theory and experiment in quantitative measure. Theory provides the framework for understanding. Experiment and data provide the means to verify and delineate that understanding. Although many disciplines rely on observational data (astronomy, geology, and paleontology, for instance), the hallmark of scientific endeavor is experiment. Clearly, the power of experimental science is its ability to design the environment in which data is gathered. And it is in the design process that modern computers play an important role.

While many believe that good experimentation depends on the skill and imagination of the designer, this is not entirely true. Insight and experience are certainly desirable to determine and optimize measurable response and procedures, but once this has been determined, it is the mathematics that dictates experimental structure, as detailed by Fisher some 70 years ago in noting that the real world is:

- noisy—repeating an experiment under identical conditions yields different results:
- multivariate—many factors potentially affect phenomena under investigation;
- interactive—the effect of one factor may depend on the level of involvement of other factors.

Computers permit extension and analysis of experimental design methodology to problems for which only crude prescriptions have been hitherto available. Computer software is now widely and economically available to automate the basic and most useful procedures. This allows the user without extensive statistical background to routinely employ methods to optimize design.

Certainly, performing numerical experiments on computers, that is, leveraging model predictions to gain insight into phenomena under study, can often provide results that give the best possible estimate of overall experimental response and behavior. The approach here is to use the smallest possible subsets of inputs to run the simulation model, thereby narrowing the focus. In designing experiments, Monte Carlo simulations are used in high energy and accelerator physics, semiconductor fabrication, material damage, neutron and photon shielding, and biomedical dose. Large deterministic modules, in excess of 100,000 lines of code, on the other hand, have been applied to the design of laser fusion target experiments. Similarly, atomistic simulations with millions and, in the future, billions of test atoms provide the opportunity for both fundamental and technological advances in material science. Nonequilibrium molecular dynamics calculations address basic scientific issues, such as interaction potentials and plastic flow. The interaction potentials developed in the last decade for metals, alloys, and ceramics can be used to model prototypical hardness experiments, such as crystal indentation. The underlying mechanisms for plastic flow are microscopic crystal defect motions, and molecular dynamics calculations yield quantitative estimates for hardness experiments. Linkages between experiment and supercomputer modeling are growing in scope and number. Consider some specifics:

- Monte Carlo Bubble Simulations

Monte Carlo calculations explicitly employ random variates, coupled to statistical sampling, to simulate physical processes and perform numerical integrations. In computational science, Monte Carlo methods play a special role because of their combination of immediacy, power, and breadth of application. The computational speed and memory capacity of supercomputers have expedited solutions of difficult physical and mathematical problems with Monte Carlo statistical trials. Although Monte Carlo is typically used to simulate a random process, it is frequently applied to problems without immediate probabilistic interpretation, thus serving as a useful computation tool in all areas of scientific endeavor. Applied to bubble formation and tissue-blood interactions, Monte Carlo methods are truly powerful supercomputing techniques.

The Monte Carlo method is different than other techniques in numerical analysis, because of the use of random sampling to obtain solutions to mathematical and physical problems. A stochastic model, which may or may not be immediately obvious, is constructed. By sampling from appropriate probability distributions, numerical solution estimates are obtained. Monte Carlo calculations simulate the physical processes at each point in an event sequence. All that is required for the simulation of the cumulative history is a probabilistic description of what happens at each point in the history. This generally includes a description of the geometrical boundaries of regions, a description of material composition within each region, and the relative probability (functional) for an *event*. With high speed computers, millions of events can be generated rapidly to provide simulation of the processes defined by the probability function. Statistically, the accuracy of the simulation increases with number of events generated.

The generation of cavitation nuclei in tissue can be effected with Monte Carlo techniques, using the Gibbs potential (bubble formation energy) across liquid-vapor interfaces as a probability function for bubble radius as the random variable. Surrounded by dissolved gas at higher tension for any ambient pressure, bubbles generated can be tracked through growth and collapse cycles in time, allowed to move with surrounding material, coalesced with each other, and removed at external boundaries. Cavitation simulations are applied to multiphase flow in nuclear reactor vessels, cavitation around ship propellors, bubbles in gels, cloud and ice condensation processes in the atmosphere, cosmic ray tracking in chambers, and boiling processes in general.

- Two Phase Porous Flow

Numerical simulations of oil-water fluid flows are a challenging problem, due in part to the complexities of interfacial dynamics and also because of the complexities of geometry. Rather than testing in the field, many oil companies have turned their efforts to the numerical study of pore spaces in oil bearing rock, with high resolution, three dimensional, X-ray scans. Traditional numerical methods have been applied to problems with simple boundaries, but none of the methods apply successfully to the arbitrary geometries found in porous media. Recent emergent numerical techniques on supercomputers, such as derivatives of cellular automata, have demonstrated such capability. Using such cellular methods, it is now possible to study the interactions between oil-water systems and porous rock media.

- HIV Analysis
  Research directed at either finding a cure or vaccine for AIDS is hampered by the extreme variability of the viral genome. Because of this variability, it is difficult to identify targets for drug and vaccine design. Exploiting the speed of modern supercomputers, methods have been developed to test for potentially distant regions in viral proteins that interact. Identifications of interacting sites can be used by experimentalists in finding a vaccine or drug preventing infection or death. Linked positions imply biological correlation of functionality, and are important sites within the virus. A map of interaction zones can be used by experimentalists trying to track and define function regions of the virus. Such maps can be generated rapidly, and in three dimensions, on modern computing platforms with graphics capabilities.

- Groundwater Remediation
  Groundwater contamination occurs commonly throughout the world. According to recent estimates, cleanup costs in the US alone are estimated at $1 trillion. Hence, any information or analysis that provides even minor cost savings for a single site, can have significant impact overall if the information is transferable to disparate sites. Computational experiments performed on modern supercomputers are useful for understanding the complex chemical migration and transformation processes that occur when hazardous substances are released into heterogeneous groundwater systems in a variety quiescent states. Simulations of this sort provide an alternative basis to study detailed behavior under natural and engineered conditions.

- Combustion Vortex Interactions
  Experiments have shown that inducing rotational motions (*vortices*) in the gases of internal combustion engines enhances both turbulence and combustion efficiency. Combustion efficiency is improved because the rotational kinetic energy breaks down into fluid turbulence when the piston approaches the cylinder head. Although a qualitative understanding of the dynamics of vortices has already been obtained, supercomputing power provides the precision and speed to determine when and where vortices develop in combustion engines, questions hitherto obscure to the engine designers.

- Molecular Dynamics
  Material phenomena, such as fracture, dislocation, plasticity, ablation, stress response, and spall are important to the development and manufacture of novel materials. Molecular dynamics simulations on supercomputers, providing

resolution on the *micron* scale, employ millions of interacting molecules to represent states of matter. In such calculations, each molecule moves in the collective force field of all other molecules, and molecular motions of all particles are tracked. This is atomistic physics at the most basic level of interaction.

Supercomputers open up new realms for investigation and enable greater problem domains to be considered. Researchers can develop solutions that treat entire problems from first principles, building from the interactions at the atomic level, all the way up to the macroscopic. As the tool of researcher imagination, new insights and approaches to problem solving are unconstrained.

- Probabilistic Decompression And Maximum Likelihood
  Maximum likelihood is a statistical technique used to fit model equations to a sample with relative probabilities for occurrence and nonoccurrence given. We can never measure any physical variable exactly, that is, without error. Progressively more elaborate experiments or theoretical representation only reduce the error in the determination. In extracting parameter estimates from data sets, it is also necessary to minimize the error (data scatter) in the extraction process. Maximum likelihood is one such technique applied to probabilistic decompression modeling.

DCI is a hit, or (hopefully) no-hit situation, and statistics are binary, as in coin tossing. As a random variable, DCI incidence is a complicated function of many physical variables, such as inert gas buildup, VGE counts, pressure reduction on decompression, volume of separated gas, number of bubble seeds, gas solubility in tissue and blood, ascent rate, nucleation rate, distribution of growing bubble sizes, and combinations thereof. Any, and all of these, can be assigned as risk functions in probabilistic decompression modeling, and associated constants deduced in the maximum likelihood fit process.

Both the LANL Data Bank associated with C&C dive operations and the DAN Project Dive Exploration are programs to collect and analyze data on real dives in real time for profiles, behavioral, and health aspects associated with recreational diving. Studies focus on actual dives and profiles recorded by depth/time computers, and verifies the general condition of the diver up to 48 hours after exiting the water, regarding health problems Upwards of a million dive profiles are anticipated for analyses, mainly because DCI incidence is low probability and many trials are necessary for meaningful modeling, statistics, correlations, and estimates. Multivariate model equations are fitted to the dive profiles and observed DCI incidence rate using maximum likelihood, a technique which minimizes the variance in fitting equations to a collected diving sample. The collected data file sizes to hundreds of gigabytes, and requires gigaflop supercomputing resources for processing. A 10 parameter risk function fit to 1 million dive profiles would take about an hour on the 256 node CRI T3D, an MPP with 16 gigabytes of memory, 65 gigabytes of fast disk, and a peak speed near 38 gigaflops. Run times scale as the number of events times the number of risk function parameters squared.

Multilevel Dive Profile Analysis

Schemes for multilevel diving are employed in the commercial, scientific, and sport sectors. In addition to validation, questions arise as to method consistency with the formulation of the US Navy Tables on critical tension principles. One approach employs back-to-back repetitive sequencing, assigning groups at the start of each multilevel dive segment based on the total bottom time (actual plus residual nitrogen) of the previous segment. Commercially, this procedure is called *repeting − up* for working ascents. At times, the method allows critical tensions, other than the controlling (repetitive) 120 minute compartment tension, to be exceeded upon surfacing. In the context of the US Navy Tables, such circumstance is not tractable. But, by tightening the exposure window and accounting for ascent and descent rates, such a multilevel technique can be made consistent with the permissible tension formulation of the US Navy Tables. Such is the case with dive computers tracking gas exchange across all compartments. Obviously, computers are a nice extension of standard dive tables for any model.

To adequately evaluate multilevel diving within any set of Tables, it is necessary to account for ascent and descent rates. While ascent and descent rates have smaller effect on ingassing and outgassing in slow tissue compartments, ascent and descent rates do impact faster tissue compartments more. And impacts on bubbles are even more pronounced with Boyle effects. Model impact is measured in nitrogen buildup and elimination in hypothetical compartments, whose halftimes denote time to double, or half, existing levels of nitrogen. Buildup and elimination of nitrogen is computed with Haldane tissue equations (exponential rate expressions), and critical tensions, are assigned to each compartment to control diving activity and exposure time. In multilevel diving, computed tissue tensions in any and all compartments must be maintained below their critical values. This is a more stringent constraint than just flooring the 120 *minute* compartment tension, the approach used in the US Navy Tables for repetitive diving.

In the context of the US Navy Tables, from which many Tables with reduced nonstop time limits derive, six compartments with 5, 10, 20, 40, 80, and 120 *minute* halftimes limit diving through maximum tensions (*M*-values) of 104, 88, 72, 58, 52, and 51 *fsw*, respectively. The 5 and 10 *minute* compartments are fast, the 80 and 120 *minute* compartments are slow, and the others are often between, depending on exposure profile. Dive exposure times, depths, ascent, and descent rates, affecting slow and fast compartments in a complicated manner, are virtually infinite in number, thus suggesting the need for both a supercomputer and meaningful representation of the results. A SGI Origin SMP supercomputer addressed the first concern, while the US Navy Tables provided a simple vehicle for representation of results.

Calculations were performed in roughly 1 *minute* time intervals, and 10 *fsw* depth increments for all possible multilevel (ascending or descending) dives up to, and including, the standard US Navy nonstop time limits, and down to a maximum depth of 130 fsw. Ascent and descent rates of 60 fsw/min were employed. Tissue tensions in all six compartments were computed and compared against their M-values. Dives for which the M-values were not violated were stored until the end of the multilevel calculations, for further processing. Dives violating any M-value, at any point in the simulation, were terminated, and the next dive sequence was initiated. The extremes in times for permissible multilevel dives form the envelope of calculations at each depth. The envelope terms out to be very close to the NAUI nonstop limits for the US Navy Tables, that is, the Tables shown in Figure 57. Within a minute, on the conservative side, the envelope tracks the reduced nonstop limits. Approximately 16 million multilevel dives were analyzed on a SGI Origin SMP in about 8 *minutes* CPU time, including construction of the envelope, with 10 fsw and 1 *minute* resolution. The SGI Origin SMP has raw speed near 400 megaflops per CPU.

Adjunct to Figure 57, one can summarize with regard to SMP calculations:

- the deeper the initial depth, the shorter the total multilevel dive time;
- maximum permissible multilevel dive times (total) vary between 100 and 60 *minutes*, depending on initial depths;
- minimum permissible multilevel increments vary from 30 fsw to 10 fsw as the depth decreases from 130 fsw to 40 fsw;
- multilevel US Navy Table dives falling within the envelope never exceed critical values, below or at the surface, in all compartments;
- the multilevel envelope is the set of reduced nonstop limits.

In terms of the modified Tables (Figure 57), multilevel dives that stay to the left of the nonstop time limits never violate critical tensions, and are (hypothetically) sanctioned. Dive computers, of course, perform the same exercise underwater, comparing instantaneous values of computed tissue tensions in all compartments, throughout the duration of the dive, against stored M-values to estimate time remaining and time at a stop.

Keyed Exercises

- *If each volume in the Library of Congress is roughly 3.84 megabytes in storage length, how much computer storage, Σ, will the 6.2 million volumes require?*

$$\Sigma = 3.84 \times 6.2 \times 10^6 = 23.8 \times 10^6 \ megabytes = 23.8 \ terabytes$$

- *Mark the following statements TRUE or FALSE.*

T F *T1 and T3 communications lines are low speed networks.*
T F *Multilevel dive computers use the 120 min tissue to limit ascents.*
T F *Maximum likelihood is a statistical technique for joining models to data.*
T F *Multilevel dive times increase with deeper initial depth*
T F *Wrist dive computers rely only on Haldane staging algorithms.*
T F *A gigaflop is a thousand million operations per second*

T	*F*	Performance growth rates for supercomputers are 50% per year
T	*F*	Latencies increase raw MPP processing speeds
T	F	In the 70s, supercomputers employed vector processing.
T	F	Primary storage has fast solid state memory.
T	*F*	Transmission bandwidth depends on network speed.
T	*F*	Scalar processors process groups of data.
T	F	Repetitive experiments performed under identical conditions yield scattered data.
T	*F*	Haldane wrist computer calculations are Grand Challenge applications.
T	F	Monte Carlo techniques use random sampling of events.
T	*F*	Parallel processors are not limited by network speed.
T	F	Limiting factors for computer speed include chip packing density.
T	F	The speed of light, c, is roughly 3×10^8 m/sec.
T	F	The bubble formation energy can be a bubble probability function.

- How long, t, does it take a signal moving at 1/10 the speed of light to traverse a fibre optic computer cable $l = 18$ m long?

$$v = \frac{1}{10}c = 0.3 \times 10^8 \ m/sec, \quad l = 18 \ m$$

$$t = \frac{l}{v} = \frac{18}{0.3 \times 10^8} \ sec = 60 \times 10^{-8} \ sec = 6 \ nsec.$$

If the signal is an electron, what is its kinetic energy, K?

$$K = E - E_0 = \frac{m_0 c^2}{(1 - v^2/c^2)^{1/2}} - m_0 c^2 \approx m_0 c^2 \left[\frac{v^2}{2c^2} \right]$$

$$K = 0.5 \times 0.01 \times 0.511 \ Mev = 2.6 \ keV$$

- If the signal is a photon, how long does it take to traverse the optic cable?

$$t = \frac{l}{c} = \frac{18}{3 \times 10^9} = 0.6 \ nsec$$

If the frequency of the photon, v, is 1.6×10^{15} sec^{-1}, what is its kinetic energy, K?

$$K = hv = 6.6 \times 10^{-34} \times 1.6 \times 10^{15} \ joule = 10.6 \times 10^{-19} \ joule = 6.6 \ eV$$

Computational Models and Algorithms

The models touched upon earlier address the coupled issues of gas uptake and elimination, bubbles, and pressure changes in different computational approaches. Application of a computational model to staging divers and aviators is often called a diving algorithm. Consider the computational model and staging regimen for 6 popular algorithms, namely, the perfusion limited, diffusion limited, thermodynamic, varying permeability, reduced gradient bubble, and tissue bubble diffusion algorithms:

- Perfusion Limited Algorithm

  Exchange of inert gas, controlled by blood flow rates across regions of varying concentration, is driven by the local gradient, that is, the difference between the arterial blood tension, p_a, and the instantaneous tissue tension, p. Such behavior is modeled in time, t, by simple classes of exponential response functions, bounded by p_a and the initial value of p, denoted p_i. These multitissue functions satisfy a differential perfusion rate equation,

  $$\frac{\partial p}{\partial t} = -\lambda (p - p_a)$$

  and take the form, tracking both dissolved gas buildup and elimination symmetrically,

  $$p - p_a = (p_i - p_a) \, exp \, (-\lambda \, t)$$

  $$\lambda = \frac{.693}{\tau}$$

  with perfusion constant, λ, defined by the tissue halftime, τ. Compartments with 1, 2.5, 5, 10, 20, 40, 80, 120, 180, 240, 360, 480, and 720 minute halftimes, τ, are employed, and halftimes are independent of pressure.

  In a series of dives or multiple stages, p_i and p_a represent extremes for each stage, or more precisely, the initial tension and the arterial tension at the beginning of the next stage. Stages are treated sequentially, with finishing tensions at one step representing initial tensions for the next step, and so on. To maximize the rate of uptake or elimination of dissolved gases the *gradient*, simply the difference between p_i and p_a, is maximized by pulling the diver as close to the surface as possible. Exposures are limited by requiring that the tissue tensions never exceed M, written,

  $$M = M_0 + \Delta M \, d$$

  as a function of depth, d, for ΔM the change per unit depth. A set of M_0 and ΔM are listed in Table 32. In absolute units, the corresponding critical gradient, G, is given by,

  $$G = \frac{M}{.79} - P$$

  with P ambient pressure, and M critical nitrogen pressure. Similarly, the critical ratio, R, takes the form,

  $$R = \frac{M}{P}$$

  At altitude, some critical tensions have been correlated with actual testing, in which case, the depth, d, is defined in terms of the absolute pressure,

  $$d = P - 33$$

  with absolute pressure, P, at altitude, z, given by (fsw),

  $$P = 33 \, exp \, (-0.0381z) = 33 \, \alpha^{-1}$$

$$\alpha = exp\ (0.0381z)$$

and z in multiples of $1000\ feet$. However, in those cases where the critical tensions have not been tested nor extended to altitude, an exponentially decreasing extrapolation scheme, called *similarity*, has been employed. Extrapolations of critical tensions, below $P = 33\ fsw$, then fall off more rapidly then in the linear case. The similarity extrapolation holds the ratio, $R = M/P$, constant at altitude. Denoting an equivalent sea level depth, δ, at altitude, z, one has for an excursion to depth d,

$$\frac{M(d)}{d+33\alpha^{-1}} = \frac{M(\delta)}{\delta+33}$$

so that the equality is satisfied when,

$$\delta = \alpha d$$

$$M(\delta) = \alpha M(d).$$

Considering the minimum surface tension pressure of bubbles, G^{min} (near $10 fsw$), as a limit point, the similarity extrapolation should be limited to 10,000 $feet$ in elevation, and neither for decompression, nor heavy repetitive diving.

As described previously, depth-time exposures are often limited by a law of the form,

$$d t_n^{1/2} = H$$

with t_n the nonstop time limit, and $400 \leq H \leq 500\ fsw\ min^{1/2}$. One can obtain the corresponding tissue constant, λ, controlling the exposure at depth d, for nonstop time t_n, by differentiating the tissue equation with respect to depth, d, and setting the result to zero. With $p_a = 0.79(d+33)$ at sea level, there results,

$$1 - exp\ (-\lambda t_n)(1 + 2\ \lambda t_n) = 0.$$

Corresponding critical tensions, M, are then easily obtained using d, λ, and t_n. In the above case, the transcendental equation is satisfied when,

$$\lambda t_n = 1.25$$

Time remaining before a stop, time at a stop, or surface interval before flying can all be obtained by inverting the tissue equation. Denoting the appropriate critical tension at some desired stage, M, and the instantaneous tension at that time, p, at stage, p_a, the time remaining, t_r, follows from,

$$t_r = \frac{1}{\lambda} \ln \left[\frac{p - p_a}{M - p_a} \right]$$

for each compartment, λ. Obviously, the smallest t_r controls the ascent.

- **Diffusion Limited Algorithm**
  Exchange of inert gas, controlled by diffusion across regions of varying concentration, is also driven by the local gradient. As before, denoting the arterial blood tension, p_a, and instantaneous tissue tension, p, the gas diffusion equation takes the form in one dimensional planar geometry,

$$D\frac{\partial^2 p}{\partial x^2} = \frac{\partial p}{\partial t}$$

with D a single diffusion coefficient appropriate to the media. Using standard techniques of separation of variables, with ω^2 the separation constant (eigenvalue), the solution is written,

$$p - p_a = (p_i - p_a) \sum_{n=1}^{\infty} W_n \, sin \, (\omega_n x) \, exp \, (-\omega_n^2 Dt)$$

assuming at the left tissue boundary, $x = 0$, we have $p = p_a$, for W_n a set of constants obtained from the initial condition. First, requiring $p = p_a$ at the right tissue boundary, $x = l$, yields,

$$\omega_n = \frac{n\pi}{l}$$

for all n. Then, taking $p = p_i$ at $t = 0$, multiplying both sides of the diffusion solution by $sin \, (\omega_m x)$, integrating over the tissue zone, l, and collecting terms gives,

$$W_{2n} = 0$$

$$W_{2n-1} = \frac{4}{(2n-1)\pi}$$

Averaging the solution over the tissue domain eliminates spatial dependence, that is $sin \, (\omega_n x)$, from the solution, giving a bulk response,

$$p - p_a = (p_i - p_a) \sum_{n=1}^{\infty} \frac{8}{(2n-1)^2 \, \pi^2} exp \, (-\omega_{2n-1}^2 Dt).$$

The expansion resembles a weighted sum over *effective* tissue compartments with time constants, $\omega_{2n-1}^2 D$, determined by diffusivity and boundary conditions. Diffusion models fit the time constant, κ,

$$\kappa = \pi^2 D l^2$$

to exposure data, with a typical value employed by the Royal Navy given by,

$$\kappa = 0.007928 \, min^{-1}.$$

The approach is aptly single tissue, with equivalent tissue halftime, τ_D,

$$\tau_D = \frac{.693}{\kappa} = 87.5 \, min$$

close to the US Navy 120 *minute* compartment used to control saturation, decompression, and repetitive diving. Corresponding critical tensions in the bulk model, take the form,

$$M = \frac{709\, P}{P + 404}$$

falling somewhere between fixed gradient and multitissue values. At the surface, $M = 53\, fsw$, while at $200 fsw$, $M = 259\, fsw$. A critical gradient, G, satisfies,

$$G = \frac{M}{.79} - P = \frac{P\,(493 - P)}{(P + 404)}.$$

The limiting features of bulk diffusion can be gleaned from an extension of the above slab model in the limit of thick tissue region, that is, $l \to \infty$. Replacing the summation over n with an integral as $l \to \infty$, we find

$$p - p_a = (p_i - p_a)\, \overline{erf}\, [l/(4Dt)^{1/2}]$$

with $\overline{erf}$ the average value of the *error − function* over l, having the limiting form (Abramowitz and Stegun),

$$\overline{erf}\, [l/(4Dt)^{1/2}] = 1 - \frac{(4Dt)^{1/2}}{l\pi^{1/2}}$$

for short times, and

$$\overline{erf}\, [l/(4Dt)^{1/2}] = \frac{l}{(4\pi Dt)^{1/2}}$$

for long times.

Unlike the perfusion case, the diffusion solution, consisting of a sum of exponentials in time, cannot be formally inverted to yield time remaining, time at a stop, nor time before flying. Such information can only be obtained by solving the equation numerically, that is, with computer or hand calculator for given M, p, and p_a.

If we wrap the above planar geometry around into a hollow cylinder of inner radius, a, and outer radius, b, we generate Krogh geometry. The hollow cylindrical model retains all the features of the planar model, and additionally includes curvature for small a and b, with $l = b - a$ from before. Assigning the same boundary conditions at a and b, namely, the tissue tension, p, equals the arterial tension, p_a, writing the diffusion equation in radial cylindrical coordinates,

$$D\frac{\partial^2 p}{\partial r^2} + \frac{D}{r}\frac{\partial p}{\partial r} = \frac{\partial p}{\partial t}$$

and solving yields,

$$p - p_a = (p_i - p_a) \sum_{n=1}^{\infty} X_n\, U_0(\varepsilon_n r)\, exp\,(-\varepsilon_n^2 Dt)$$

with X_n a constant satisfying initial conditions, U_0 the cylinder functions (Abramowitz and Stegun), and ε_n the eigenvalues satisfying,

$$U_0(\varepsilon_n a) = \frac{\partial U_0(\varepsilon_n b/2)}{\partial r} = 0$$

Averaging over the tissue region, $a \leq r \leq b$, finally gives,

$$p - p_a = (p_i - p_a) \frac{4}{(b/2)^2 - a^2} \sum_{n=1}^{\infty} \frac{1}{\varepsilon_n^2} \frac{J_1^2(\varepsilon_n b/2)}{J_0^2(\varepsilon_n a) - J_1^2(\varepsilon_n b/2)} \ exp \ (-\varepsilon_n^2 Dt)$$

with J_1 and J_0 Bessel functions, order 1 and 0. Typical vascular parameters are bounded,

$$0 < a \leq 4 \ microns$$

$$10 \leq b \leq 32 \ microns.$$

- Thermodynamic Algorithm
  The thermodynamic model couples both the tissue diffusion and blood perfusion equations. Cylindrical symmetry is assumed in the model. From a boundary vascular zone of thickness, a, gas diffuses into the extended extravascular region, bounded by b. The radial diffusion equation is given by,

$$D\frac{\partial^2 p}{\partial r^2} + \frac{D}{r}\frac{\partial p}{\partial r} = \frac{\partial p}{\partial t}$$

with the tissue tensions, p, equal to the venous tensions, p_v, at the vascular interfaces, a and b. The solution to the tissue diffusion equation is given previously,

$$p - p_v = (p_i - p_v) \frac{4}{(b/2)^2 - a^2} \sum_{n=1}^{\infty} \frac{1}{\varepsilon_n^2} \frac{J_1^2(\varepsilon_n b/2)}{J_0^2(\varepsilon_n a) - J_1^2(\varepsilon_n b/2)} \ exp \ (-\varepsilon_n^2 Dt)$$

with ε_n eigenvalue roots of the boundary conditions,

$$J_0(\varepsilon_n a) \, Y_1(\varepsilon_n b/2) - Y_0(\varepsilon_n a) \, J_1(\varepsilon_n b/2) = 0$$

for J and Y Bessel and Neumann functions, order 1 and 0. Perfusion limiting is applied as a boundary condition through the venous tension, p_v, by enforcing a mass balance across both the vascular and cellular regions at a,

$$\frac{\partial p_v}{\partial t} = -\kappa \ (p_v - p_a) - \frac{3}{a} S_p \ D \left[\frac{\partial p}{\partial r}\right]_{r=a}$$

with S_p the ratio of cellular to blood gas solubilities, κ the perfusion constant, and p_a the arterial tension. The coupled set relate tension, gas flow, diffusion and perfusion, and solubility in a complex feedback loop.

The thermodynamic trigger point for decompression sickness is the volume fraction, χ, of separated gas, coupled to mass balance. Denoting the separated gas partial pressure, P_{N_2}, under worse case conditions of zero gas elimination upon decompression, the separated gas fraction is estimated,

$$\chi \, P_{N_2} = S_c \, (p - P_{N_2})$$

with S_c the cellular gas solubility. The separated nitrogen partial pressure, P_{N_2} is taken up by the inherent unsaturation, and given by (fsw),

$$P_{N_2} = P + 3.21$$

in the original Hills formulation, but other estimates have been employed. Mechanical fluid injection pain, depending on the injection pressure, δ, can be related to the separated gas fraction, χ, through the tissue modulus, K,

$$K\chi = \delta$$

so that a decompression criteria requires,

$$K\chi \leq \delta$$

with δ in the range, for $K = 3.7 \times 10^4 \, dyne \, cm^{-2}$,

$$0.34 \leq \delta \leq 1.13 \, fsw.$$

Identification of the separated phase volume as a critical indicator is a significant development in decompression theory.

- Varying Permeability Algorithm
  The critical radius, r_i, at fixed pressure, P_0, represents the cutoff for growth upon decompression to lesser pressure. Nuclei larger than r_i will all grow upon decompression. Additionally, following an initial compression, $\Delta P = P - P_0$, a smaller class of micronuclei of critical radius, r, can be excited into growth with decompression. If r_i is the critical radius at P_0, then, the smaller family, r, excited by decompression from P, obeys,

$$\frac{1}{r} = \frac{1}{r_i} + \frac{\Delta P}{158}$$

with ΔP measured in fsw, and r in $microns$. Table 32 lists critical radii, r, excited by sea level compressions ($P_0 = 33 \, fsw$), assuming $r_i = .8 \, microns$. Entries also represent the equilibrium critical radius at pressure, P.
The permissible gradient, G, is written for each compartment, τ, using the standard formalism,

$$G = G_0 + \Delta G d$$

at depth $d = P - 33 \, fsw$. A nonstop bounce exposure, followed by direct return to the surface, thus allows G_0 for that compartment. Both G_0 and ΔG are tabulated in Table 2, with ΔG suggested by Buhlmann. The minimum excitation, G^{min}, initially probing r, and taking into account regeneration of nuclei over time scales τ_r, is (fsw),

$$G^{min} = \frac{2\,\gamma\,(\gamma_c - \gamma)}{\gamma_c\,r(t)} = \frac{11.01}{r(t)}$$

with,

$$r(t) = r + (r_i - r)\,[1 - exp\,(-\lambda_r t)]$$

γ, γ_c film, surfactant surface tensions, that is, $\gamma = 17.9\,dyne/cm$, $\gamma_c = 257\,dyne/cm$, and λ_r the inverse of the regeneration time for stabilized gas micronuclei (many days). Prolonged exposure leads to saturation, and the largest permissible gradient, G^{sat}, takes the form (fsw), in all compartments,

$$G^{sat} = \frac{58.6}{r} - 49.9 = .372\,P + 11.01.$$

On the other hand, G^{min} is the excitation threshold, the amount by which the surrounding tension must exceed internal bubble pressure to just support growth. Although the actual size distribution of gas nuclei in humans is unknown, experiments *in vitro* suggest that a decaying exponential is reasonable,

$$n = N\,exp\,(-\beta r)$$

with β a constant, and N a convenient normalization factor across the distribution. For small values of the argument, βr,

$$exp\,(-\beta r) = 1 - \beta r$$

as a nice simplification. For a stabilized distribution, n_0, accommodated by the body at fixed pressure, P_0, the excess number of nuclei, Λ, excited by compression-decompression from new pressure, P, is,

$$\Lambda = n_0 - n = N\,\beta\,r_i\,\left[1 - \frac{r}{r_i}\right].$$

For large compressions- decompressions, Λ is large, while for small compressions-decompressions, Λ is small. When Λ is folded over the gradient, G, in time, the product serves as a critical volume indicator and can be used as a limit point in the following way.

The rate at which gas inflates in tissue depends upon both the excess bubble number, Λ, and the gradient, G. The critical volume hypothesis requires that the integral of the product of the two must always remain less than some limit point, $\alpha\,V$, with α a proportionality constant,

$$\int_0^\infty \Lambda G dt = \alpha V$$

for V the limiting gas volume. Assuming that gradients are constant during decompression, t_d, while decaying exponentially to zero afterwards, and taking the limiting condition of the equal sign, yields simply for a bounce dive, with λ the tissue constant,

$$\Lambda G \left(t_d + \lambda^{-1}\right) = \alpha V.$$

In terms of earlier parameters, one more constant, δ, closes the set, defined by,

$$\delta = \frac{\gamma_c \, \alpha \, V}{\gamma \, \beta \, r_i \, N} = 7180 \; fsw \; min$$

so that,

$$\left[1 - \frac{r}{r_i}\right] G \left(t_d + \lambda^{-1}\right) = \delta \, \frac{\gamma}{\gamma_c} = 500.8 \; fsw \; min.$$

The five parameters, γ, γ_c, δ, λ_r, r_i, are five of the six fundamental constants in the varying permeability model. The remaining parameter, λ_m, interpolating bounce and saturation exposures, represents the inverse time constant modulating multidiving. Bubble growth experiments suggest that λ_m^{-1} is in the neighborhood of an hour. Discussion of λ follows in the next section (RGBM).

The depth at which a compartment controls an exposure, and the excitation radius as a function of halftime, τ, in the range, $12 \leq d \leq 220 \; fsw$, satisfy,

$$\frac{r}{r_i} = 0.90 - 0.43 \; exp \left(-\zeta \tau\right)$$

with $\zeta = 0.0559 \; min^{-1}$. The regeneration constant, λ_r, is on the order of inverse days, that is, $\lambda_r = 0.0495 \; days^{-1}$. Characteristic halftimes, τ_r and τ_h, take the values $\tau_r = 14 \; days$ and $\tau_h = 12.4 \; min$. For large τ, r is close to r_i, while for small τ, r is on the order of $0.5 \, r_i$. At sea level, $r_i = 0.8 \; microns$ as discussed.

- Reduced Gradient Bubble Algorithm

  The phase integral for multiexposures is written,

$$\sum_{j=1}^{J} \left[\Lambda G \, t_{d_j} + \int_0^{t_j} \Lambda G dt\right] \leq \alpha V$$

with the index j denoting each dive segment, up to a total of J, and t_j the surface interval after the jth segment. For the inequality to hold, that is, for the sum of all growth rate terms to total less than αV, obviously each term must be less the αV. Assuming that $t_J \rightarrow \infty$, gives,

$$\sum_{j=1}^{J-1} \left[\Lambda G \left[t_{d_j} + \lambda^{-1} - \lambda^{-1} exp \left(-\lambda t_j\right)\right]\right] + \Lambda G \left(t_{d_J} + \lambda^{-1}\right) \leq \alpha V.$$

Defining G_j,

$$\Lambda G_j \left(t_{d_j} + \lambda^{-1}\right) = \Lambda G \left(t_{d_j} + \lambda^{-1}\right) - \Lambda G \, \lambda^{-1} exp \left(-\lambda t_{j-1}\right)$$

for $j = 2$ to J, and,

$$\Lambda G_1 = \Lambda G$$

for $j = 1$, it follows that

$$\sum_{j=1}^{J} \Lambda\, G_j\, (t_{d_j} + \lambda^{-1}) \leq \alpha\, V$$

with the important property,

$$G_j \leq G.$$

This implies we employ reduced gradients extracted from bounce gradients by writing,

$$G_j = \xi_j\, G$$

with ξ_j a *multidiving* fraction requisitely satisfying,

$$0 \leq \xi_j \leq 1$$

so that, as needed,

$$\Lambda G_j \leq \Lambda G.$$

The fractions, ξ, applied to G always reduce them. As time and repetitive frequency increase, the body's ability to eliminate excess bubbles and nuclei decreases, so that we restrict the permissible bubble excess in time by writing,

$$\Lambda(t_{j-1}^{cum}) = N r_i \left[1 - \frac{r(t_{j-1}^{cum})}{r_i} \right] = \Lambda\, exp\, (-\lambda_r t_{j-1}^{cum})$$

$$t_{j-1}^{cum} = \sum_{i=1}^{j-1} t_i$$

with t_{j-1}^{cum} cumulative dive time. A reduction factor, η_j^{rg}, accounting for creation of new micronuclei is taken to be the ratio of present excess over initial excess, written,

$$\eta_j^{rg} = \frac{\Lambda(t_{j-1}^{cum})}{\Lambda} = exp\, (-\lambda_r t_{j-1}^{cum})$$

For reverse profile diving, the gradient is restricted by the ratio (minimum value) of the bubble excess on the present segment to the bubble excess at the deepest point over segments. The gradient reduction, η_j^{rd}, is then written,

$$\eta_j^{rd} = \frac{(\Lambda)_{max}}{(\Lambda)_j} = \frac{(rd)_{max}}{(rd)_j}$$

with rd the product of the appropriate excitation radius and depth. Because bubble elimination periods are shortened over repetitive dives, compared to intervals for bounce dives, the gradient reduction, η_j^{rp}, is proportional to the difference between maximum and actual surface bubble inflation rate, that is,

$$\eta_j^{rp} = 1 - \left[1 - \frac{G^{min}}{G} \right] exp\, (-\lambda_m t_{j-1})$$

with t_{j-1} consecutive total dive time, λ_m^{-1} on the order of an hour, and G^{min} the smallest G_0 in Table 2.

Finally, for multidiving, the gradient reduction factor, ξ, is defined by the product of the three η,

$$\xi_j = \eta_j^{rd} \, \eta_j^{rp} \, \eta_j^{rg} = \frac{(\Lambda)_{max}}{(\Lambda)_j} \left[1 - \left(1 - \frac{G^{min}}{G} \right) exp \left(-\lambda_m t_{j-1} \right) \right] exp \left(-\lambda_r t_{j-1}^{cum} \right)$$

with t_{j-1} consecutive dive time, and t_{j-1}^{cum} cumulative dive time, as noted. Since bubble numbers increase with depth, reduction in permissible gradient is commensurate. Multiday diving is mostly impacted by λ_r, while repetitive diving mostly by λ_m. Obviously, an equivalent critical tension, M, takes the form,

$$M = \xi (G_0 + \Delta Gd) + P.$$

- Tissue Bubble Diffusion Algorithm
  Bubbles shrink or grow according to a simple radial diffusion equation linking total gas tension, Π, ambient pressure, P, and surface tension, γ, to bubble radius, r,

$$\frac{\partial r}{\partial t} = \frac{DS}{r} \left[\Pi - P - \frac{2\gamma}{r} \right]$$

with D the gas diffusion coefficient, and S the gas solubility. Bubbles grow when the surrounding gas tension exceeds the sum of ambient plus surface tension pressure, and vice versa. Higher gas solubilities and diffusivities enhance the rate. Related bubble area, A, and volume, V, changes satisfy,

$$\frac{\partial A}{\partial t} = 8\pi r \frac{\partial r}{\partial t}$$

$$\frac{\partial V}{\partial t} = 4\pi r^2 \frac{\partial r}{\partial t}$$

Using Fick's law, a corresponding molar current, J, of gas into, or out of, the bubble is easily computed assuming an ideal gas,

$$J = -\frac{DS}{RTh} \left[\Pi - P - \frac{2\gamma}{r} \right]$$

for R the ideal gas constant, T the temperature, and h an effective diffusion barrier thickness. And the molal flow rate is just the molal current times the interface area, that is,

$$\frac{\partial n}{\partial t} = JA$$

for n the number of moles of gas. The change in pressure and volume of the bubble, due to gas diffusion, follows simply from the ideal gas law,

$$\frac{\partial (PV + 2\gamma r^{-1}V)}{\partial t} = R \frac{\partial (nT)}{\partial t}$$

for V the bubble volume.

Certainly, the above constitute a coupled set of differential equations, solvable for a wide range of boundary and thermodynamic conditions connecting the state variables, namely, P, V, Π, r, n, and T.

A bubble dose, based on the hypothetical volume of an expanding test bubble, is linked to decompression data for the exposure. Maximum likelihood regression is used to correlate bubble dose with DCI risk, as seen in Figure 5.

Model and Table Reverse Profile Comparisons

Though the manifestations of DCI are statistically distributed, tables and meters use deterministic models to stage divers, with models broadly categorized as Haldane (dissolved phase) or bubble (combinations of dissolved and free phases). And model differences depend on profiles, exposures, and model assumptions. For diversity, we will focus on reverse diving profiles (RPs), wherein the second dive is deeper than the previous in any repetitive sequence. A summary of models, their underpinnings, correlations with data, and predictions for 100/60 and 60/100 RPs with variable surface intervals are first presented, and then for deeper and greater reverse profile increments.

Diving models address the coupled issues of gas uptake and elimination, bubbles, and pressure changes in different computational frameworks. Application of a computational model to staging divers, recall, is called a diving algorithm. Consider the foregoing computational models and staging regimens for the popular algorithms, namely, the perfusion limited, diffusion limited, thermodynamic, varying permeability, reduced gradient bubble, and tissue bubble diffusion algorithms The first two are Haldane models (workhorse algorithms in most tables and meters), while the remaining four are bubble models in the generic sense (coming online in tables and meters, often driven by tech diving). The first two track just dissolved gas transfer, using *critical tissue tensions* as limit points, while the latter four treat both dissolved and free phase transfer, using *free phase volumes* as limit points.

- Comparative Model Reverse Profiles
  Employing the above described algorithms, we consider model predictions for RPs, extract underlying features and tendencies, and draw comparisons. The code, *DECOMP*, containing a number of model kernels, is employed for calculations.

  The RPs (100/60 and 60/100) are normalized to roughly the same NDLs so that the nonstop time limits at 100 *fsw* and 60 *fsw* are 15 *min* and 50 *min*, respectively. This normalization leans slightly toward the conservative side as far as NDLs are concerned. Table 28 encapsulates the results for the MTM, BDM, TM, VPM, RGBM, and TBDM. Typically, tracking bubble growth and dissolved gas buildup and elimination, phase models require slightly more decompression times for the RPs. The MTM and BDM are comparable, the TM, VPM, and TBDM also track closely, and the RGBM is most conservative. These profiles are relatively shallow, and the RP increment is small ($\Delta d =$

40 *fsw*). Generally, bubble models affect deep and prolonged exposures the most, requiring deeper stops, but usually shorter overall decompression times. The effect is not seen here trendwise, but will reappear as the RP increments increase. Bubble and Haldane models overlap for short and shallow exposures, such as these RPs, and entries in Table 28 are no exception. The observation has often been made that not much free gas phase has been excited during short and shallow exposures, and then, bubble models should collapse to dissolved gas phase models in the limit.

When exposures are deeper and RP increments are greater than 40 *fsw*, model differentiations between dissolved gas and dual phase models appear in the staging regimens, as seen in Table 29, contrasting the MTM and RGBM only for 160/40 and 40/160 RPs. Clearly phase models (RGBM) require deeper staging but shorter times, as seen in Table 29 for the same surface intervals in Table 28. The bottom times are 7 *min* and 100 *min* at 160 *fsw* and 40 *fsw* respectively in Table 29.

- NEST Reverse Profile Data
  The Nuclear Emergency Strategy Team (NEST) is involved in counterterrorism and countermeasures related to nuclear and biological threats. Exercises and tests have yielded scattered data about RPs across a spectrum of breathing gas mixtures (nitrox, heliox, trimix). Recent activities have settled on trimix as the bottom and ascent gas, with pure oxygen breathed at 20 *fsw*. Mixtures range 13–40% helium, 44–64% nitrogen, and 16–30% oxygen. RP increments, Δd, vary from 40–120 *fsw*, and surface intervals are nominally greater than 60 *min*. The RGBM is the staging algorithm.
  Table 30 tabulates results of NEST field activities, with nominal surface intervals of an hour or more. Maximum bottom depth is 250 *fsw*, and exposures are near trimix NDLs. Dives are grouped in RP categories of 40 *fsw*. The NDLs computed from the RGBM for trimix in the range down to 250 *fsw* are roughly:

100 *fsw*	8–10 *min*
150 *fsw*	5–7 *min*
200 *fsw*	4–6 *min*
250 *fsw*	2–3 *min*

similar in duration to Haldane trimix NDLs. The ascent profile is different under the RGBM, as compared to standard Haldane staging. And this is well known, especially in technical diving circles where mixed gas diving pushes the exposure envelope.

Table 28. Comparative RPs And Algorithms

Algorithm	Dive 1	Deco 1	Surface Interval	Dive 2	Deco 2
MTM	100/15	none	30	60/30	10/2
BDM		none			10/2
TM		none			10/1
VPM		none			10/2
RGBM		none			10/4
TBDM		none			10/3
MTM	60/30	none		100/15	10/2
BDM		none			10/2
TM		none			10/2
VPM		none			10/3
RGBM		none			10/5
TBDM		none			10/3
MTM	100/15	none	60	60/30	10/1
BDM		none			10/1
TM		none			10/1
VPM		none			10/2
RGBM		none			10/4
TBDM		none			10/2
MTM	60/30	none		100/15	10/1
BDM		none			10/1
TM		none			10/1
VPM		none			10/3
RGBM		none			10/6
TBDM		none			10/2
MTM	100/15	none	120	60/30	none
BDM		none			none
TM		none			10/1
VPM		none			10/1
RGBM		none			10/3
TBDM		none			10/1
MTM	60/30	none		100/15	10/1
BDM		none			10/1
TM		none			10/1
VPM		none			10/2
RGBM		none			10/4
TBDM		none			10/2
MTM	100/15	none	240	60/30	none
BDM		none			none
TM		none			none
VPM		none			none
RGBM		none			10/1
TBDM		none			10/1
MTM	60/30	none		100/15	none
BDM		none			none
TM		none			none
VPM		none			10/1
RGBM		none			10/2
TBDM		none			10/1

Table 29. Comparative MTM And RGBM (Deep) RPs

Algorithm	Dive 1	Deco 1	Surface Interval	Dive 2	Deco 2
MTM	160/7	10/3	30	40/100	none
RGBM		10/1			10/4
MTM	40/100	none		160/7	10/11
RGBM		none			30/1,20/1,10/2
MTM	160/7	10/3	60	40/100	none
RGBM		10/1			10/3
MTM	40/100	none		160/7	10/3
RGBM		none			20/1,10/2
MTM	160/7	10/3	120	40/100	none
RGBM		10/1			10/2
MTM	40/100	none		160/7	10/3
RGBM		none			20/1,10/1
MTM	160/7	10/3	240	40/100	none
RGBM		10/1			10/1
MTM	40/100	none		160/7	10/3
RGBM		none			20/1,10/1

The incidence rate, p, in Table 30 is 6.7%, with highest count in the 40–120 fsw increment range. There are many variables here, such as staging depth, gas mixture, exposure time, and surface interval not tabulated separately.

Table 30. NEST RP Risk Table

Dives	RP Increment (fsw)	Probable Hits
36	0 - 40	0
18	40 -80	2
6	80 - 120	2

Practices for the deeper increments may border the yo-yo category, though no prior history of repetitive diving existed. Exercises continue, and data will grow. Trends are apparent in the above Table 6, but further analysis is required.

- Comparative NAUI Table Reverse Profiles
  NAUI Training adopts a conservative view on RPs, contraindicated over many hour time intervals. Within the NAUI Tables (US Navy Tables with reduced NDLs), implications of this approach are discussed and quantified. NAUI Training has an admirable record of diving safety and surety, and statistics underscore this fact. And so do other Training Agencies (PADI, SSI, YMCA, NASDS, TDI).

  The US Navy Tables with reduced NDLs and the NAUI modifications based on consideration of multilevel activity (ascending or descending profiles) were discussed. For reference and comparison, a set of NAUI (modified) US Navy Tables is given in Figure 57, exhibiting reduced nonstop time limits, consistent with present safety margins associated with lower Doppler scores (Spencer reduction). But there is much more to the NAUI modification of the basic US Navy Tables, based on multilevel considerations. And that modification, coupled to recommended 1 *hr* surface intervals (SI) for repetitive diving, also impacts RPs favorably, as will be shown.

For the modified Tables (Figure 57), multilevel dives that stay to the left of the nonstop time limits never violate critical tensions, and are (hypothetically) sanctioned. Dive computers, of course, perform the same exercise underwater, comparing instantaneous values of computed tissue tensions in all compartments, throughout the duration of the dive, against stored M-values to estimate time remaining and time at a stop.
The set of NAUI NDLs corresponds to a reduced set of critical tensions, M_0, ΔM, given by,

$$M_0 = 102,\ 86,\ 70,\ 57,\ 51,\ 50\ fsw$$

$$\Delta M = 2.27,\ 2.01,\ 1.67,\ 1.34,\ 1.26,\ 1.19$$

in round numbers for the same set of tissue halftimes, τ. With risk analysis performed by US Navy investigators, the relative probability, p, of DCI in (always) diving to the NAUI NDLs limits is bounded by,

$$1\% < p < 5\%$$

yet remembering that divers never dive consistently to (any) Table limits. Interpolating between bounding NDLs, the estimated probability, p, is

$$p < 2.5\%$$

at the limit point of diving to NAUI NDLs. Simple difference weighting between bounding NDLs and NAUI NDLs was invoked for the estimate. Consider the scripted RPs within the NAUI Table framework. In a rather simple sense, these RPs represent multilevel diving with nonzero surface intervals, at least when only dissolved gases are tracked. However, with bubble growth under decompression fueled by high tissue tensions, such extensions and analogies probably breakdown. Profiles are 100 *fsw* and 60 *fsw* for 15 *min* and 30 *min* as also contrasted in Table 28.

Table 31. NAUI Tables and RPs

Algorithm	Dive 1	Deco 1	Surface Interval	Dive 2	Deco 2
NAUI Tables	100/15	none	30	60/30	15/5
	60/30	none		100/15	15/15
	100/15	none	60	60/30	none
	60/30	none		100/15	15/15
	100/15	none	120	60/30	none
	60/30	none		100/15	15/5
	100/15	none	240	60/30	none
	60/30	none		100/15	none

Clearly the step nature of Table decompression formats is evident in Table 31. The decompression stops at 15 fsw do not smoothly decrease in time as surface interval time increases. NAUI, of course, requires all training to be nonstop diving, so such profiles would not occur routinely.

- NAUI Reverse Profile Statistics
In the 10 years since NAUI introduced these Tables, nearly 1,000,000 divers were certified at an entry level. This represents some 5,000,000 actual dives, mainly performed above 60 fsw, with surface intervals beyond 60 min, and no more than 2 dives per day. Reverse profiles are not suggested, and training regimens also mandate minimum 60 min surface intervals, depth floors at 60 fsw, and less than 3 dives per day. To build diver confidence, much activity occurs at depths in the 20–30 fsw range. All recreational NAUI diving is limited to 130 fsw, as are the NAUI Tables. These limits and mandates restrict all diving, and certainly impact RPs favorably.

Accident reports gathered by NAUI in this time average 50 per year (required for insurance and liability coverage). Of these 50 reports, only 5 relate (average) to DCI afflictions. This suggests an incidence rate, p, on the order of 1×10^{-5}, certainly a very low annual rate. Other Training Agencies (PADI, SSI, YMCA, NASDS, TDI) should echo the same ballpark figure, since training regimens across recreational diving are roughly the same.

Thus, any RPs probably range 30–40 fsw as far as depth increment, Δd, in training maneuvers. This is small, as are actual training depths. Based on low DCI incidence rate, NAUI Table conservatism, small RP increment, and shallow staging depths, RPs appear to have not been a major problem for NAUI Training Operations. But as RP depths and increments increase, the situation becomes less clear and riskier.

Keyed Exercises

- *Solve the perfusion rate equation for the tissue tension, p, as a function of time?*

$$\frac{\partial p}{\partial t} = -\lambda(p - p_a)$$

$$y = p - p_a, \quad dy = dp$$

$$\frac{dy}{y} = -\lambda dt$$

$$\ln y = -\lambda t + \ln c \quad (c \text{ is integration constant})$$

$$y = c \exp(-\lambda t), \quad t = 0, \quad p = p_i, \quad y = p_i - p_a = c$$

$$p - p_a = (p_i - p_a) \exp(-\lambda t)$$

- *For a depth-time law of the form, $dt_n^{1/2} = C$, what is the nonstop time limit for compartment, $\tau = 45$ min, and what is the depth, d, for $C = 450$ fsw $min^{1/2}$?*

$$\lambda t_n = 1.25, \quad \tau = 45 \text{ min}$$

$$t_n = \frac{1.25}{\lambda} = \frac{1.25\tau}{.693} = \frac{1.25 \times 45}{.693} \text{ min} = 81.2 \text{ min}$$

$$dt_n^{1/2} = C = 450 \text{ fsw } min^{1/2}$$

$$d = \frac{C}{t_n^{1/2}} = \frac{450}{81.2^{1/2}} \text{ fsw} = 49.9 \text{ fsw}$$

- *Average the diffusion limited tissue response over length, l, to eliminate spatial dependences?*

$$p - p_a = (p_i - p_a) \sum_{n=1}^{\infty} W_n \frac{1}{l} \int_0^l \sin(\omega_n x) dx \exp(-\omega_n^2 Dt)$$

$$p - p_a = (p_i - p_a) \sum_{n=1}^{\infty} \frac{2W_n}{\omega_n} \exp(-\omega_n^2 Dt)$$

$$p - p_a = (p_i - p_a) \sum_{n=1}^{\infty} \frac{8}{(2n-1)^2 \pi^2} \exp(-\omega_{2n-1}^2 Dt)$$

- *Given temporal diffusion length, $\zeta = l/D^{1/2} = 10 \ sec^{1/2}$, what are short and long time values of the bulk diffusion response function?*

$$p - p_a = (p_i - p_a) \left[1 - \frac{(4Dt)^{1/2}}{l\pi^{1/2}} \right] \ (short)$$

$$p - p_a = (p_i - p_a) \left[1 - \frac{.4t^{1/2}}{\pi^{1/2}} \right]$$

$$p - p_a = (p_i - p_a) \frac{l}{(4\pi Dt)^{1/2}} \ (long)$$

$$p - p_a = (p_i - p_a) \frac{10}{(4\pi t)^{1/2}}$$

- In the VPM and RGBM, a normalized distribution of bubble seeds, n, in radii r, is assumed to be excited by compression-decompression, and takes the form,

$$n = N\beta \ exp \ (-\beta r)$$

with N and β distribution constants. If the excess, Λ, excited into growth by compression-decompression is just the difference between the total number at r_0 and the total number at r, with r and r_0 linked by the magnitude of the pressure change, ΔP, compute Λ for r and r_0, normalizing over all radii?

$$\Lambda = \int_r^\infty n dr - \int_{r_0}^\infty n dr = N \left[\int_r^\infty exp \ (-\beta r) dr - \int_{r_0}^\infty exp \ (-\beta r) dr \right]$$

$$\Lambda = N \left[exp \ (-\beta r) - exp \ (-\beta r_0) \right]$$

For small argument, a, one has, $exp \ (-a) = 1 - a$, so obtain a small argument expression for the bubble excess, Λ?

$$\Lambda = N \left[1 - \beta r - 1 + \beta r_0 \right] = N \left[\beta r_0 - \beta r \right]$$

- Formally evaluate the phase volume integral, assuming constant gradients, G, during decompression, and exponentially decaying gradients afterwards, with tissue decay constant, λ, assuming λt_d is small?

$$G \rightarrow G \ 0 \le t \le t_d, \ G \rightarrow G \ exp \ (-\lambda t) \ t_d < t$$

$$\int_0^\infty \Lambda G dt = \int_0^{t_d} \Lambda G dt + \int_{t_d}^\infty \Lambda G dt = \alpha V$$

$$\int_0^\infty \Lambda G dt = \Lambda G \int_0^{t_d} dt + \Lambda G \int_{t_d}^\infty exp \ (-\lambda t) dt = \Lambda G t_d + \lambda^{-1} \Lambda G \ exp \ (-\lambda t_d)$$

$$\int_0^\infty \Lambda G dt = \Lambda G \left[t_d + \lambda^{-1} \ exp \ (-\lambda t_d) \right]$$

$$exp \ (-\lambda t_d) \rightarrow 1, \ \lambda t_d << 1$$

$$\int_0^\infty \Lambda G dt \rightarrow \Lambda G \left[t_d + \lambda^{-1} \right] \rightarrow \alpha V$$

- *What is the minimum excitation gradient, G^{min}, and saturation gradient, G^{sat}, for seeds of radius, $r = .5$ microns, according to the VPM and RGBM?*

$$G^{min} = \frac{11.01}{r}, \quad G^{sat} = \frac{58.6}{r} - 49.9$$

$$G^{min} = \frac{11.01}{.5} \, fsw = 22.02 \, fsw$$

$$G^{sat} = \frac{58.6}{.5} - 49.9 \, fsw = 67.3 \, fsw$$

What is the corresponding pressure, P, for this saturation gradient?

$$G^{sat} = .372P + 11.01$$

$$P = \frac{G^{sat}}{.372} + 26.6 = \frac{67.3}{.372} + 26.6 \, fsw = 207.5 \, fsw$$

- *Using the TBDM, couple the bubble volumetric growth rate to corresponding molal diffusion current and rate of pressure change for constant temperature?*

$$\frac{\partial(PV + 2V\gamma r^{-1})}{\partial t} = R\frac{\partial(nT)}{\partial t}$$

$$V\frac{\partial P}{\partial t} + P\frac{\partial V}{\partial t} + \frac{2\gamma}{r}\frac{\partial V}{\partial t} - \frac{2V\gamma}{r^2}\frac{\partial r}{\partial t} = TR\frac{\partial n}{\partial t}$$

$$\frac{\partial r}{\partial t} = \frac{1}{4\pi r^2}\frac{\partial V}{\partial t}$$

- *In the TM, assuming $J_0(a) \to 1$ and $J_1(a) \to a$, for small a, expand the tissue response function?*

$$p - p_v = (p_i - p_v)\frac{16}{b^2 - 4a^2}\sum_{n=1}^{\infty}\frac{1}{\varepsilon_n^2}\frac{J_1^2(\varepsilon_n b/2)}{J_0^2(\varepsilon_n a) - J_1^2(\varepsilon_n b/2)} \, exp\left(-\varepsilon_n^2 Dt\right)$$

$$p - p_v = (p_i - p_a)\frac{16}{b^2 - 4a^2}\sum_{n=1}^{\infty}\frac{1}{\varepsilon_n^2}\frac{(\varepsilon_n b/2)^2}{1 - (\varepsilon_n b/2)^2} \, exp\left(-\varepsilon_n^2 Dt\right)$$

$$p - p_v = (p_i - p_v)\sum_{n=1}^{\infty}\left[\frac{16}{(\varepsilon_n b)^2 - (2\varepsilon_n a)^2}\right]\left[\frac{(\varepsilon_n b)^2}{4 - (\varepsilon_n b)^2}\right] \, exp\left(-\varepsilon_n^2 Dt\right)$$

Protocols

Operational diving requires arbitrary numbers of dives to various depths over periods of hours, and often days. Once a standard set of decompression tables has been constructed, with bounce diving the simple case of nonstop decompression, a repetitive dive procedure is a necessity. After any air dive, variable amounts of dissolved and free residual nitrogen remain in body tissues for periods of 24 *hr*, and more. Similarly, elevated tissue tensions can promote, or sustain, bubble growth over the same time scales. This residual gas buildup (dissolved and free) will shorten the exposure time for subsequent repetitive dives. The longer and deeper the first dive, the greater the amount of residual tissue nitrogen affecting decompression on subsequent dives. Nonstop depth-time allowances for repetitive dives are reduced in such circumstance. Within bubble models, residual free gas phases are also included in procedures, imposing additional constraints on repetitive diving. The many possibilities are easily tracked in continuous time mode by computers, as mentioned, but tables face a more difficult task.

Tables

Considering only dissolved gases, one standard table approach, developed by Workman, groups combinations of depth and exposure times according to the surfacing tension in the slowest compartment. Then it is possible to account for desaturation during any arbitrary surface interval. The remaining excess nitrogen at the start of the next dive can always be converted into equivalent time spent at the deepest point of the dive. So called penalty time is then added to actual dive time to updated appropriate tissue tensions. Surfacing tensions in excess of 33 fsw (absolute) in the slowest compartment are assigned letter designations (groups), A to O, for each 2 fsw over 33 fsw. Any, and all, exposures can be treated in this manner. To credit outgassing, a Surface Interval Table, accounting for 2 fsw incremental drops in tensions in the slowest compartment, is also constructed. Such procedures are bases for the US Navy Air Decompression and Repetitive Surface Interval Tables, with the 120 min compartment (the slowest) controlling repetitive activity. Standard US Navy Tables provide safe procedures for dives up to 190 fsw for 60 min. Dives between 200 and 300 fsw were tested and reported in the exceptional exposure US Navy tables, including a 240 min compartment. The Swiss tables, compiled by Buhlmann, incorporate the same basic procedures, but with a notable exception. While the US Navy tables were constructed for sea level usage, requiring some safe extrapolation procedure to altitude, the Swiss tables are formulated and tested over a range of reduced ambient pressure. The controlling repetitive tissue in the Buhlmann compilation is the 635 min compartment. Similar approaches focusing on deep and saturation diving have resulted in decompression tables for helium-oxygen (heliox), helium-oxygen-nitrogen (trimix), and recent mixtures with some hydrogen (hydrox). Clearly, the USN and Swiss Repetitive Tables can be easily converted to other (longer or shorter) controlling tissues by arithmetic scaling of the 120 min or 635 min compartment to the desired controlling tissue halftime (simple ratio). To scale the USN Tables to 720 min, for instance, the repetitive intervals need only be multiplied by $720/120 = 6$.

While it is true that the table procedures just described are quite easily encoded in digital meters, and indeed such devices exist, digital meters are capable of much more than table recitations. Pulsing depth and pressure at short intervals, digital meters can monitor diving almost continuously, providing rapid estimates of any model parameter. When employing the exact same algorithms as tables, meters provide additional means to control and safety beyond table lookup. When model equations can be inverted in time, meters can easily compute time remaining before decompression, time at a stop, surface interval before flying, and optimal ascent procedure. Profiles can be stored for later analysis, and the resulting data bank used to tune and improve models and procedures. Considering utility and functionality, meter usage is increasing in diving, supported by technological advance in computing power, algorithmic sophistication, and general acceptance, though it will probably be some time before tables are eliminated, particularly in the training and technical diving arena.

A set of (modified) USN Tables is given in Figure 57. The set has reduced nonstop time limits, consistent with present safety margins associated with lower Doppler scores (Spencer reduction).

Meters

On the heels of growing interest in underwater science and exploration following World War II, monitoring devices have been constructed to control diver exposure and decompression procedures. Devices, with records of varying success, include mechanical and electrical analogs, and within the past 15 years, microprocessor based digital computers. With inexpensive microprocessor technology, recent years have witnessed explosive growth in compact digital meters usage. All use the simple dissolved tissue gas model proposed by Haldane some 100 years ago, but given the sophistication of these devices, many feel that broader models can be incorporated into meter function today, increasing their range and flexibility. Although the biophysics of bubble formation, free and dissolved phase buildup and elimination is formidable, and not fully understood yet, contemporary models treating both dissolved and free phases, correlated with existing data, and consistent with diving protocols might extend the utility of diving computers. An approach treating bubble nucleation, excitation, and growth in tissue and blood is needed. In the industry, such new models are termed bubble mechanical, because they focus on bubbles and their interactions with dissolved gas in tissue and blood.

Decompression computers are moderately expensive items these days. Basically a decompression meter is a microprocessor computer consisting of a power source, pressure transducer, analog to digital signal converter, internal clock, microprocessor chip with RAM (random access memory) and ROM (read only memory), and pixel display screen. Pressure readings from the transducer are converted to digital format by the converter, and sent to memory with the elapsed clock time for model calculations, usually every 1–3 *sec.* Results are displayed on the screen, including time remaining, time at a stop, tissue gas buildup, time to flying, and other model flag points, usually Haldanian (perfusion) tissue control variables. Some 3–9 volts is sufficient power to drive the computer for a couple of years, assuming about 100 dives per year. The ROM contains the model program (step application of model equations), all constants, and queries the transducer and clock. The RAM maintains storage registers for all dive calculations ultimately sent to the display screen. Dive computers can be worn on the wrist, incorporated in consoles, or even integrated into *heads – up* displays in masks. A typical dive computer is schematized in Figure 58.

Statistics point to an enviable track record of decompression meter usage in nominal diving activities, as well as an expanding user community. When coupled to slow ascent rates and safety stops, computer usage has witnessed a very low incidence rate of decompression sickness, below 0.01% according to some reports. Computers for nitrox are presently online today, with heliox and trimix units a rather simple modification of any nitrox unit, using existing decompression algorithms. Technical divers, on mixed gases and making deep decompression dives on OC and RB systems use modern dive computers based on bubble models as backup for their activities. The modern technical diver relies mostly on wrist slates for decompression schedules extracted from Tables and software, and blended with a particular brand of personal safety gained from knowledge and experience. Deep stops are integral part of their diving activities, whether bubble models propose them exactly or are juxta positioned on their ascent profiles by diver choice. These computer units are not inexpensive, but their use is expanding across both technical and recreational diving. So is decompression diving across all sectors of exploration, scientific, military, and related endeavors.

Model History

Tables and schedules for diving at sea level can be traced to a model proposed in 1908 by the eminent English physiologist, John Scott Haldane. He observed that goats, saturated to depths of 165 feet of sea water (*fsw*), did not develop decompression sickness (DCS) if subsequent decompression was limited to half the ambient pressure. Extrapolating to humans, researchers reckoned that tissues tolerate elevated dissolved gas pressures (tensions), greater than ambient by factors of two, before the onset of symptoms. Haldane then constructed schedules which limited the critical supersaturation ratio to two in hypothetical tissue compartments. Tissue compartments were characterized by their halftime, τ. Halftime is also termed *halflife* when linked to exponential processes, such as radioactive decay. Five compartments (5, 10, 20, 40, 75 *min*) were employed in decompression calculations and staged procedures for fifty years. The paradigm used by Haldane to stage divers was to bring them as close as possible to the surface and decompress in the shallow zone. Most of his testing followed such procedure. However, and not well known, is the fact that Haldane also tested deeper staging, where divers were not brought to the shallow zone, instead making deep stops on their way to the surface. This deep stop procedure was requisite to adequately and safely decompress divers. Unfortunately, in subsequent years, as world Navies tested new schedules, the deep stop regimen escaped further testing, completely replaced by the shallow staging approach. This is changing today and more will follow on the subject of deep stops.

Some years following, in performing deep diving and expanding existing table ranges in the 1930s, US Navy investigators assigned separate limiting tensions (*M*-values) to each tissue compartment.

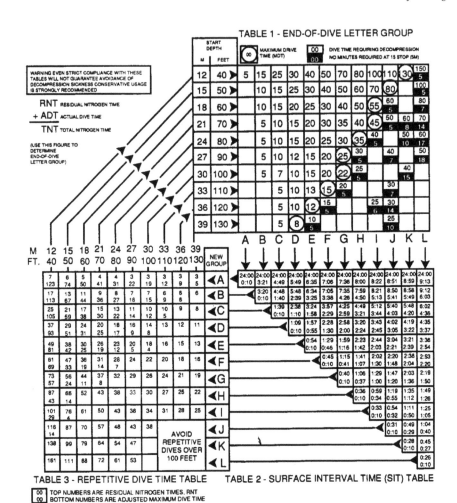

Figure 57. Modified Multilevel USN Tables

The Tables below have reduced nonstop time limits (NDLs), consistent with present safety margins assigned by lowering Doppler scores. The NDLs are also the permissible envelope for USN Table multilevel diving, with back-to-back repetitive sequencing. Computer simulations show that the NDLs are the limit points, in that no USN critical tensions are violated by multilevel diving, not just the 120 min tissue compartment. Multilevel dives must stay to the right of the modified NDLs. In the commercial diving industry, this is the repet — up procedure for systematic working ascents.

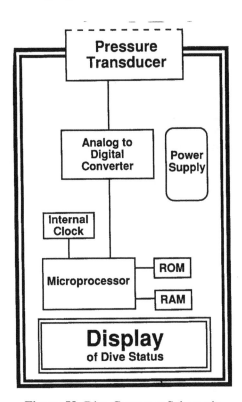

Figure 58. Dive Computer Schematic

Dive computers are fairly rapid microprocessors these days, consisting of pressure transducer, analog to digital signal converter (for pressure reading), internal clock, power supply, ROM and RAM for processing information and performing rapid calculations online.

Later in the 1950s and early 1960s, other USN investigators and divers, in addressing repetitive exposures and staging regimens for the first time, advocated the use of six tissues (5, 10, 20, 40, 80, 120 *min*) in constructing decompression schedules, with each tissue compartment again possessing its own limiting tension. Temporal uptake and elimination of inert gas was based on mechanics addressing only the macroscopic aspects of gas exchange between blood and tissue. Exact bubble production mechanisms, interplay of free and dissolved gas phases, and related transport phenomena were not quantified, since they were neither known nor understood. Today, we know more about dissolved and free phase dynamics, bubbles, and transport mechanisms, but still rely heavily on the Haldane model. Inertia and simplicity tend to sustain its popularity and use, and it has been a workhorse.

Bulk Diffusion Model

Diffusion limited gas exchange is modeled in time by a sum of exponential response functions, bounded by arterial and initial tissue tensions. However, instead of many tissue compartments, a single bulk tissue is assumed for calculations, characterized by a gas diffusion constant, D. Tissue is separated into intravascular (blood) and extravascular (cells) regions. Blood containing dissolved inert and metabolic gases passes through the intravascular zone, providing initial and boundary conditions for subsequent gas diffusion into the extravascular zone. Diffusion is driven by the difference between arterial and tissue tensions, according to the strength of a single diffusion coefficient, D, appropriate to the media. Diffusion solutions, averaged over the tissue domain, resemble a weighted sum over effective tissue compartments with time constants, $\lambda_{2n-1} = \alpha_{2n-1}^2 D$, determined by diffusivity and boundary conditions, with $\alpha_{2n-1} = (2n-1)\pi/l$ for tissue thickness, l.

Applications fit the time constant, $K = \pi^2 D/l^2$, to exposure data, with a typical value employed by the Royal Navy given by, $K = 0.007928\ min^{-1}$, approximating the US Navy 120 *min* compartment used to control saturation, decompression, and repetitive diving. Corresponding critical tensions in the bulk model,

$$M = \frac{709P}{P+404},$$

fall somewhere between fixed gradient and multitissue values. At the surface, $M = 53\ fsw$, while at 200 fsw, $M = 259\ fsw$. A critical gradient,

$$G = \frac{P(493-P)}{(P+404)},$$

also derives from the above. Originally, a critical gradient, G, near 30 fsw was used to limit exposures. Such value is too conservative for deep and bounce exposures, and not conservative enough for shallow exposures. Hempleman introduced the above relationship, providing the means to parameterize bounce and saturation diving.

Bulk diffusion models (BDM) are attractive because they permit the whole dive profile to be modeled with one equation, and because they predict a $t^{1/2}$ behavior of gas uptake and elimination. Nonstop time limits, t_n, are related to depth, d, by the bulk diffusion relationship,

$$dt_n^{1/2} = C,$$

with approximate range, $400 \leq C \leq 500\ fsw\ min^{1/2}$, linking nonstop time and depth simply through the value of C. For the US Navy nonstop limits, $C \approx 500\ fsw\ min^{1/2}$, while for the Spencer reduced limits, $C \approx 465\ fsw\ min^{1/2}$. In the Wienke-Yount model, $C \approx 400\ fsw\ min^{1/2}$.

Multitissue Model

Multitissue models (MTM), variations of the original Haldane model, assume that dissolved gas exchange, controlled by blood flow across regions of varying concentration, is driven by the local gradient, that is, the difference between the arterial blood tension and the instantaneous tissue tension. Tissue response is modeled by exponential functions, bounded by arterial and initial tensions, and perfusion constants, λ, linked to the tissue halftimes, τ, for instance, 1, 2, 5, 10, 20, 40, 80, 120, 180, 240, 360, 480, and 720 *min* compartments assumed to be independent of pressure.

In a series of dives or multiple stages, initial and arterial tensions represent extremes for each stage, or more precisely, the initial tension and the arterial tension at the beginning of the next stage. Stages are treated sequentially, with finishing tensions at one step representing initial tensions for the next step, and so on. To maximize the rate of uptake or elimination of dissolved gases the gradient, simply the difference between arterial and tissue tensions is maximized by pulling the diver as close to the surface as possible. Exposures are limited by requiring that the tissue tensions never exceed

$$M = M_0 + \Delta M \, d,$$

as a function of depth, d, for ΔM the change per unit depth. A set of M_0 and ΔM are listed in Table 32.

Table 32. Classical US Navy Surfacing Ratios and Critical Tensions.

Halftime τ (*min*)	Critical ratio R_0	Critical tension M_0 (*fsw*)	Tension change ΔM
5	3.15	104	2.27
10	2.67	88	2.01
20	2.18	72	1.67
40	1.76	58	1.34
80	1.58	52	1.26
120	1.55	51	1.19

At altitude, some critical tensions have been correlated with actual testing, in which case, an effective depth, d, is referenced to the absolute pressure, P (in *fsw*),

$$d = P - 33$$

with surface pressure, P_h, at elevation, h, given by,

$$P_h = 33 \, exp \, (-0.0381h)$$

for h in multiples of 1,000 *ft*. However, in those cases where critical tensions have not been tested, nor extended, to altitude, an exponentially decreasing extrapolation scheme, called similarity, has been employed. Extrapolations of critical tensions, below $P = 33$ *fsw*, then fall off more rapidly then in the linear case. A similarity extrapolation holds the ratio, $R = M/P$, constant at altitude. Estimating minimum surface tension pressure of bubbles near 10 *fsw*, as a limit point, the similarity extrapolation might be limited to 10,000 ft in elevation, and neither for decompression nor heavy repetitive diving.

Models of dissolved gas transport and coupled bubble formation are not complete, and all need correlation with experiment and wet testing. Extensions of basic (perfusion and diffusion) models can redress some of the difficulties and deficiencies, both in theory and application. Concerns about microbubbles in the blood impacting gas elimination, geometry of the tissue region with respect to gas exchange, penetration depths for gas diffusion, nerve deformation trigger points for pain, gas uptake and elimination asymmetry, effective gas exchange with flowing blood, and perfusion versus diffusion limited gas exchange, to name a few, motivate a number of extensions of dissolved gas models.

The multitissue model addresses dissolved gas transport with saturation gradients driving the elimination. In the presence of free phases, free-dissolved and free-blood elimination gradients can compete with dissolved-blood gradients. One suggestion is that the gradient be split into two weighted parts, the free-blood and dissolved-blood gradients, with the weighting fraction proportional to the amount of separated gas per unit tissue volume. Use of a split gradient is consistent with multiphase flow partitioning, and implies that only a portion of tissue gas has separated, with the remainder dissolved. Such a split representation can replace any of the gradient terms in tissue response functions.

If gas nuclei are entrained in the circulatory system, blood perfusion rates are effectively lowered, an impairment with impact on all gas exchange processes. This suggests a possible lengthening of tissue halftimes for elimination over those for uptake, for instance, a 10 *min* compartment for uptake becomes a 12 *min* compartment on elimination. Such lengthening procedure and the split elimination gradient obviously render gas uptake and elimination processes asymmetric. Instead of both exponential uptake and elimination, exponential uptake and linear elimination response functions can be used. Such modifications can again be employed in any perfusion model easily, and tuned to the data.

Thermodynamic Model

The thermodynamic model (TM) suggested by Hills, and extended by others, is more comprehensive than earlier models, addressing a number of issues simultaneously, such as tissue gas exchange, phase separation, and phase volume trigger points. This model is based on phase equilibration of dissolved and separated gas phases, with temporal uptake and elimination of inert gas controlled by perfusion and diffusion. From a boundary (vascular) thin zone, gases diffuse into the cellular region. Radial, one dimensional, cylindrical geometry is assumed as a starting point, though the extension to higher dimensionality is straightforward. As with all dissolved gas transfer, diffusion is controlled by the difference between the instantaneous tissue tension and the venous tension, and perfusion is controlled by the difference between the arterial and venous tension. A mass balance for gas flow at the vascular cellular interface, enforces the perfusion limit when appropriate, linking the diffusion and perfusion equations directly. Blood and tissue tensions are joined in a complex feedback loop. The trigger point in the thermodynamic model is the separated phase volume, related to a set of mechanical pain thresholds for fluid injected into connective tissue.

The full thermodynamic model is complex, though Hills has performed massive computations correlating with the data, underscoring basic model validity. One of its more significant features can be seen in Figure 59. Considerations of free phase dynamics (phase volume trigger point) require deeper decompression staging formats, compared to considerations of critical tensions, and are characteristic of phase models. Full blown bubble models require the same, simply to minimize bubble excitation and growth.

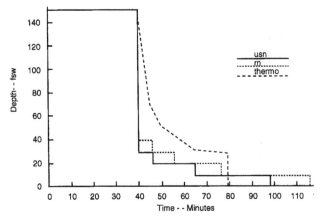

Figure 59. Thermodynamic And Phase Model Decompression Profiles

Decompression profiles after a dive to 150 fsw for 40 min are depicted for supersaturation and phase decompression formats. The supersaturation schedules (labeled USN and RN) differ from phase format (labeled thermo). Such differences are generic to phase and bubble models versus critical tension models, and are based on fundamental pressure differences between eliminating free and dissolved gas phases. Increasing pressure is necessary to eliminate free phases, while decreasing pressure more optimally eliminates dissolved gas phases. Decompression staging is really a tricky playoff in trying to eliminate both, something of a minimax problem as it is called in mathematical circles.

Varying Permeability Model

The varying permeability model (VPM) treats both dissolved and free phase transfer mechanisms, postulating the existence of gas seeds (micronuclei) with permeable skins of surface active molecules, small enough to remain in solution and strong enough to resist collapse. The model is based upon laboratory studies of bubble growth and nucleation.

Inert gas exchange is driven by the local gradient, the difference between the arterial blood tension and the instantaneous tissue tension. Compartments with 1,

2, 5, 10, 20, 40, 80, 120, 240, 480, and 720 halftimes, τ, are again employed. While, classical (Haldane) models limit exposures by requiring that the tissue tensions never exceed the critical tensions, fitted to the US Navy nonstop limits, for example, the varying permeability model, however, limits the supersaturation gradient, through the phase volume constraint. An exponential distribution of bubble seeds, falling off with increasing bubble size is assumed to be excited into growth by compression-decompression. A critical radius, r_c, separates growing from contracting micronuclei for given ambient pressure, P_c. At sea level, $P_c = 33\ fsw$, $r_c = .8\ microns$. Deeper decompressions excite smaller, more stable, nuclei.

Within this phase volume constraint, a set of nonstop limits, t_n, at depth, d, satisfy a modified law, $dt_n^{1/2} = 400\ fsw\ min^{1/2}$, with gradient, G, extracted for each compartment, τ, using the nonstop limits and excitation radius, at generalized depth, $d = P - 33\ fsw$. Tables 33 and 13 summarize t_n, G_0, ΔG, and δ, the depth at which the compartment begins to control exposures.

Table 33. Critical Phase Volume Time Limits.

Depth d (fsw)	Nonstop limit t_n (min)	Depth d (fsw)	Nonstop limit t_n (min)
30	250.	130	9.0
40	130.	140	8.0
50	73.	150	7.0
60	52.	160	6.5
70	39.	170	5.8
80	27.	180	5.3
90	22.	190	4.6
100	18.	200	4.1
110	15.	210	3.7
120	12.	220	3.1

Gas filled crevices can also facilitate nucleation by cavitation. The mechanism is responsible for bubble formation occurring on solid surfaces and container walls. In gel experiments, though, solid particles and ragged surfaces were seldom seen, suggesting other nucleation mechanisms. The existence of stable gas nuclei is paradoxical. Gas bubbles larger than 1 μm should float to the surface of a standing liquid or gel, while smaller ones should dissolve in a few *sec*. In a liquid supersaturated with gas, only bubbles at the critical radius, r_c, would be in equilibrium (and very unstable equilibrium at best). Bubbles larger than the critical radius should grow larger, and bubbles smaller than the critical radius should collapse. Yet, the Yount gel experiments confirm the existence of *stable* gas phases, so no matter what the mechanism, effective surface tension must be zero. Although the actual size distribution of gas nuclei in humans is unknown, these experiments in gels have been correlated with a decaying exponential (radial) distribution function. For a stabilized distribution accommodated by the body at fixed pressure, P_c, the excess number of nuclei excited by compression-decompression must be removed from the body. The rate at which gas inflates in tissue depends upon both the excess bubble number, and the supersaturation gradient, G. The critical volume hypothesis requires that the integral of the product of the two must always remain less than some volume limit point, αV, with α a proportionality constant.

Reduced Gradient Bubble Model

The reduced gradient bubble model (RGBM) extends the earlier VPM naturally. The full blown RGBM treats coupled perfusion-diffusion transport as a two step flow process, with blood flow (perfusion) serving as a boundary condition for tissue gas penetration by diffusion. Depending on time scales and rate coefficients, one or another (or both) processes dominate the exchange. However, for most meter implementations, perfusion is assumed to dominate, simplifying matters and permitting online calculations. Additionally, tissues and blood are naturally undersaturated with respect to ambient pressure at equilibration through the mechanism of biological inherent unsaturation (oxygen window), and the model includes this debt in calculations.

The RGBM assumes that a size distribution of seeds (potential bubbles) is always present, and that a certain number is excited into growth by compression-decompression. An iterative process for ascent staging is employed to control the inflation rate of these growing bubbles so that their collective volume never exceeds a phase volume limit point. Gas mixtures of helium, nitrogen, and oxygen contain bubble distributions of different sizes, but possess the same phase volume limit point.

The RGBM postulates bubble seeds with varying skin structure. Bubble skins are assumed permeable under all crushing pressure. The size of seeds excited into growth is inversely proportional to the supersaturation gradient. At increasing pressure, bubble seeds permit gas diffusion at a slower rate. The model assumes bubble skins are stabilized by surfactants over calculable time scales, producing seeds with variable persistent in the body. Bubble skins are probably molecularly activated, complex, biosubstances found throughout the body. Whatever the formation process, the model assumes the size distribution is exponentially decreasing in size, that is, more smaller seeds than larger seeds in exponential proportions. The RGBM also employs an equation-of-state (EOS) for bubble skin response (Boyle-like) to free phase compression-decompression, unlike the VPM.

The model incorporates a spectrum of tissue compartments, ranging from 1 *min* to 720 *min*, depending on gas mixture (helium, nitrogen, oxygen). Phase separation and bubble growth in slower compartments is a central focus in calculations, and the model uses nonstop time limits tuned to recent Doppler measurements, conservatively reducing them along the lines originally suggested by Spencer (and others), but within the phase volume constraint.

The RGBM reduces the phase volume limit in multidiving by considering free phase elimination and buildup during surface intervals, depending on altitude, time, and depth of previous profiles. Repetitive, multiday, and reverse profile exposures are tracked and impacted by critical phase volume reductions over appropriate time scales. The model generates replacement bubble seed distributions on time scales of days, adding new bubbles to existing bubbles in calculations. Phase volume limit points are also reduced by the added effects of new bubbles.

The reduced gradient bubble model extends the varying permeability model to repetitive diving, by conservatively reducing the gradients, *G*. A conservative set of bounce gradients, *G*, can always be used for multiday and repetitive diving, provided they are multiplicatively reduced by a set of bubble factors, all less than one. Three bubble factors reduce the driving gradients to maintain the phases volume constraint. The first bubble factor reduces *G* to account for creation of new stabilized micronuclei over time scales of days. The second factor accounts for additional micronuclei excitation on reverse profile dives. The third bubble factor accounts for bubble growth over repetitive exposures on time scales of hours. Their behavior is depicted in Figures 41, 42, and 43.

The RGBM and VPM are both diveware implementations, accessible on the Internet at various sites. Additionally, the RGBM has been encoded into a number of commercial decompression meter products. Specific comparisons between RGBM and Haldane predictions for staging will be presented, with resultants generic to phase versus dissolved gas models. NAUI employs RGBM Tables for trimix, helitrox, EANx, and altitude dive training.

Tissue Bubble Diffusion Model

The tissue bubble diffusion model (TBDM), according to Gernhardt and Vann, considers the diffusive growth of an extravascular bubble under arbitrary hyperbaric and hypobaric loadings. The approach incorporates inert gas diffusion across the tissue-bubble interface, tissue elasticity, gas solubility and diffusivity, bubble surface tension, and perfusion limited transport to the tissues. Tracking bubble growth over a range of exposures, the model can be extended to oxygen breathing and inert gas switching. As a starting point, the TBDM assumes that, through some process, stable gas nuclei form in the tissues during decompression, and subsequently tracks bubble growth with dynamical equations. Diffusion limited exchange is invoked at the tissue-bubble interface, and perfusion limited exchange is assumed between tissue and blood, very similar to the thermodynamic model, but with free phase mechanics. Across the extravascular region, gas exchange is driven by the pressure difference between dissolved gas in tissue and free gas in the bubble, treating the free gas as ideal. Initial nuclei in the TBDM have assumed radii near 3 *microns* at sea level, to be compared with .8 *microns* in the VPM and RGBM.

As in any free phase model, bubble volume changes become more significant at lower ambient pressure, suggesting a mechanism for enhancement of hypobaric bends, where constricting surface tension pressures are smaller than those encountered in hyperbaric cases. Probabilistically, the model has been bootstrapped to statistical likelihood, correlating bubble size with decompression risk, a topic discussed in a few chapters. So, seen in Figure 60, a theoretical bubble dose of 5 *ml* correlates with a 20% risk of decompression sickness, while a 35 *ml* dose correlates with a 90% risk, with the bubble dose representating an unnormalized measure of the separated phase volume. Coupling bubble volume to risk represents yet another extension of the phase volume hypothesis, a viable trigger point mechanism for bends incidence.

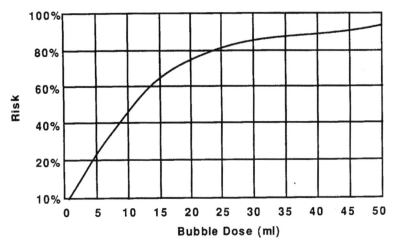

Figure 60. Decompression Risk And Bubble Size

It is possible to correlate model parameters across experimental diving and exposure data. The curve below correlates risk with computed model bubble size, that is, theoretically computed bubble dose (ml) is linked to incidence of decompression sickness in a sigmoidal dose curve. Dose is a measure of separated gas volume, a natural trigger point in phase models, such as the TM, VPM, RGBM, and TBDM.

Empirical Practices

Utilitarian procedures, entirely consistent with phase mechanics and bubble dissolution time scales, have been developed under duress, and with trauma, by Australian pearl divers and Hawaiian diving fishermen, for both deep and repetitive diving with possible in-water recompression for hits. While the science behind such procedures was not initially clear, the operational effectiveness was always noteworthy and could not be discounted easily. Later, the rationale, essentially recounted in the foregoing, became clearer.

Pearling fleets, operating in the deep tidal waters off northern Australia, employed Okinawan divers who regularly journeyed to depths of 300 *fsw* for as long as one hour, two times a day, six days per week, and ten months out of the year. Driven by economics, and not science, these divers developed optimized decompression schedules empirically. As reported by Le Messurier and Hills, deeper decompression stops, but shorter decompression times than required by Haldane theory, were characteristics of their profiles. Such protocols are entirely consistent with minimizing bubble growth and the excitation of nuclei through the application of increased pressure, as are shallow safety stops and slow ascent rates. With higher incidence of surface decompression sickness, as might be expected, the Australians devised a simple, but very effective, in-water recompression procedure. The stricken diver is taken back down to 30 fsw on oxygen for roughly 30 *minutes* in mild cases, or 60 *minutes* in severe cases. Increased pressures help to constrict bubbles, while breathing pure oxygen maximizes inert gas washout (elimination). Recompression time scales are consistent with bubble dissolution experiments.

Similar schedules and procedures have evolved in Hawaii, among diving fishermen, according to Farm and Hayashi. Harvesting the oceans for food and profit, Hawaiian divers make between 8 and 12 dives a day to depths beyond 350 fsw. Profit incentives induce divers to take risks relative to bottom time in conventional tables. Three repetitive dives are usually necessary to net a school of fish. Consistent with bubble and nucleation theory, these divers make their deep dive first, followed by shallower excursions. A typical series might start with a dive to 220 fsw, followed by 2 dives to 120 fsw, and culminate in 3 or 4 more excursions to less than 60 fsw. Often, little or no surface intervals are clocked between dives. Such types of profiles literally clobber conventional tables, but, with proper reckoning of bubble and phase mechanics, acquire some credibility. With ascending profiles and suitable application of pressure, gas seed excitation and any bubble growth are constrained within the body's capacity to eliminate free and dissolved gas phases. In a broad sense, the final shallow dives have been tagged as prolonged safety stops, and the effectiveness of these procedures has been substantiated *in vivo* (dogs) by Kunkle and Beckman. In-water recompression procedures, similar to the Australian regimens, complement Hawaiian diving practices for all the same reasons.

While the above practices developed by trial-and-error, albeit with seeming principle, venous gas emboli measurements, performed off Catalina by Pilmanis on divers making shallow safety stops, fall into the more *scientific* category perhaps. Contrasting bubble counts following bounce exposures near 100 fsw, with and without zonal stops in the 10–20 fsw range, marked reductions (factors of 4 to 5) in venous gas emboli, as seen in Figure 61, were noted when stops were made. If, as some suggest, venous gas emboli in bounce diving correlate with bubbles in sites such as tendons and ligaments, then safety stops probably minimize bubble growth in such extravascular locations. In these tests, the sample population was small, so additional validation and testing is warranted.

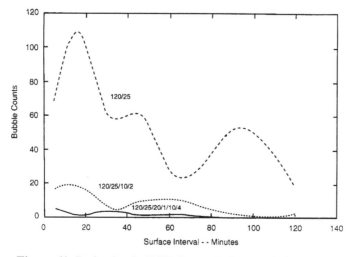

Figure 61. Reduction in VGE Counts Following Safety Stops

Safety stops have considerable impact on Doppler sounded VGE measurements, according to Pilmanis, Neuman, and Linaweaver. Following a dive to 100 fsw for 25 min, the top curve registers VGE counts over increasing surface interval time. The lower two curves depict the count after a brief stop for 2 min at 10 fsw, and then 1 min at 20 fsw followed by 4 min at 10 fsw. Reductions by factors of 4-6 are apparent. Whether VGE correlate with overall susceptibility to DCI, or not, or only in certain cases, free phase reduction in the pulmonary circulation is impressive with shallow safety stops.

Phase and Haldane Model Comparisons

Suunto, Abysmal Diving, HydroSpace Engineering, and ConnecXon have released meters and software incorporating a modern phase algorithm, the above Reduced Gradient Bubble Model (RGBM), for diving. An iterative approach to staging diver ascents, the RGBM employs separated phase volumes as limit points, instead of the usual Haldane (maximum) critical tensions across tissue compartments. The model is inclusive (altitude, repetitive, mixed gas, decompression, saturation, nonstop exposures), treating both dissolved and free gas phase buildup and elimination. NAUI Technical Diving employs the RGBM to schedule nonstop and decompression training protocols on trimix, heliox, and nitrox while also testing gas switching alternatives for deep exposures. The RGBM has its roots in the earlier work of the Tiny Bubble Group at the University of Hawaii, drawing upon and extending the so-called Varying Permeability Model (VPM) to multidiving, altitude, and mixed gas applications. While certainly not radical, the RGBM is both different and new on the diving scene. And not unexpectedly, the RGBM recovers the Haldane approach to decompression modeling in the limit of relatively safe (tolerably little) separated phase, with *tolerably little* a qualitative statement here.

The Suunto D9 and Mares M1 are RGBM decometers for competent divers while GAP/RGBM is a licensed Gas Absorption Program software product. All are serious and modern commercial products with a realistic implementation of a diving phase algorithm across a wide spectrum of exposure extremes. And both accommodate user knobs for additional conservatism. Other Suunto and Mares computers targeted for the RGBM are in development stages. HydroSpace has also released the mixed gas EXPLORER, while Steam Machines is contemplating a constant oxygen partial decometer for rebreathers. Atomic Aquatics similarly markets the COBALT, a full up RGBM computer for air and nitrox. Free Phase Diving developed a downloadable RGBM application for the Liquivision XEO OC and RB computer. More are in the works from other meter vendors.

Here, our intent is to (just) look at the underpinnings of both meter and diveware implementations of the RGBM algorithm, one with extended range of applicability based on simple dual phase principles. Haldane approaches have dominated decompression algorithms for a very long time, and the RGBM has been long in coming on the commercial scene. With recent technical diving interest in deep stop modeling, and concerns with repetitive diving in the recreational community, phase modeling is timely and pertinent. And, of course, since the RGBM extends the VPM, much of the following applies to the VPM directly.

Recent years have witnessed many changes and modifications to diving protocols and table procedures, such as shorter nonstop time limits, slower ascent rates, discretionary safety stops, ascending repetitive profiles, multilevel techniques, both faster and slower controlling repetitive tissues, smaller critical tensions (M-values), longer flying-after-diving surface intervals, and others. Stimulated by observation, Doppler technology, decompression meter development, theory, statistics, or safer diving consensus, these modifications affect a gamut of activity, spanning bounce to multiday diving. Of these changes, conservative nonstop time limits, no decompression safety stops, and slower ascent rates (around $30 \ fsw/min$) are in vogue, and have been incorporated into many tables and meters. As you might expect, recent developments support them on operational, experimental, and theoretical grounds.

But there is certainly more to the story as far as table and meter implementations. To encompass such far reaching (and often diverse) changes in a unified framework requires more than the simple Haldane models we presently rely upon in 99% of our tables and dive computers. To model gas transfer dynamics, modelers and table designers need address both free and dissolved gas phases, their interplay, and their impact on diving protocols. Biophysical models of inert gas transport and bubble formation all try to prevent decompression sickness. Developed over years of diving application, they differ on a number of basic issues, still mostly unresolved today:

- the rate limiting process for inert gas exchange, blood flow rate (perfusion) or gas transfer rate across tissue (diffusion);
- composition and location of critical tissues (bends sites);
- the mechanistics of phase inception and separation (bubble formation and growth);

- the critical trigger point best delimiting the onset of symptoms (dissolved gas buildup in tissues, volume of separated gas, number of bubbles per unit tissue volume, bubble growth rate to name a few);
- the nature of the critical insult causing bends (nerve deformation, arterial blockage or occlusion, blood chemistry or density changes).

Such issues confront every modeler and table designer, perplexing and ambiguous in their correlations with experiment and nagging in their persistence. And here comments are confined just to Type I (limb) and II (central nervous system) bends, to say nothing of other types and factors. These concerns translate into a number of what decompression modelers call dilemmas that limit or qualify their best efforts to describe decompression phenomena. Ultimately, such concerns work their way into table and meter algorithms, with the same caveats. The RGBM treats these issues in a natural way, gory details of which are found in the References.

The establishment and evolution of gas phases, and possible bubble trouble, involves a number of distinct, yet overlapping, steps:

- nucleation and stabilization (free phase inception);
- supersaturation (dissolved gas buildup);
- excitation and growth (free-dissolved phase interaction);
- coalescence (bubble aggregation);
- deformation and occlusion (tissue damage and ischemia).

Over the years, much attention has focused on supersaturation. Recent studies have shed much light on nucleation, excitation and bubble growth, even though *in vitro*. Bubble aggregation, tissue damage, ischemia, and the whole question of decompression sickness trigger points are difficult to quantify in any model, and remain obscure. Complete elucidation of the interplay is presently asking too much. Yet, the development and implementation of better computational models is necessary to address problems raised in workshops, reports and publications as a means to safer diving.

The computational issues of bubble dynamics (formation, growth, and elimination) are mostly outside the traditional framework, but get folded into halftime specifications in a nontractable mode. The very slow tissue compartments (halftimes large, or diffusivities small) might be tracking both free and dissolved gas exchange in poorly perfused regions. Free and dissolved phases, however, do not behave the same way under decompression. Care must be exercised in applying model equations to each component. In the presence of increasing proportions of free phases, dissolved gas equations cannot track either species accurately. Computational algorithms tracking both dissolved and free phases offer broader perspectives and expeditious alternatives, but with some changes from classical schemes. Free and dissolved gas dynamics differ. The driving force (gradient) for free phase elimination increases with depth, directly opposite to the dissolved phase elimination gradient which decreases with depth. Then, changes in operational procedures become necessary for optimality. Considerations of excitation and growth invariably require deeper staging procedures than supersaturation methods. Though not as dramatic, similar constraints remain operative in multiexposures, that is, multilevel, repetitive, and multiday diving.

Other issues concerning time sequencing of symptoms impact computational algorithms. That bubble formation is a predisposing condition for decompression sickness is universally accepted. However, formation mechanisms and their ultimate physiological effect are two related, yet distinct, issues. On this point, most hypotheses makes little distinction between bubble formation and the onset of bends symptoms. Yet we know that silent bubbles have been detected in subjects not suffering from decompression sickness. So it would thus appear that bubble formation, per se, and bends symptoms do not map onto each other in a one-to-one manner. Other factors are truly operative, such as the amount of gas dumped from solution, the size of nucleation sites receiving the gas, permissible bubble growth rates, deformation of surrounding tissue medium, and coalescence mechanisms for small bubbles into large aggregates, to name a few. These issues are the pervue of bubble theories, but the complexity of mechanisms addressed does not lend itself easily to table, nor even meter, implementation. But implement and improve we must, so consider the bubble issues taken in RGBM computer implementations (and issues for all bubble models):

• Perfusion and Diffusion
  Perfusion and diffusion are two mechanisms by which inert and metabolic gases exchange between tissue and blood. Perfusion denotes the blood flow rate in simplest terms, while diffusion refers to the gas penetration rate in tissue, or across tissue-blood boundaries. Each mechanism has a characteristic rate constant for the process. The smallest rate constant limits the gas exchange process. When diffusion rate constants are smaller than perfusion rate constants, diffusion dominates the tissue-blood gas exchange process, and vice-versa. In the body, both processes play a role in real exchange process, especially considering the diversity of tissues and their geometries. The usual Haldane tissue halftimes are the inverses of perfusion rates, while the diffusivity of water, thought to make up the bulk of tissue, is a measure of the diffusion rate.

  Clearly in the past, model distinctions were made on the basis of perfusion or diffusion limited gas exchange. The distinction is somewhat artificial, especially in light of recent analyses of coupled perfusion-diffusion gas transport, recovering limiting features of the exchange process in appropriate limits. The distinction is still of interest today, however, since perfusion and diffusion limited algorithms are used in mutually exclusive fashion in diving. The obvious mathematical rigors of a full blown perfusion-diffusion treatment of gas exchange mitigate table and meter implementation, where model simplicity is a necessity. So one or another limiting models is adopted, with inertia and track record sustaining use. Certainly Haldane models fall into that categorization.

Inert gas transfer and coupled bubble growth are subtly influenced by metabolic oxygen consumption. Consumption of oxygen and production of carbon dioxide drops the tissue oxygen tension below its level in the lungs (alveoli), while carbon dioxide tension rises only slightly because carbon dioxide is 325 times more soluble than oxygen. Figure 32 compares the partial pressures of oxygen, nitrogen, water vapor, and carbon dioxide in dry air, alveolar air, arterial blood, venous blood, and tissue (cells).

Arterial and venous blood, and tissue, are clearly unsaturated with respect to dry air at 1 *atm*. Water vapor content is constant, and carbon dioxide variations are slight, though sufficient to establish an outgradient between tissue and blood. Oxygen tensions in tissue and blood are considerably below lung oxygen partial pressure, establishing the necessary ingradient for oxygenation and metabolism. Experiments also suggest that the degree of unsaturation increases linearly with pressure for constant composition breathing mixture, and decreases linearly with mole fraction of inert gas in the inspired mix.

Since the tissues are unsaturated with respect to ambient pressure at equilibrium, one might exploit this window in bringing divers to the surface. By scheduling the ascent strategically, so that nitrogen (or any other inert breathing gas) supersaturation just takes up this unsaturation, the total tissue tension can be kept equal to ambient pressure. This approach to staging is called the zero supersaturation ascent.

The full blown RGBM treats coupled perfusion-diffusion transport as a two step flow process, with blood flow (perfusion) serving as a boundary condition for tissue gas penetration by diffusion. Depending on time scales and rate coefficients, one or another (or both) processes dominate the exchange. However, for all recreational implementations, perfusion is assumed to dominate, simplifying matters and permitting online calculations. Additionally, tissues and blood are naturally undersaturated with respect to ambient pressure at equilibration through the mechanism of biological inherent unsaturation (oxygen window), and the RGBM includes this debt in calculations.

- Bubbles
We do not really know where bubbles form nor lodge, their migration patterns, their birth and dissolution mechanisms, nor the exact chain of physico-chemical insults resulting in decompression sickness. Many possibilities exist, differing in the nature of the insult, the location, and the manifestation of symptoms. Bubbles might form directly (*de novo*) in supersaturated sites upon decompression, or possibly grow from preformed, existing seed nuclei excited by compression-decompression. Leaving their birth sites, bubbles may move to critical sites elsewhere. Or stuck at their birth sites, bubbles may grow locally to pain-provoking size. They might dissolve locally by gaseous diffusion to surrounding tissue or blood, or passing through screening filters, such as the lung complex, they might be broken down into smaller aggregates,

or eliminated completely. Whatever the bubble history, it presently escapes complete elucidation. But whatever the process, the end result is very simple, both separated and dissolved gas must be treated in the transfer process, as depicted in Figures 34 and 35.

Bubbles may hypothetically form in the blood (intravascular) or outside the blood (extravascular). Once formed, intravascularly or extravascularly, a number of critical insults are possible. Intravascular bubbles may stop in closed circulatory vessels and induce ischemia, blood sludging, chemistry degradations, or mechanical nerve deformation. Circulating gas emboli may occlude the arterial flow, clog the pulmonary filters, or leave the circulation to lodge in tissue sites as extravascular bubbles. Extravascular bubbles may remain locally in tissue sites, assimilating gas by diffusion from adjacent supersaturated tissue and growing until a nerve ending is deformed beyond its pain threshold. Or, extravascular bubbles might enter the arterial or venous flows, at which point they become intravascular bubbles.

Spontaneous bubble formation in fluids usually requires large decompressions, like hundreds of atmospheres, somewhere near fluid tensile limits. Many feel that such circumstance precludes direct bubble formation in blood following decompression. Explosive, or very rapid decompression, of course is a different case. But, while many doubt that bubbles form in the blood directly, intravascular bubbles have been seen in both the arterial and venous circulation, with vastly greater numbers detected in venous flows (venous gas emboli). Ischemia resulting from bubbles caught in the arterial network has long been implied as a cause of decompression sickness. Since the lungs are effective filters of venous bubbles, arterial bubbles would then most likely originate in the arteries or adjacent tissue beds. The more numerous venous bubbles, however, are suspected to first form in lipid tissues draining the veins. Lipid tissue sites also possess very few nerve endings, possibly masking critical insults. Veins, thinner than arteries, appear more susceptible to extravascular gas penetration.

Extravascular bubbles may form in aqueous (watery) or lipid (fatty) tissues in principle. For all but extreme or explosive decompression, bubbles are seldom observed in heart, liver, and skeletal muscle. Most gas is seen in fatty tissue, not unusual considering the five-fold higher solubility of nitrogen in lipid tissue versus aqueous tissue. Since fatty tissue has few nerve endings, tissue deformation by bubbles is unlikely to cause pain locally. On the other hand, formations or large volumes of extravascular gas could induce vascular hemorrhage, depositing both fat and bubbles into the circulation as noted in animal experiments. If mechanical pressure on nerves is a prime candidate for critical insult, then tissues with high concentrations of nerve endings are candidate structures, whether tendon or spinal cord. While such tissues are usually aqueous, they are invested with lipid cells whose propensity reflects total body fat. High nerve density and some lipid content supporting bubble formation and growth would appear a conducive environment for a mechanical insult.

To satisfy thermodynamic laws, bubbles assume spherical shapes in the absence of external or mechanical (distortion) pressures. Bubbles entrain free gases because of a thin film, exerting surface tension pressure on the gas. Hydrostatic pressure balance requires that the pressure inside the bubble exceed ambient pressure by the amount of surface tension, γ. Figure 34 depicts the pressure balance in a spherical (air) bubble. At small radii, surface tension pressure is greatest, and at large radii, surface tension pressure is least.

Gases will also diffuse into or out of a bubble according to differences in gas partial pressures inside and outside the bubble, whether in free or dissolved phases outside the bubble. In the former case, the gradient is termed free-free, while in the latter case, the gradient is termed free-dissolved. Unless the surface tension is identically zero, there is always a gradient tending to force gas out of the bubble, thus making the bubble collapse on itself because of surface tension pressure. If surrounding external pressures on bubbles change in time, however, bubbles may grow or contract. Figure 35 sketches bubble gas diffusion under instantaneous hydrostatic equilibrium for an air bubble.

Bubbles grow or contract according to the strength of the free-free or free-dissolved gradient, and it is the latter case which concerns divers under decompression. The radial rate at which bubbles grow or contract depends directly on the diffusivity and solubility, and inversely on the bubble radius. A critical radius, r_c, separates growing from contracting bubbles. Bubbles with radius $r > r_c$ will grow, while bubbles with radius $r < r_c$ will contract. Limiting bubble growth and adverse impact upon nerves and circulation are issues when decompressing divers and aviators.

The RGBM assumes that a size distribution of seeds (potential bubbles) is always present, and that a certain number is excited into growth by compression-decompression. An iterative process for ascent staging is employed to control the inflation rate of these growing bubbles so that their collective volume never exceeds a phase volume limit point. Gas mixtures of helium, nitrogen, and oxygen contain bubble distributions of different sizes, but possess the same phase volume limit point.

- Bubble Seeds
Bubbles, which are unstable, are thought to grow from micron size, gas nuclei which resist collapse due to elastic skins of surface activated molecules (surfactants), or possibly reduction in surface tension at tissue interfaces or crevices. If families of these micronuclei persist, they vary in size and surfactant content. Large pressures (somewhere near 10 *atm*) are necessary to crush them. Micronuclei are small enough to pass through the pulmonary filters, yet dense enough not to float to the surfaces of their environments, with which they are in both hydrostatic (pressure) and diffusion (gas flow) equilibrium. When

nuclei are stabilized, and not activated to growth or contraction by external pressure changes, the skin (surfactant) tension offsets both the Laplacian (film) tension and any mechanical help from surrounding tissue. Then all pressures and gas tensions are equal. However, on decompression, the seed pockets are surrounded by dissolved gases at high tension and can subsequently grow (bubbles) as surrounding gas diffuses into them. The rate at which bubbles grow, or contract, depends directly on the difference between tissue tension and local ambient pressure, effectively the bubble pressure gradient. At some point in time, a critical volume of bubbles, or separated gas, is established and bends symptoms become statistically more probable. On compression, the micronuclei are crunched down to smaller sizes across families, apparently stabilizing at new reduced size. Bubbles are also crunched by increasing pressure because of Boyle's law, and then additionally shrink if gas diffuses out of them. As bubbles get smaller, they probably restabilize as micronuclei.

The RGBM postulates bubble seeds with varying skin structure. Bubble skins are assumed permeable under all crushing pressure. The size of seeds excited into growth is inversely proportional to the supersaturation gradient. At increasing pressure, bubble seeds permit gas diffusion at a slower rate. The RGBM assumes bubble skins are stabilized by surfactants over calculable time scales, producing seeds with variable persistent in the body. Bubble skins are probably molecularly activated, complex, biosubstances found throughout the body. Whatever the formation process, the RGBM assumes the size distribution is exponentially decreasing in size, that is, more smaller seeds than larger seeds in exponential proportions.

• Slow Tissue Compartments
Based on concerns in multiday and heavy repetitive diving, with the hope of controlling staircasing gas buildup in exposures through critical tensions, slow tissue compartments (halftimes greater than 80 minutes) have been incorporated into some algorithms. Calculations, however, show that virtually impossible exposures are required of the diver before critical tensions are even approached, literally tens of hours of near continuous activity. As noted in many calculations, slow compartment cannot really control multidiving through critical tensions, unless critical tensions are reduced to absurd levels, inconsistent with nonstop time limits for shallow exposures. That is a model limitation, not necessarily a physical reality. The physical reality is that bubbles in slow tissues are eliminated over time scales of days, and the model limitation is that the arbitrary parameter space does not accommodate such phenomena.

And that is no surprise either, when one considers that dissolved gas models are not suppose to track bubbles and free phases. Repetitive exposures do provide fresh dissolved gas for excited nuclei and growing free phases, but it is not the dissolved gas which is the problem just by itself. When bubble growth is considered, the slow compartments appear very important, because, therein, growing free phases are mostly left undisturbed insofar as surrounding tissue tensions are concerned. Bubbles grow more gradually in slow compartments because the gradient there is typically small, yet grow over longer time scales. When coupled to free phase dynamics, slow compartments are necessary in multidiving calculations.

The RGBM incorporates a spectrum of tissue compartments, ranging from 1 min to 720 min, depending on gas mixture (helium, nitrogen, oxygen). Phase separation and bubble growth in slower compartments is a central focus in calculations.

- Venous Gas Emboli
  While the numbers of venous gas emboli detected with ultrasound Doppler techniques can be correlated with nonstop limits, and the limits then used to fine tune the critical tension matrix for select exposure ranges, fundamental issues are not necessarily resolved by venous gas emboli measurements. First of all, venous gas emboli are probably not the direct cause of bends per se, unless they block the pulmonary circulation, or pass through the pulmonary traps and enter the arterial system to lodge in critical sites. Intravascular bubbles might first form at extravascular sites. According to studies, electron micrographs have highlighted bubbles breaking into capillary walls from adjacent lipid tissue beds in mice. Fatty tissue, draining the veins and possessing few nerve endings, is thought to be an extravascular site of venous gas emboli. Similarly, since blood constitutes no more than 8% of the total body capacity for dissolved gas, the bulk of circulating blood does not account for the amount of gas detected as venous gas emboli. Secondly, what has not been established is the link between venous gas emboli, possible micronuclei, and bubbles in critical tissues. Any such correlations of venous gas emboli with tissue micronuclei would unquestionably require considerable first-hand knowledge of nuclei size distributions, sites, and tissue thermodynamic properties. While some believe that venous gas emboli correlate with bubbles in extravascular sites, such as tendons and ligaments, and that venous gas emboli measurements can be reliably applied to bounce diving, the correlations with repetitive and saturation diving have not been made to work, nor important correlations with more severe forms of decompression sickness, such as chokes and central nervous system (CNS) hits.

Still, whatever the origin of venous gas emboli, procedures and protocols which reduce gas phases in the venous circulation deserve attention, for that matter, anywhere else in the body. The moving Doppler bubble may not be the bends bubble, but perhaps the difference may only be the present site. The propensity of venous gas emboli may reflect the state of critical tissues where decompression sickness does occur. Studies and tests based on Doppler detection of venous gas emboli are still the only viable means of monitoring free phases in the body.

The RGBM uses nonstop time limits tuned to recent Doppler measurements, conservatively reducing them along the lines originally suggested by Spencer (and others), but within the phase volume constraint. The D9 implementation penalizes ascent violations by requiring additional safety stop time dictated by risk analysis of the violation.

• Multidiving
Concerns with multidiving can be addressed through variable critical gradients, then tissue tensions in Haldane models. While variable gradients or tensions are difficult to codify in table frameworks, they are easy to implement in digital meters. Reductions in critical parameters also result from the phase volume constraint, a constraint employing the separated volume of gas in tissue as trigger point for the bends, not dissolved gas buildup alone in tissue compartments. The phase volume is proportional to the product of the dissolved-free gas gradient times a bubble number representing the number of gas nuclei excited into growth by the compression-decompression, replacing just slow tissue compartments in controlling multidiving.

In considering bubbles and free-dissolved gradients within critical phase hypotheses, repetitive criteria develop which require reductions in Haldane critical tensions or dissolved-free gas gradients. This reduction simply arises from lessened degree of bubble elimination over repetitive intervals, compared to long bounce intervals, and need to reduce bubble inflation rate through smaller driving gradients. Deep repetitive and spike exposures feel the greatest effects of gradient reduction, but shallower multiday activities are impacted. Bounce diving enjoys long surface intervals to eliminate bubbles while repetitive diving must contend with shorter intervals, and hypothetically reduced time for bubble elimination. Theoretically, a reduction in the bubble inflation driving term, namely, the tissue gradient or tension, holds the inflation rate down. Overall, concern is bubble excess driven by dissolved gas. And then both bubbles and dissolved gas are important. Here, multidiving exposures experience reduced permissible tensions through lessened free phase elimination over time spans of two days. Parameters are consistent with bubble experiments, with both slow and fast compartments considered.

The RGBM reduces the phase volume limit in multidiving by considering free phase elimination and buildup during surface intervals, depending on altitude, time, and depth of previous profiles, Repetitive, multiday, and reverse profile exposures are tracked and impacted by critical phase volume reductions over appropriate time scales.

• Adaptation
Divers and caisson workers have long contended that tolerance to decompression sickness increases with daily diving, and decreases after a few weeks layoff, that in large groups of compressed air workers, new workers were at higher risk than those who were exposed to high pressure regularly. This acclimatization

might result from either increased body tolerance to bubbles (physiological adaptation), or decreased number and volume of bubbles (physical adaptation). Test results are totally consistent with physical adaptation.

Yet, there is slight inconsistency here. Statistics point to slightly higher bends incidence in repetitive and multiday diving. Some hyperbaric specialists confirm the same, based on experience. The situation is not clear, but the resolution plausibly links to the kinds of first dives made and repetitive frequency in the sequence. If the first in a series of repetitive dives are kept short, deep, and conservative with respect to nonstop time limits, initial excitation and growth are minimized. Subsequent dives would witness minimal levels of initial phases. If surface intervals are also long enough to optimize both free and dissolved gas elimination, any nuclei excited into growth could be efficiently eliminated outside repetitive exposures, with adaptation occurring over day intervals as noted in experiments. But higher frequency, repetitive and multiday loading may not afford sufficient surface intervals to eliminate free phases excited by earlier exposures, with additional nuclei then possibly excited on top of existing phases. Physical adaptation seems less likely, and decompression sickness more likely, in the latter case. Daily regimens of a single bounce dive with slightly increasing exposure times are consistent with physical adaptation, and conservative practices. The regimens also require deepest dives first. In short, acclimatization is as much a question of eliminating any free phases formed as it is a question of crushing or reducing nuclei as potential bubbles in repetitive exposures. And then time scales on the order of a day might limit the adaptation process.

The RGBM generates replacement bubble seed distributions on time scales of hours, adding new bubbles to existing bubbles in calculations. Phase volume limit points are also reduced by the added effects of new bubbles.

So, having waded through the foregoing, a next question is how does the RGBM compare with classical Haldane models as far as staging ascents, limiting multiexposures, and treating mixed gases? Generally, for short nonstop air diving, the RGBM reproduces the Spencer limits. For multidiving in spans shorter than 1–3 *hr*, the RGBM reduces nonstop limits by 10% to 20% depending on surface interval, depth, altitude, and duration of present and previous dive. Multiday diving is impacted to lesser degree. Some comparisons appear in Table 34 for 3 days of repetitive air diving (120 *fsw*/10 *min* twice a day with 45 *min* surface interval). Computer choices are illustrative, not indictive.

Table 34. Nonstop Limits For D9/RGBM And Haldane Air Multidiving

Computer/Algorithm	Dive 1 (*min*)	Dive 2 (*min*)	Dive 3 (*min*)	Dive 4 (*min*)	Dive 5 (*min*)	Dive 6 (*min*)
D9/RGBM	10	6	9	5	9	5
SPYDER/Haldane	10	9	10	9	10	9
DATA PLUS/Haldane	12	6	12	6	12	6
DELPHI/Haldane	10	10	10	10	10	10
DC11/Haldane	6	6	6	6	6	6
DC12/Haldane	9	7	9	7	9	7
ALADIN/Haldane	8	8	8	8	8	8
ALADIN PRO/Haldane	10	7	10	7	10	7
SOURCE/Haldane	12	9	12	9	12	9

The D9/RGBM (first dive) nonstop limits (depth/time) are 150/6, 140/7, 130/9, 120/10, 110/13, 100/17, 90/22, 80/28, 70/36, 60/51, 50/69, and 40/120. In the mixed gas arena, Table 35 lists nonstop time limits for ranged trimix, that is, 13% to 17% helium, 61% to 53% nitrogen, and 26% to 30% oxygen, according to GAP/RGBM and GAP/ZHL (Buhlmann).

Table 35. Trimix Nonstop Limits For GAP/RGBM And GAP/ZHL (Haldane).

Depth (*fsw*)	GAP/RGBM (*min*)	GAP/ZHL (*min*)
80	28	26
90	23	22
100	19	18
110	16	15
120	14	13
130	12	11
140	11	10
150	10	9

These limits are used by NAUI Technical Diving for training purposes. While both sets of nonstop time limits are different in Tables 3 and 4, the more dramatic effects of the RGBM show up for deep staging, as seen in Table 36. Comparative deep schedules for a trimix dive to 250 *fsw* for 30 *min* are contrasted, following a switch to air at 100 *fsw* and a switch to pure oxygen at 20 *fsw* on the way up. GAP/RGBM and GAP/ZHL are again employed, but with and without conservative safety knobs. In the case of GAP/ZHL, the outgassing tissue halftimes are increased by 1.5 in the conservative case, while for GAP/RGBM the bubble excitation radius is increased by 1.2 for comparison. Deeper stops are noticeably requisite in GAP/RGBM, but total decompression times are less than GAP/ZHL. The trimix is 33% helium, 51% nitrogen, and 16% oxygen.

Table 36. Deep Schedules According To GAP/RGBM And GAP/ZHL (Haldane)

Stop	Depth (*fsw*)	GAP/ZHL (*min*) (*standard*)	GAP/RGBM (*min*) (*standard*)	GAP/ZHL (*min*) (*safer*)	GAP/RGBM (*min*) (*safer*)
1	180	0	0	0	1
2	170	0	1	0	1
3	160	0	1	0	1
4	150	0	1	0	1
5	140	0	1	0	2
6	130	0	2	0	2
7	120	0	2	0	2
8	110	0	2	1	2
9	100	0	2	2	2
10	90	2	2	3	3
11	80	2	2	4	3
12	70	2	3	5	4
13	60	5	5	8	6
14	50	7	6	12	7
15	40	12	9	18	19
16	30	18	12	28	13
17	20	16	10	28	11
18	10	28	16	48	18
		93	77	147	98

That in a nutshell is a comparison of major differences between phase and dissolved gas models. The phase models recover dissolved gas models for short and nominal exposures, but require deeper stops and shorter decompression times for longer and exceptional exposures. A rundown of the software configuration of the RGBM used in full blown simulations follows. The package is under constant refinement and updating.

- Module: Three major routines (RGBMNX, RGBMHX, RGBMTMX) for nitrox, heliox, and trimix.
- Source Code: 1640 Lines
- Language/Compiler: FORTRAN 77/90, BASIC.
- SGI Origin SMP Running Time: 1 *sec* for deep trimix profile with 5 gas switches on way up.
- Input: altitude, bottom mixture, ascent/descent rate, switch levels and gas mixtures, predive breathing gas, safety knobs, previous dive history.
- Output: controlling tissue compartments, stop depth and times, supersaturation gradient, permissible supersaturation, effective bubble and gas parameters, critical phase volume, dive profile.

278   *Science of Diving*

RGBM Field Data

Models need validation and field testing. Often, strict hyperbaric chamber tests are not possible, economically nor otherwise, and models employ a number of benchmarks and regimens to underscore viability. The following are some supporting the RGBM phase model and (released) nitrox, heliox, and trimix diving tables and meters. Profiles are recorded in the RGBM Data Bank, and are representative of entries in terms of dive counts and technical diving applications. How this data is specifically manipulated to validate the model follows in the next major section, along with statistical correlations.

- Counterterror and Countermeasures Team (C & C) RB and OC exercises have used the RGBM (iterative deep stop version) for a number of years, logging some 2245 dives on mixed gases (trimix, heliox, nitrox) with 0.4% incidence of DCS – 85% were deco dives, and 55% were repets with at least 2 hr SIs, with most in the forward direction (deepest dives first). Some 9 cases of DCS were logged by the Team, mainly in the deep reverse profile category on nitrox and trimix, plus RB hits on heliox;

- NAUI Technical Diving has been diving the deep stop version for the past 9 yrs, some estimated 22,000 dives, on mixed gases down to 300 fsw, with 2 reported cases of DCS, both on trimix. Some 15 divers, late 1999, in France used the RGBM to make 2 mixed gas dives a day, without mishap, in cold water and rough seas. Same thing in the warm waters of Roatan in 2000 and 2001;

- NAUI Worldwide released a set of RGBM Tables for air, EAN32, and EAN36 recreational diving, from sea level to 10,000 ft, a few years ago. Minimum SIs of 1 hour are supported for repetitive diving in all Tables, and safety stops for 2 *min* in the 15 fsw zone, plus 1 min deep stops at half bottom depth, are required always. Tables were tested by NAUI Instructor Trainers, Instructors, and Divemasters over a 2 year period without mishap, and continue so today as the the mainstay teaching Tables in NAUI basic air and nitrox courses;

- modified RGBM recreational algorithms (Haldane imbedded with bubble reduction factors limiting reverse profile, repetitive, and multiday diving), as coded in Suunto, Mares, Dacor, UTC, Zeagle, Steam Machines, Atomic Aquatics, Liquivision, GAP, ABYSS, HydroSpace, ConneXon decometers, maintain an already low DCS incidence rate of approximately 1/50,000 or less. More RGBM decompression meters, including mixed gases, are in the works;

- a cadre of divers and instructors in mountainous New Mexico, Utah, and Colorado have been diving the modified RGBM at altitude, an estimated 1,200 dives, without peril. Again, not surprising since the altitude RGBM is slightly more conservative than the usual Cross correction used routinely up to about 8,000 ft elevation, and with estimated DCS incidence less than 1/10,000;

- within decometer implementations of the RGBM, only a few scattered DCS hits have been reported in nonstop and multidiving categories, beyond 1,300,000 dives or more, up to now, according to statistics furnished the author (BRW) by meter vendors;

- extreme hyperbaric chamber tests for mixed gas RGBM protocols are in the works, and less stressful exposures will be addressed also – extreme here means 300 *fsw* and beyond;

- as seen, probabilistic decompression analysis of selected recreational air RGBM profiles, calibrated against similar calculations of the same profiles by Duke, help validate the RGBM on computational bases, suggesting the RGBM has no more theoretical risk than other bubble or dissolved gas models (Weathersby, Vann, Gerth methodology at USN and Duke);

- all divers and Instructors using RGBM decometers, tables, or Internet software have been asked to report individual profiles to DAN Project Dive Exploration (Vann, Denoble at Duke), plus to the RGBM Data Bank (Wienke, O'Leary at LANL and NAUI);

- GAP, Free Phase Diving, HydroSpace RGBM Simulator, and ABYSS are NET software packages that offer the modified RGBM (folded Buhlmann ZHL) and, especially, the full up, deep stop version for any gas mixture, have a fairly large contingent of tech divers already using the RGBM and have not received any reports of DCS to date. The EXPLORER RGBM Simulator is furnished to meter owners of the HydroSpace EXPLORER;

- extreme WKPP profiles in the 300 *fsw* range on trimix were used to calibrate the RGBM. WKPP profiles are the most impressive application of RGBM staging, with as much as 12 hours less decompression time for WKPP helium based diving on RGBM schedules versus Haldane schedules, with estimated 200 dives;

- Ellyat, a TDI Instructor, dived the Baden in the North Sea to 540 *fsw* on RGBM schedules on two different occasions, and 3 hours were shaved off conventional hang time by RGBM application. Unfortunately, with diver error and mismatched gas switching strategies from helium to nitrogen, dives to 840 *fsw* likely resulted in vestibular DCS;

- NAUI Worldwide released sets of deep stop RGBM nitrox, heliox, and trimix technical and recreational Tables that have been tested by NAUI Technical Diving Operations over the past 9 years, with success and no reported cases of DCS, for open circuit regulators and rebreathers;

- Doppler and imaging tests in the laboratory, and analyses by Bennett, Marroni, Brubakk and Wienke, and Neuman all suggest reduction in free phase counts with deep stop staging;

- deep air RGBM Tables with surface oxygen decompression are employed by American oil patch diving companies;

- Scorese, a NAUI instructor, and his students made a total of 234 dives on the Andrea Doria using rebreathers and RGBM (constant ppo_2) RB Tables, and various nitrogen and trimix diluents. Dive abortions off rebreathers employed ranged RGBM (open circuit) Tables as bailouts, and witnessed no mishaps;

- Freauf, a Navy SEAL in Hawaii, logged 20 trimix decompression dives beyond $250\ fsw$ on consecutive days using RGBM Tables (pure oxygen switch at 20 fsw);

- Melton, owner of HydroSpace Engineering and developer of the RGBM EXPLORER (OC plus RB) dive computer reports 100s of dives in the $400\ fsw$ range on the RGBM EXPLORER;

- GAP, Gas Absorption Program, an RGBM software product out of the Netherlands, supports brisk and sustained use of the RGBM within the tec and rec diving community and has been implemented in the Atomic Aquatics COBALT computer;

- NEDU in Panama City performed deep stop man trials in a test pod using a US Navy bubble model;

- heliox RGBM Tables are being used by a commercial diving operation in Argentina;

- McMillan implemented the full RGBM for OC and RB diving in the Liquivision XEO computer;

- Raine, a wreck diver in California, reports 100s of RGBM dives in the $250\ fsw$ range with low Doppler counts;

- the RGBM site, *RGBMdiving.com*, receives 100s of hits weekly, and provides custom RGBM Tables;

- ANDI, a training agency, has adopted a custom version of GAP for diver training on mixed gases, OC and RBs;

- NAUI similarly employs a custom version of GAP for dive planning, with nominal GAP parameter settings recovering released and published NAUI RGBM Tables;

- O'Leary, Director NAUI Technical Operations, has made over 70 dives on OC and RB systems using RGBM Table and the Hydrospace EXPLORER to depths beyond $250\ fsw$, with anywhere from 6–9 other divers;

- O'Leary, Sharp, Scorese, Bell, Hunley and 6 other NAUI Instructors used RGBM during NAUI Technical Instructor Training Courses; and RB Tables to dive the USS Perry in Anguar in very strong currents, down to $260\ fsw$, logging 2 repetitive deco dives a day for a week or so;

- the Finnish Diving Federation (FDF) has adopted RGBM Tables for recreational air and nitrox diver training, as well as light decompression exposures down to $130\ fsw$.

With DCS binomially distributed in incidence probability, many trials are needed (or other close profiles) to fully validate any model at the 1% level. Additionally, full validation requires DCS incidences, the higher the number, the better, contrary to desired dive outcomes. While the foregoing list of field tests and profiles are not controlled scientific experiments with attendant data collection, the shear number of diving events and diversity of exposure spectrum ought not be discounted nor treated lightly. Collective information has been dubbed a *living laboratory* by segments of the technical, scientific, and operational diving community.

Bubble Model Computer Implementation

The following details the coupling (fitting) of the RGBM across critical parameters and nonstop time limits of the ZHL algorithm. The RGBM (Reduced Gradient Bubble Model) is a phase algorithm that iteratively stages diver ascents for arbitrary exposures and times on any gas mixture. Some of its dual phase features can be ported to Haldane models, such as the ZHL, through profile and parameter fitting techniques (maximum likelihood). Extensive computer fitting of profiles and recalibration of parameters to maintain the RGBM within the ZHL limits is requisite here.

- Critical Parameters (a, b)
  Haldane approaches use a simple dissolved gas (tissue) transfer equation, and a set of critical parameters to dictate diver staging through the gas transfer equation. In the Workman approach, the critical parameters are called M-values, while in the Buhlmann formulation they are called a and b. They are equivalent sets, just slightly different in representation, but not content. First consider the transfer equation, assuming air (79/21 nitrox).
  Tissue tensions (nitrogen partial pressures), p, for ambient nitrogen partial pressure, p_a, and initial tissue tension, p_i, evolve in time, t, in standard fashion in compartment, τ, according to,

$$p - p_a = (p - p_a) \, exp \, (-\lambda t)$$

for,

$$\lambda = \frac{.693}{\tau}$$

with τ tissue halftime, and, for air,

$$p_a = .79 \, P = .79 \, (d + P_0)$$

and with ambient pressure, P, given as a function of depth, d, and surface atmospheric pressure, P_0 , in units of fsw. Staging is controlled in the Buhlmann ZHL algorithm through sets of tissue parameters, a and b, listed below in Table 38 for 14 tissue compartments, τ, through the minimum permissible (tolerable) ambient pressure, P_{min}, according to,

$$P_{min} = (p - a)b$$

across all tissue compartments, τ, with the largest P_{min} limiting the allowable ambient pressure, P_{min}. Recall that,

$$1 \, bar = 1.013 \, atm, \quad 1 \, atm = 33 \, fsw$$

as conversion metric between *bar* and *fsw* in pressure calculations. Linear extrapolations across tissue compartments are used for different sets of halftimes and critical parameters, *a* and *b*.

Table 37. Nitrogen ZHL Critical Parameters (a, b)

Halftime τ (*min*)	Critical intercept a (*bar*)	Critical slope b
5.0	1.198	.542
10.0	.939	.687
20.0	.731	.793
40.0	.496	.868
65.0	.425	.882
90.0	.395	.900
120.0	.372	.912
150.0	.350	.922
180.0	.334	.929
220.0	.318	.939
280.0	.295	.944
350.0	.272	.953
450.0	.255	.958
635.0	.236	.966

In terms of critical tensions, M, according to the USN, the relationship linking the two sets is simply,

$$M = \frac{P}{b} + a = \Delta M \, P + M_0$$

so that,

$$\Delta M = \frac{1}{b}$$

$$M_0 = a$$

in units of *bar*, though the usual representation for M is *fsw*. The above set, *a* and *b*, hold generally for nitrox, and, to low order, for heliox (and trimix too). Tuned modifications for heliox and trimix are also presented below.

Corresponding nonstop time limits, t_n, are listed in Table 38, and the nonstop limits follow the Hempleman square root law, roughly,

$$dt_n^{1/2} = 475 \, fsw \, min^{1/2}$$

in a least squares fit. The square root law also follows directly from the form of the bulk diffusion transfer equation, but not from any Haldane assumptions nor limiting forms of the tissue equation.

Table 38. Air ZHL Nonstop Time Limits

Depth $d\ (fsw)$	Time $t_n\ (min)$
30	290
40	130
50	75
60	54
70	38
80	26
90	22
100	20
110	17
120	15
130	11
140	9
150	8
160	7
170	6
180	5
190	4
200	3

- Likelihood Profile and Model Analysis
  Over ranges of depths, tissue halftimes, and critical parameters of the ZHL algorithm, approximately 2,300 dive profiles were simulated using both the RGBM and Haldane ZHL algorithms. To correlate the two as closely as possible to the predictions of the RGBM across these profiles, maximum likelihood analysis is used, that is, extracting the temporal features of three bubble parameters mating the RGBM and ZHL algorithms extending critical parameters of the ZHL Haldane model to more complete bubble dynamical framework and physical basis. These factors, f, are described next, with their linkages to a and b, and are the well known *reduction factors* of the RGBM.

- Multidiving Fractions
  According to the RGBM fits across the ZHL profiles (2,300), a correlation can be established through multidiving reduction factors, f, such that for any set of nonstop gradients, G,

$$G = M - P$$

a reduced set, G_f, obtains from the nonstop set, G, for multidiving through the reduction factors, $f \leq 1$,

$$G_f = fG$$

so that,

$$M_f = \frac{P}{b_f} + a_f = G_f + P = fG + P$$

but, since,

$$fG = f(M - P) = f \left[\frac{P}{b} + a - P \right]$$

we have,

$$a_f = fa$$

$$b_f = \frac{b}{f(1-b)+b}$$

with a and b the standard set above.

The new (reduced) staging regimen is then simply,

$$P_{min} = (p - a_f) b_f$$

using the *reduced* critical parameters, a_f and b_f. Certainly, as $f \to 1$, then $a_f \to a$, and $b_f \to b$, as requisite. Now all that remains is specification of f, particularly in terms of repetitive, reverse profile, and multiday diving, as limited by the bubble dynamical RGBM.

The full factor, f, depends on tissue halftime, τ, generally through the relationship (for nitrox),

$$f = (1 - f_0) \frac{\tau}{180} + f_0 \quad (f = 1, \ \tau \geq 180 \, min)$$

as the tissue scaling up through the 180 *min* nitrogen compartment, with multidiving weighting,

$$f_0 = .45 \, f_{rp} + .30 \, f_{rd} + .25 \, f_{rg}$$

where f_{rp}, f_{rd}, and f_{rg} are reduction factors for repetitive, reverse profile (deeper than previous), and multiday (time spans of 30 *hr* or more) diving. These forms for multidiving f are dependent on time between dives, t_{sur}, ambient pressure difference between reverse profile dives, ΔP, ambient pressure, P, and multiday diving frequency, n, over 24 *hr* time spans. Specifically, they take the form,

$$f_{rp} = 1 - 0.45 \, exp \left[-\frac{(t_{sur} - 30)^2}{3600} \right]$$

$$f_{rd} = 1 - 0.45 \left[1 - exp \left(-\frac{\Delta P}{P} \right) \right] exp \left[-\frac{(t_{sur} - 60)^2}{14400} \right]$$

$$f_{rg} = 0.70 + 0.30 \, exp \left(-\frac{n}{20} \right)$$

with t_{sur} measured in *min*, and n the number of consecutive days of diving within 30 *hr* time spans. These factors are applied after 1 *min* of surface interval (otherwise, previous dive continuation). The difference, ΔP, is the time averaged difference between depths on the present and previous dives (computed on the fly).

Again, the reduction factors are consistent (folded in maximum likelihood in the RGBM) with the following:

- Doppler bubble scores peak in an hour or so after a dive;
- reverse profiles with depth increments beyond 50 fsw incur increasing DCI risk, somewhere between 5% and 8% in the depth increment range of 40 fsw–120 fsw;
- Doppler bubble counts are reduced an order of magnitude when ascent rates are cut from 60 fsw/min to 30 fsw/min;
- multiday diving risks increase by factors of 2 -3 (though still small) over risk associated with a single dive.

- Nitrox
  The standard set, a, b, and τ, given in Table 37 hold across nitrox exposures, and the tissue equation remains the same. The obvious change for a nitrox mixture with nitrogen fraction, f_{N_2}, occurs in the nitrogen ambient pressure, p_{aN_2}, at depth, d, in analogy with the air case,

$$p_{aN_2} = f_{N_2} P = f_{N_2} (d + P_0)$$

with P ambient pressure (fsw). All else is unchanged. The case, $f_{N_2} = 0.79$, obviously represents an air mixture.

- Heliox
  The standard set, a, b, and τ is modified for helium mixtures, with basic change in the set of halftimes, τ, used for the set, a and b. To lowest order set, a and b for helium are the same as those for nitrogen, though we will list the modifications in Table 39 below. The halftimes for helium are approximately 2.65 times faster than those for nitrogen, by Graham's law (molecular diffusion rates scale inversely with square root of atomic masses). That is to say,

$$\tau_{He} = \frac{\tau_{N_2}}{2.65}$$

because helium is approximately 7 times lighter than nitrogen, and diffusion rates scale with square root of the ratio of atomic masses.
The tissue equation is the same as the nitrox tissue equation, but with helium constants, λ, defined by the helium tissue halftimes. Denoting the helium fraction, f_{He}, the helium ambient pressure, p_{aHe}, is given by,

$$p_{aHe} = f_{He} P = f_{He} (d + P_0)$$

as before with nitrox. The multidiving fractions are the same, but the tissue scaling is different across the helium set,

$$f = (1 - f_0) \frac{\tau}{67.8} + f_0 \quad (f = 1, \ \tau \geq 67.8 \ min)$$

though in analogy with the nitrox case. All else remains the same.

Table 39. Helium ZHL Critical Parameters (a, b)

Halftime τ (min)	Critical intercept a (bar)	Critical slope b
1.8	1.653	.461
3.8	1.295	.604
7.6	1.008	.729
15.0	.759	.816
24.5	.672	.837
33.9	.636	.864
45.2	.598	.876
56.6	.562	.885
67.8	.541	.892
83.0	.526	.901
105.5	.519	.906
132.0	.516	.914
169.7	.510	.919
239.6	.495	.927

- Trimix

For trimix, both helium and nitrogen must be tracked with tissue equations, and appropriate average of helium and nitrogen critical parameters used for staging. Thus, denoting nitrogen and helium fractions, f_{N_2}, and f_{He}, ambient nitrogen and helium pressures, p_{aN_2} and p_{aHe}, take the form,

$$p_{aN_2} = f_{N_2} P = f_{N_2} (d + P_0)$$

$$p_{aHe} = f_{He} P = f_{He} (d + P_0)$$

Tissue halftimes are mapped exactly as listed in Tables 5 and 6, and used appropriately for nitrogen and helium tissue equations. Additionally,

$$f_{O_2} + f_{N_2} + f_{He} = 1$$

and certainly in Tables 5 and 6, one has the mapping,

$$\tau_{He} = \frac{\tau_{N_2}}{2.65}$$

Then, total tension, Π, is the sum of nitrogen and helium components,

$$\Pi = (p_{aN_2} + p_{aHe}) + (p_{iN_2} - p_{aN_2}) \, exp \, (-\lambda_{N_2} t) + (p_{iHe} - p_{aHe}) \, exp \, (-\lambda_{He} t)$$

with λ_{N_2} and λ_{He} decay constant for the nitrogen and helium halftimes in Tables 5 and 6. Critical parameters for trimix, α_f and β_f, are just weighted averages of critical parameters, a_{N_2}, b_{N_2}, a_{He} b_{He}, from Tables 5 and 6, that is, generalizing to the reduced set, a_f and b_f,

$$\alpha_f = \frac{f_{N_2} a_{fN_2} + f_{He} a_{fHe}}{f_{N_2} + f_{He}}$$

$$\beta_f = \frac{f_{N_2} b_{fN_2} + f_{He} b_{fHe}}{f_{N_2} + f_{He}}$$

The staging regimen for trimix is,

$$P_{min} = (\Pi - \alpha_f)\beta_f$$

as before. The corresponding critical tension, M_f, generalizes to,

$$M_f = \frac{P}{\beta_f} + \alpha_f$$

- Risk Estimates
  Overall, the ZHL/RGBM algorithm is conservative with safety imparted to the Haldane ZHL model through multidiving f factors. Estimated DCI incidence rate from likelihood analysis is 0.001% at the 95% confidence level for the overall air ZHL/RGBM. Table and meter implementations with consistent coding should reflect this estimated risk. Similar estimates and comments apply to the ZHL mixed gas synthesis.

Keyed Exercises

- *Match model features to the BDM, MTM, TM, VPM, RGBM, and TBDM: Dissolved gas phase treatment only?*

  MTM, BDM

Many perfusion tissue compartments?

  MTM, TM, VPM, RGBM, TBDM

Single bulk tissue compartment?
  BDM

Exponential distributions of bubble seeds?

  VPM, RGBM

Critical tension, ratio, or gradient limit points?

  BDM, MTM

Critical separated phase volume or dose limit points?

  TM, VPM, RGBM, TBDM

Pain thresholds?
  TM

Multidiving limitations?

RGBM

Commercial meter implementations?

MTM, RGBM

Seed regeneration?

VPM, RGBM

Dissolved and free gas phase treatment?

TM, VPM, RGBM, TBDM

• *Match the following problematic profiles to model issues addressed by the BDM, MTM, TM, VPM, RGBM, or TBDM:*
Deepest dive not first?

Additional bubble seed excitation

Yo, yo diving?

Rapid bubble growth

Multiple inert gas switches during dive?

Isobaric counterdiffusion

Multilevel diving?

Bubble growth and gas elimination

Rapid ascents?

VGE elimination

Short interval repetitive diving?

Bubble growth and gas elimination

Multiday diving?

Seed regeneration

Saturation exposures?

Very slow tissue compartments

Altitude diving?

Larger bubble seed excitation radii

- Link the MTM, BDM, TM, VPM, RGBM, and TBDM to the 5 overlapping steps leading to bubble trouble:
  Nucleation and stabilization?

VPM and RGBM

Supersaturation?

MTM, BDM, TM, VPM, RGBM, and TBDM

Bubble excitation and growth?

TM, VPM, RGBM, and TBDM

Coalescence?

TM, VPM, and RGBM

Tissue deformation and occlusion?

TM

- According to the Wienke-Yount bulk diffusion law, what is the nonstop time limit, t_n, at a depth of 155 fsw?

$$dt_n^{1/2} = C, \quad C = 400 \ fsw \ min^{1/2}$$

$$t_n = \left[\frac{C}{d}\right]^2 = \left[\frac{400}{155}\right]^2 \ min = 6.4 \ min$$

- According to USN Tables (modified), what is the surfacing Group for a photographer at 67 fsw for 35 min, assuming the ascent rate is standard, $r = 60 \ fsw/min$?

$Group = G$

If 68 min are spent on the surface, what is the new Group?

$Group = F$

On the next dive to 46 fsw, what is the penalty time, t?

$Penalty \ Time = t = 47 \ min$

If bottom time at 46 fsw is 15 min, what is the new surfacing Group?

$Group = I$

- A Group F diver sustains what overpressure, ΔP, in nitrogen loading (absolute) in the 120 min compartment?

$$\Delta P = 6 \times 2 \ fsw = 12 \ fsw$$

What is the nitrogen tension, p, in the 120 min compartment of that (surface) F diver after 160 min?

$$\Delta P = 12\ fsw, \quad p_i - p_a = f_{N_2}\Delta P = .79 \times 12\ fsw = 9.48\ fsw$$

$$\lambda = \frac{.693}{120}\ min^{-1} = .0058\ min^{-1}$$

$$p = p_a + (p_i - p_a)\ exp\ (-\lambda t)$$

$$p = 26.1 + 9.48 \times exp\ (-.0058 \times 160) = 29.8\ fsw$$

Into what Group does the diver now fall?

$$\Delta P = \frac{(p - p_a)}{f_{N_2}} = \frac{(29.8 - 26.1)}{.79} = 4.68\ fsw$$

$$Group = C$$

- *If a Park Ranger lugs his dive gear to Lake Catherine above Santa Fe (New Mexico) at an elevation of 9,560 ft and plans a dive to 40 ft, what is the altitude correction factor, β, and what is the equivalent sea level depth, δ, for the dive?*

$$\beta = \eta\ exp\ (0.038h) = .975 \times exp\ (0.038 \times 9.65) = 1.40$$

$$\delta = \beta d = 1.40 \times 40\ fsw = 56.2\ fsw$$

If the ascent rate, r_0, in the Tables at sea level is 60 fsw/min, what is the altitude rate, r?

$$r = \frac{r_0}{\beta} = \frac{60}{1.4}\ ft/min = 42.8\ ft/min$$

If the excursion to Lake Catherine is launched from Sante Fe, elevation 6,860 ft, taking 15 min, what Group should the Ranger diver assign to the start of the dive?

$$\Delta z = 9650 - 6860\ ft = 2790\ ft$$

$$Altitude\ Group = B$$

If the dive lasts 20 min, in what group does the diver surface?

$$Group\ B\ Penalty\ Time\ (60\ fsw) = 11\ min$$

$$Total\ Dive\ Time = 20 + 11\ min = 31\ min$$

$$Surfacing\ Group = G$$

As a Group G diver, what is the maximum change in altitude permitted?

$$Permitted\ Altitude\ Change = 6,000\ ft$$

How long before a mountain Group G diver drops into Group A?

$$Surface\ Interval\ Time = 7.6\ hr$$

How long before a Group G diver can ascend 7,000 ft in elevation, according to the 24 hr rule?

$$Surface\ Interval\ Time\ = 3.7\ hr$$

- *According to the USN Tables at sea level, the nonstop limit at 100 fsw is 22 min. What is the nonstop limit, t_n, at elevation of 5,600 ft, using the similarity method?*

$$\beta = \eta \ exp \ (0.038h) = .975 \times exp \ (0.038 \times 5.6)$$

$$\beta = .975 \times 1.23 = 1.20$$

$$\delta = 100 \times 1.20 \ fsw = 120 \ fsw$$

$$t_n = 12 \ min$$

- *If the surfacing critical tension for the $\tau = 90$ min compartment is, $M_0 = 55$ fsw, what is the compartment limit, t_n, for 79/21 nitrox (air) at, $d = 50$ fsw?*

$$f_{N_2} = .79, \quad p_i = f_{N_2} \times 33 \ fsw = .79 \times 33 \ fsw = 26.1 \ fsw$$

$$p_a = f_{N_2}(33+50) \ fsw = .79 \times 83 \ fsw = 65.6 \ fsw$$

$$\lambda = \frac{.693}{90} \ min^{-1} = .0077 \ min^{-1}, \quad t_n = \frac{1}{\lambda} \ln \frac{p_i - p_a}{M_0 - p_a}$$

$$t_n = \frac{1}{.0077} \times \ln \left[\frac{26.1 - 65.6}{55 - 65.6} \right] \ min = 121.6 \ min$$

What is the compartment limit, t_n, for 79/21 heliox at, $d = 50$ fsw?

$$\lambda = \frac{.693}{90/2.65} \ min^{-1} = .0204 \ min^{-1}$$

$$t_n = \frac{1}{.0204} \times \ln \left[\frac{26.1 - 65.6}{55 - 65.6} \right] = 45.8 \ min$$

- *Invert the tissue equation,*

$$(M_0 - p_a) = (p_i - p_a) \ exp \ (-\lambda t_n), \quad \lambda = \frac{.693}{\tau}$$

for nitrogen surfacing M-values, M_0, and tissues, τ, in the table, and compute the NDLs, t_n, for EAN$_{21}$ (air) at sea level and down to 150 fsw.

$$p_i = .79 \times 33 \ fsw = 26.1 \ fsw, \quad p_a = .79 \times (d+33) \ fsw$$

τ (min)	$\tau/3$ (min)	M_0 (fsw)
3	1	119
6	2	102
12	4	82
24	8	69
36	12	59
48	16	57
60	20	55
84	28	48
120	40	44

The NDLs are given below, with τ the controlling (shortest NDL) compartment.

depth (fsw)	t_n (min)	τ (min)
40	146	120
50	94	36
60	62	36
70	47	36
80	37	12
90	27	12
100	21	12
110	18	12
120	14	6
130	10	3
140	8	3
150	7	3

- *Repeat the exercise for EAH_{21} (heliair) assuming surface equilibration with heliair before descent using the surfacing M-values, M_0, and tissues, $\tau/3$, in the same table above at sea level and down to 100 fsw.*

$$(M_0 - p_a) = (p_i - p_a) \, exp \, (-3\lambda t_n)$$

$$p_i = .79 \times 33 \, fsw = 26.1 \, fsw, \quad p_a = .79 \times (d + 33) \, fsw$$

The NDLs and controlling compartments are listed below. Taking heliair saturation at the surface is an academic exercise and not usual for real diving. Air saturation at the surface for any mixture is the usual case, resulting in shorter NDLs than below because of surface nitrogen loading.

depth (fsw)	t_n (min)	$\tau/3$ (min)
40	82	20
50	31	12
60	21	12
70	16	12
80	12	4
90	9	4
100	7	4

- *Repeat the foregoing for 20/40 trimix using the nitrogen and helium M-values and tissues listed and averaged over the helium and nitrogen gas fractions at sea level and down to 200 fsw. The equation cannot be inverted analytically but can be solved iteratively. This is not a trivial exercise and is done on the fly by decompression meters for dive planning. Also take the diver as saturated on air (not heliair) on the surface. Therefore, we have,*

$$p_{iN_2} = .79 \times 33 \, fsw = 26.1 \, fsw, \quad p_{iHe} = 0 \, fsw$$

$$p_{aN_2} = .40 \times (d + 33) \, fsw, \quad p_{He} = .40 \times (d + 33) \, fsw$$

$$f_{N_2} = f_{He} = .40, \quad \bar{M}_0 = \frac{f_{N_2} M_{0N_2} + f_{He} M_{0He}}{f_{N_2} + f_{He}} = \frac{1}{2}(M_{0N_2} + M_{0He})$$

with the appropriate 2 species tissue equation,

$$\bar{M}_0 = p_{aN_2} + p_{aHe} + (p_{iN_2} - p_{aN_2})\, exp\,(-\lambda t_n) + (p_{iHe} - p_{aHe})\, exp\,(-3\lambda t_n)$$

nitrogen		helium		mixed
$\tau\,(min)$	$M_{0N_2}\,(fsw)$	$\tau/3\,(min)$	$M_{0He}\,(fsw)$	$\bar{M}_0\,(fsw)$
1.0	119.6	0.3	153.3	136.6
2.0	115.2	0.7	147.4	131.2
5.0	100.5	1.7	129.8	115.2
10.0	81.7	3.3	103.5	92.6
20.0	68.3	6.7	83.8	76.1
40.0	60.2	13.3	72.0	66.1
80.0	53.9	26.7	63.0	58.4
120.0	51.1	40.0	59.3	55.2
160.0	49.4	53.3	57.3	53.3
240.0	47.1	80.0	55.5	51.3
320.0	45.8	106.7	55.0	50.4
400.0	44.9	133.3	54.7	49.8
480.0	44.2	160.0	54.5	49.4
560.0	43.7	186.7	54.4	49.0
720.0	42.7	240.0	54.1	48.4

Resulting NDLs for controlling compartments are given below.

depth (fsw)	$t_n\,(min)$	$\tau\,(min)$	$\tau/3\,(min)$
40	156.9	120.0	40.0
50	78.2	80.0	26.7
60	54.5	80.0	26.7
70	32.3	40.0	13.3
80	25.5	40.0	13.3
90	21.3	40.0	13.3
100	13.4	20.0	6.7
110	11.5	20.0	6.7
120	10.0	20.0	6.7
130	9.0	20.0	6.7
140	6.4	10.0	3.3
150	5.7	10.0	3.3
160	5.2	10.0	3.3
170	4.8	10.0	3.3
180	4.4	10.0	3.3
190	3.3	5.0	1.7
200	3.0	5.0	1.7

On this mixture, a dive is planned to 200 fsw for 20 min. What is the equivalent air depth, δ, for this dive?

$$\delta = \frac{f_{N_2}}{.79}\,(P_0 + d) = 0.503 \times (33 + 200)\, fsw = 117.9\, fsw$$

For maximum oxygen partial pressure, p_{O_2}, of 1.4 atm, what is the maximum oxygen depth, d_{max}, for this mixture?

$$p_{O_2} = f_{O_2}\left[1 + \frac{d_{max}}{33}\right],\quad f_{O_2} = 1. - f_{N_2} - f_{He} = 1. - .80 = .20$$

$$d_{max} = 33 \left[\frac{p_{O_2}}{f_{O_2}} - 1. \right] = 33 \times \left[\frac{1.4}{.20} - 1. \right] fsw = 198 \, fsw$$

Is this mixture suitable for a decompression dive to 200 fsw for 20 min?

Yes And Many Others

- *Listed below are NDLs, t_n, for EAN_{21} and EAH_{21}, using the same M-values and assuming air saturation of the diver at the surface.*

depth (fsw)	EAN_{21} t_n (min)	EAH_{21} t_n (min)
40	146.2	22.8
60	61.9	13.0
80	36.8	7.4
100	21.1	5.1
120	13.9	3.0
140	8.0	2.0
160	5.8	1.6
180	4.6	1.3
200	3.8	1.1

Why are helium NDLs shorter than nitrogen NDLs for the same fraction of oxygen?

Helium Ingasses Faster Than Nitrogen

Why are nitrogen decompression times longer than helium decompression times for deep diving?

Nitrogen Outgasses Slower Than Helium

- *What is the decompression schedule for an air dive to 120 fsw for 15 min at sea level neglecting ascent and descent rates? As a helping shortcut, the 10 min compartment controls decompression at the 10 fsw stop and this light decompression dive only requires a 10 fsw stop. So for the bottom exposure, we have,*

$\lambda = 0.0693 \, min^{-1}$, $p_i = .79 \times 33 \, fsw = 26.1 \, fsw$, $p_a = .79 \times (33 + 120) \, fsw = 120.$

$p = p_a + (p_i - p_a) \exp(-\lambda t) = 120.9 + (26.1 - 120.9) \exp(-.0693 \times 15) \, fsw = 87.$

For the 10 fsw decompression stop, followed by surfacing, decompression time, t_d, is,

$$M_0 = 81.3 \, fsw, \quad p_i = p = 87.3 \, fsw, \quad p_a = .79 \times (33 + 10) \, fsw = 34.0 \, fsw$$

$$(M_0 - p_a) = (p_i - p_a) \exp(-\lambda t_d)$$

$$t_d = \frac{1}{\lambda} \ln\left[\frac{p_i - p_a}{M_0 - p_a} \right] = \frac{1}{.0693} \ln\left[\frac{87.3 - 34}{81.3 - 34} \right] min = 1.72 \, min$$

Beyond the examples above, decompression calculations are tedious and computer software is requisite, as detailed in the Part 7. Plus ascent and descent rates become important.

Part 5

STATISTICS, RISK, COMPARATIVE PROFILES, AND MALADIES

Systematics and Issues

The systematics of gas exchange, nucleation, bubble growth and elimination, and decompression are so complicated that theories only reflect pieces of the puzzle. Computational algorithms, tables, and manned testing are requisite across a spectrum of activities. And the potential of electronic devices to process tables of information or detailed equations underwater is near maturity, with virtually any algorithm or model amenable to digital implementation. Pressures for even more sophisticated algorithms are expected to grow.

Still computational models enjoy varying degrees of success or failure. More complex models address a greater number of issues, but are harder to codify in decompression tables. Simpler models are easier to codify, but are less comprehensive. Some models are based on first principles, but many are not. Application of models can be subjective in the absence of definitive data, the acquisition of which is tedious, sometimes controversial, and often ambiguous. If deterministic models are abandoned, statistical analysis can address the variability of outcome inherent to random occurrences, but only in manner indifferent to specification of controlling mechanisms. The so called dose-reponse characteristics of statistical analysis are very attractive in the formulation of risk tables. Applied to decompression sickness incidence, tables of comparative risk offer a means of weighing contributing factors and exposure alternatives. At the basis of statistical and probabilistic analyses of decompression sickness is the binomial distribution. The binomial distribution is the fundamental frequency distribution governing random events.

Binomial Distribution

Decompression sickness is a hit, or no hit, situation. Statistics are binary, as in coin tossing. Probabilities of occurrence are determined from the binomial distribution, which measures the numbers of possibilities of occurrence and nonoccurrence in any number of events, given the incidence rate. Specifically, the probability, P, in a random sample of size, N, for n occurrences of decompression sickness and m nonoccurrences, takes the form,

$$P(n) = \frac{N!}{n!\,m!}\,p^n q^m,$$

with,

$$n + m = N,$$

p the underlying incidence rate (average number of cases of decompression sickness), and q,

$$q = 1 - p,$$

the underlying nonincidence. The discrete probability distributions, P, are the individual terms of the binomial expansion of $(p+q)^N$,

$$(p+q)^N = \sum_{n=0}^{N} P(n) = 1.$$

In risk analysis, p and q are also the failure and success rates, gleaned, for instance, from random or strategic sampling of arbitrary lot sizes. Obviously, the larger the sample size, the better are the estimates of p or q. Once p or q is determined, the binomial statistics and probabilities are also fixed. The statistical mean, M, and variance, s, are given by,

$$M = \sum_{n=1}^{N} nP(n) = pN,$$

$$s = \sum_{n=1}^{N} (n - M)^2\, P(n) = pqN,$$

the usual measures of a statistical distribution. The square root of the variance is the standard deviation. The cumulative probability for more than n cases of decompression sickness, $P_>(n)$, is written,

$$P_>(n) = \sum_{j=n+1}^{N} P(j) = 1 - \sum_{j=0}^{n} P(j),$$

and the probability of less than n cases, $P_<(n)$, is similarly,

$$P_<(n) = \sum_{j=0}^{n-1} P(j) = 1 - \sum_{j=n}^{N} P(j).$$

The probability of nonoccurrence in any set of N trials is simply,

$$P(0) = q^N,$$

while the probability of total occurrence in the same number, N, of trials is given by,

$$P(N) = p^N.$$

The binomial distribution is a special case of the multinomial distribution describing processes in which several results having fixed probabilities, p_l, q_l, for $l = 1$, L, are possible. Separate probabilities are given by the individual terms in the general multinomial expansion,

$$(p_1 + q_1 + ... + p_L + q_L)^N = \sum_{n_1,...,n_{L-1}=0}^{N} P(n_1, ..., n_{L-1}) = 1,$$

as in the binomial case. The normal distribution is a special case of the binomial distribution when N is very large and variables are not necessarily confined to integer values. The Poisson distribution is another special case of the binomial distribution when the number of events, N, is also large, but the incidence, p, is small.

Normal Distribution

The normal distribution is an analytic approximation to the binomial distribution when N is very large, and n, the observed value (success or failure rate), is not confined to integer values, but ranges continuously,

$$-\infty \leq n \leq \infty.$$

Normal distributions thus apply to continuous observables, while binomial and Poisson distributions apply to discontinuous observables. Statistical theories of errors are ordinarily based on normal distributions.

For the same mean, $M = pN$, and variance, $s = pqN$, the normal distribution, P, written as a continuously varying function of n,

$$P(n) = \frac{1}{(2\pi s)^{1/2}} \, exp\left[-(n-M)^2/2s\right],$$

is a good approximation to the binomial distribution in the range,

$$\frac{1}{N+1} < p < \frac{N}{N+1},$$

and within three standard deviations of the mean,

$$pN - 3\,(pqN)^{1/2} \leq n \leq pN + 3\,(pqN)^{1/2}.$$

The distribution is normalized to one over the real infinite interval,

$$\int_{-\infty}^{\infty} P dn = 1.$$

The probability that a normally distributed variable, n, is less than or equal to b is,

$$P_<(b) = \int_{-\infty}^{b} P dn,$$

while the corresponding probability that n is greater than or equal to b is,

$$P_>(b) = \int_b^\infty P\,dn.$$

The normal distribution is extremely important in statistical theories of random variables. By the central limit theorem, the distribution of sample means of identically distributed random variables is approximately normal, regardless of the actual distribution of the individual variables.

Poisson Distribution

The Poisson distribution is a special case of the binomial distribution when N becomes large, and p is small, and certainly describes all discrete random processes whose probability of occurrence is small and constant. The Poisson distribution applies substantially to all observations made concerning the incidence of decompression sickness in diving, that is, $p \ll 1$ as the desired norm. The reduction of the binomial distribution to the Poisson distribution follows from limiting forms of terms in the binomial expansion, that is, $P(n)$.

In the limit, $N \to \infty$, and, $p \ll 1$, we have,

$$\frac{N!}{(N-n)!} \approx N^n,$$

$$q^m = (1-p)^{N-n} \approx exp\,(-pN),$$

and therefore the binomial probability reduces to,

$$P(n) = \frac{N^n p^n}{n!}\,exp\,(-pN) = \frac{M^n}{n!}\,exp\,(-M),$$

which is the discrete Poisson distribution. The mean, M, is given as before,

$$M = pN$$

and the variance, s, has the same value,

$$s = pN,$$

because q is approximately one. The cumulative probabilities, $P_>(n)$ and $P_<(n)$, are the same as those defined in the binomial case, a summation over discrete variable, n. It is appropriate to employ the Poisson approximation when $p \le 0.10$, and $N \ge 10$ in trials. Certainly, from a numerical point of view, the Poisson distribution is easier to use than binomial distribution. Computation of factorials is a lesser task, and bookkeeping is minimal for the Poisson case.

In addition to the incidence of decompression sickness, the Poisson distribution describes the statistical fluctuations in such random processes as the number of cavalry soldiers kicked and killed by horses, the disintegration of atomic nuclei, the emission of light quanta by excited atoms, and the appearance of cosmic ray bursts. It also applies to most rare diseases.

Probabilistic Decompression

Table 40 lists corresponding binomial decompression probabilities, $P(n)$, for 1% and 10% underlying incidence (99% and 90% nonincidence), yielding 0, 1, and 2 or more cases of decompression sickness. The underlying incidence, p, is the (fractional) average of hits.

As the number of trials increases, the probability of 0 or 1 occurrences drops, while the probability of 2 or more occurrences increases. In the case of 5 dives, the probability might be as low as 5%, while in the case of 50 dives, the probability could be 39%, both for $p = 0.01$. Clearly, odds even percentages would require testing beyond 50 cases for an underlying incidence near 1%. Only by increasing the number of trials for fixed incidences can the probabilities be increased. Turning that around, a rejection procedure for 1 or more cases of decompression sickness at the 10% probability level requires many more than 50 dives. If we are willing to lower the confidence of the acceptance, or rejection, procedure, of course, the number of requisite trials drops. Table 40 also shows that the test practice of accepting an exposure schedule following 10 trials without incidence of decompression sickness is suspect, merely because the relative probability of nonincidence is high, near 35%.

Questions as to how safe are decompression schedules have almost never been answered satisfactorily. As seen, large numbers of binary events are required to reliably estimate the underlying incidence. One case of decompression sickness in 30 trials could result from an underlying incidence, p, bounded by 0.02 and 0.16 roughly. Tens more of trials are necessary to shrink those bounds.

Table 40. Probabilities Of Decompression Sickness For Underlying Incidences.

N (dives)	n (hits)	$P(n)$ $p = .01$ $q = .99$	$P(n)$ $p = .10$ $q = .90$
5	0	.95	.59
	1	.04	.33
	2 or more	.01	.08
10	0	.90	.35
	1	.09	.39
	2 or more	.01	.26
20	0	.82	.12
	1	.16	.27
	2 or more	.02	.61
50	0	.61	.01
	1	.31	.03
	2 or more	.08	.96

Biological processes are highly variable in outcome. Formal correlations with outcome statistics are then generally requisite to validate models against data. Often, this correlation is difficult to firmly establish (couple of percent) with fewer than 1,000 trial observations, while ten percent correlations can be obtained with 30 trials, assuming binomial distributed probabilities. For decompression analysis, this works as a disadvantage, because often the trial space of dives is small. Not discounting the possibly small trial space, a probabilistic approach to the occurrence of decompression sickness is useful and necessary. One very successful approach, developed and tuned by Weathersby, and others for decompression sickness in diving, called maximum likelihood, applies theory or models to diving data and adjusts the parameters until theoretical prediction and experimental data are in as close agreement as possible.

Validation procedures require decisions about uncertainty. When a given decompression procedure is repeated with different subjects, or the same subjects on different occasions, the outcome is not constant. The uncertainty about the occurrence of decompression sickness can be quantified with statistical statements, though, suggesting limits to the validation procedure. For instance, after analyzing decompression incidence statistics for a set of procedures, a table designer may report that the procedure will offer an incidence rate below 5%, with 90% confidence in the statement. Alternatively, the table designer can compute the probability of rejecting a procedure using any number of dive trials, with the rejection criteria any arbitrary number of incidences. As the number of trials increases, the probability of rejecting a procedure increases for fixed incidence criteria. In this way, relatively simple statistical procedures can provide vital information as to the number of trials necessary to validate a procedure with any level of acceptable risk, or the maximum risk associated with any number of incidences and trials.

One constraint usually facing the statistical table designer is a paucity of data, that is, number of trials of a procedure. Data on hundreds of repetitions of a dive profile are virtually nonexistent, excepting bounce diving perhaps. As seen, some 30–50 trials are requisite to ascertain procedure safety at the 10% level. But 30–50 trials is probably asking too much, is too expensive, or generally prohibitive. In that case, the designer may try to employ global statistical measures linked to models in a more complex trial space, rather than a single profile trial space. Integrals of risk parameters, such as bubble number, supersaturation, separated phase, etc., over exposures in time, can be defined as probability measures for incidence of decompression sickness, and the maximum likelihood method then used to extract appropriate constants.

Maximum Likelihood

We can never measure any physical variable exactly, that is, without error. Progressively more elaborate experimental or theoretical efforts only reduce the possible error in the determination. In extracting parameter estimates from data sets, it is necessary to also try to minimize the error (or data scatter) in the extraction process. A number of techniques are available to the analyst, including the well known maximum likelihood approach.

The measure of any random occurrence, p, can be a complicated function of many parameters, $x = (x_k, k = 1, K)$, with the only constraint,

$$0 \leq p(x) \leq 1,$$

for appropriate values of the set, x. The measure of nonoccurrence, q, is then by conservation of probability,

$$q(x) = 1 - p(x),$$

over the same range,

$$0 \leq q(x) \leq 1.$$

Multivalued functions, $p(x)$, are often constructed, with specific form dictated by theory or observation over many trials or tests. In decompression applications, the parameters, x, may well be the bubble-nucleation rate, number of venous gas emboli, degree of supersaturation, amount of pressure reduction, volume of separated gas, ascent rate, or combinations thereof. Parameters may also be integrated in time in any sequence of events, as a global measure, though such measures are more difficult to analyze over arbitrary trial numbers.

The likelihood of any outcome, Φ, of N trials is the product of individual measures of the form,

$$\Phi(n) = p^n q^m = p^n (1-p)^m,$$

given n cases of decompression sickness and m cases without decompression sickness, and,

$$n + m = N.$$

The natural logarithm of the likelihood, Ψ, is easier to use in applications, and takes the form,

$$\Psi = \ln \Phi = n \ln p + m \ln (1-p),$$

and is maximized when,

$$\frac{\partial \Psi}{\partial p} = 0.$$

In terms of the above, we then must have,

$$\frac{n}{p} - \frac{m}{1-p} = 0,$$

trivially requiring,

$$p = \frac{n}{n+m} = \frac{n}{N},$$

$$1 - p = q = \frac{m}{n+m} = \frac{m}{N}.$$

Thus, the likelihood function is maximized when p is the actual incidence rate, and q is the actual nonincidence rate. The multivalued probability functions, $p(x)$, generalize in the maximization process according to,

$$\frac{\partial \Psi}{\partial p} = \sum_{k=1}^{K} \frac{\partial \Psi}{\partial x_k} \frac{\partial x_k}{\partial p} = 0,$$

satisfied when,

$$\frac{\partial \Psi}{\partial x_k} = 0 \ \ for \ k = 1, \ K.$$

In application, such constraints are most easily solved on computers, with analytical or numerical methods.

In dealing with a large number of decompression procedures, spanning significant range in depth, time, and environmental factors, an integrated approach to maximum likelihood and risk is necessary. Integral measures, $p(x,t)$ and $q(x,t)$, can be defined over assumed decompression risk, $\zeta(x,t)$,

$$p(x,t) = 1 - exp\left[-\int_0^t \zeta(x,t')dt'\right],$$

$$q(x,t) = exp\left[-\int_0^t \zeta(x,t')dt'\right],$$

with t' any convenient time scale, and ζ any assumed risk, such as bubble number, saturation, venous emboli count, etc. as mentioned. Employing $p(x,t)$ and $q(x,t)$ in the likelihood function, and then maximizing according to the data, permits maximum likelihood estimation of $\zeta(x,t)$. Such an approach can be employed in decompression table fabrication, yielding good statistical estimates on incidence rates as a function of exposure factors.

Saturation Bends Probability

Many factors contribute to bends susceptibility. Age, obesity, temperature, physical condition, alcohol, and cigarettes are a few. Whatever the contributing factors, the distribution of bends depths for saturation exposures has been characterized in terms of the saturation tension, Q, and ambient pressure, P, by Hills. This characterization is not only of academic interest, but is also useful in assigning formal risk to decompression formats.

The distribution of saturation bends depths, χ, fits a Weibull function. This is true for all breathing mixtures, nitrox, heliox, trimix, etc. If cumulative fraction of air bends cases up to G is χ, the survivor fraction, $1 - \chi$, satisfies,

$$\ln (1 - \chi) = -\left[\frac{G - 14.3}{25.1}\right]^{4.73}$$

for cumulative bends probability, χ, the usual integral over bends risk, ζ, as a function of gradient, G,

$$\chi = \int_0^G \zeta(G')dG'$$

with saturation bends gradient, G, measured in fsw,

$$G = Q - P$$

As the gradient grows, the survivor function approaches zero exponentially. The smallest bends gradient is 14.3 fsw, which can be contrasted with the average value of 26.5 fsw. The root mean square gradient is 27.5 fsw. At 27 fsw, the survivor fraction is 0.96, while 67% of survivors fall in the range, 26.5 ± 7.6 fsw, with 7.6

fsw the standard deviation. For gas mixtures other than air, the general form is given by,

$$\ln\,(1-\chi) = -\varepsilon \left[\frac{(P_f - 20.5)}{(P_i - 33.0)} - \frac{1}{f_i} \right]^{\delta}$$

where f_i is the total volume fraction of inert breathing gases, for $G = P_f - P_i$, and with ε, δ constants.

The efficiency of the Weibull distribution in providing a good fit to the saturation data is not surprising. The Weibull distribution enjoys success in reliability studies involving multiplicities of fault factors. It obviously extends to any set of hyperbaric or hypobaric exposure data, using any of the many parameter risk variables described above.

Table and Profile Risks

A global statistical approach to table fabrication consists of following a risk measure, or factor p, throughout and after sets of exposures, tallying the incidence of DCI, and then applying maximum likelihood to the risk integral in time, extracting any set of risk constants optimally over all dives in the maximization procedure. In analyzing air and helium data, Weathersby assigned risk as the difference between tissue tension and ambient pressure divided by ambient pressure. One tissue was assumed, with time constant ultimately fixed by the data in ensuing maximum likelihood analysis. The measure of nonincidence, q, was taken to be the exponential of risk integrated over all exposure time,

$$q(\kappa,\tau) = exp \left[- \int_0^{\infty} \zeta(\kappa,\tau,t')dt' \right],$$

$$\zeta(\kappa,\tau,t') = \kappa \, \frac{p(t') - p_a}{p_a},$$

with κ a constant determined in the likelihood maximization, p_a ambient pressure, and $p(t')$ the instantaneous Haldane tension for tissue with halftime, τ, also determined in the maximization process, corresponding to arbitrary tissue compartments for the exposure data. Other more complex likelihood functions can also employed, for instance, the separated phase volume according to the varying permeability and reduced gradient bubble models,

$$\zeta(\kappa,\xi,\tau,t') = \kappa\Lambda(t')G(t'),$$

$$\Lambda(t') = \left[1 - \frac{r(t')}{\xi} \right],$$

with Λ the permissible bubble excess, r the bubble radius, G the bubble diffusion gradient (dissolved-free gas), and κ and ξ constants determined in the fit maximization of the data. Another risk possibility is the tissue ratio,

$$\zeta(\kappa,\tau,t') = \kappa \, \frac{p(t')}{p_a},$$

a measure of interest in altitude diving applications.

Hundreds of air dives were analyzed using this procedure, permitting construction of decompression schedules with 95% and 99% confidence (5% and 1% bends probability). These tables were published by US Navy investigators, and Table 41 tabulates the corresponding nonstop time limits ($p = 0.05, 0.01$), and also includes the standard US Navy (Workman) limits for comparison. Later re-evaluations of the standard set of nonstop time limits estimate a probability rate of 1.25% for the limits. In actual usage, the incidence rates are below 0.001%, because users do not dive to the limits generally.

Table 41. Nonstop Time Limits For 1% And 5% DCI Probability.

Depth d (*fsw*)	Nonstop limit t_n (*min*) $p = .05$	Nonstop limit t_n (*min*) $p = .01$	Nonstop limit t_n (*min*) US Navy
30	240	170	
40	170	100	200
50	120	70	100
60	80	40	60
70	80	25	50
80	60	15	40
90	50	10	30
100	50	8	25
110	40	5	20
120	40	5	15
130	30	5	10

For the past 10–15 years, this probabilistic approach to assessing risk in diving has been in vogue. Sometimes this can be confusing, or misleading, since definitions or terms, as presented, are often mixed. Also confusing are risk estimates varying by factors of 10 to 1,000, and distributions serving as basis for analysis, also varying in size by the same factors. So, before continuing with a risk analysis of recreational profiles, a few comments are germane.

Any set of statistical data can be analyzed directly, or sampled in smaller chunks. The smaller sets (samples) may or may not reflect the parent distribution, but if the analyst does his work correctly, samples reflecting the parent distribution can be extracted for study. In the case of dive profiles, risk probabilities extracted from sample profiles try to reflect the incidence rate, p, of the parent distribution (N profiles, and p underlying DCI rate). The incidence rate, p, is the most important metric, followed by the shape of the distribution in total as measured by the variance, s. For smaller sample of profile size, $K < N$, we have mean incidences, Q, for sample incidence rate, r,

$$Q = rK$$

and variance, v,

$$v = r(1 - r)K$$

By the central limit theorem, the distribution of sample means, Q, is normally distributed about parent (actual) mean, M, with variance, $v = s/K$. Actually, the distribution of sample means, Q, is normally distributed no matter what the distribution of samples. This important fact is the basis for error estimation with establishment of confidence intervals, χ, for r, with estimates denoted, $r_{\pm}$,

$$r_{\pm} = r \pm \chi \left[\frac{s}{K}\right]^{1/2}$$

$$0 < \chi < 1$$

The sample binomial probability, $B(k)$, is analogously,

$$B(k) = \frac{K!}{k!\, j!} r^k (1 - r)^j$$

constrained, $k + j = K$, for k number of DCI hits, and normalized,

$$\sum_{k=1}^{K} B(k) = 1$$

with important limiting property, if $K \to \infty$, then $B(k) \to 0$, when, $r << 1$.

For example, if 12 cases of DCI are reported in a parent set of 7,896 profiles, then,

$$N = 7896$$

$$p = \frac{12}{7896} = .0015$$

Smaller samples might be used to estimate risk, via sample incidence, r, with samples possibly chosen to reduce computer processing time, overestimate p for conservancy sake, focus on a smaller subregion of profiles, or any other reason. Thus, one might nest all 12 DCI incidence profiles in a smaller sample, $K = 1,000$, so that the sample risk, $r = 12/1,000 = 0.012$, is larger than p. Usually though the analyst wishes to mirror the parent distribution in the sample. If the parent is a set of benign, recreational, no decompression, no multiday dive profiles, and the sample mirrors the parent, then both risks, p and r, are are reasonably true measures of actual risk associated with recreational diving. If sample distributions chosen are not representative of the class of diving performed, risk estimates are not trustworthy. For instance, if a high risk set of mixed gas decompression profiles were the background against which recreational dive profiles were compared, all estimates would be skewed and faulty (actually underestimated in relative risk, and overestimated in absolute risk). For this parent set, N is large, p is small, with mean, $M = pN = 0.0015 \times 7896 = 12$, and the applicable binomial statistics smoothly transition to Poisson representation, convenient for logarithmic and covariant numerical analysis (on a computer). Additionally, any parent set may be a large sample of a megaset, so that p is itself an estimate of risk in the megaset.

Turns out that our parent distribution above is just that, a subset of larger megaset, namely, the millions and millions of recreational dives performed and logged over the past 30 years, or so. The above set of profiles was collected in training and vacation diving scenarios. The set is recreational (no decompression, no multiday, light, benign) and representative, with all the distribution metrics as listed. For reference and perspective, sets of recreational profiles collected by others (Gilliam, NAUI, PADI, YMCA, DAN) are similar in context, but larger in size, N, and smaller in incidence rate, p. Data and studies reported by many sources quote, $N > 1,000,000$, with, $p < 0.00001 = 0.001\%$. Obviously our set has higher rate, p, though still nominally small, but the same shape. So our estimates will be liberal (overestimate risk).

To perform risk analysis, a risk estimator need be employed. For diving, dissolved gas and phase estimators are useful. Two, detailed earlier, are used here. First is the dissolved gas supersaturation ratio, historically coupled to Haldane models, ϕ,

$$\phi = \kappa \, \frac{p - \lambda p_a}{p_a}$$

and second, ψ, is the separated phase, invoked by phase models,

$$\psi = \gamma \left[1 - \frac{r}{\xi} \right] G$$

For simplicity, the asymptotic exposure limit is used in the likelihood integrals for both risk functions,

$$1 - r(\kappa,\lambda) = exp \left[- \int_0^\infty \phi(\kappa,\lambda,t)dt \right]$$

$$1 - r(\gamma,\xi) = exp \left[- \int_0^\infty \psi(\gamma,\xi,t)dt \right]$$

with $hit - no\ hit$, likelihood function, Ω, of form,

$$\Omega = \prod_{k=1}^{K} \Omega_k$$

$$\Omega_k = r_k^{\delta_k} (1 - r_k)^{1-\delta_k}$$

where, $\delta_k = 0$ if DCI does not occur in profile, k, or, $\delta_k = 1$ if DCI does occur in profile, k. To estimate κ, λ, γ, and ξ in maximum likelihood, a modified Levenberg-Marquardt algorithm is employed (*SNLSE*, Common Los Alamos Applied Mathematical Software Library), just a nonlinear least squares data fit to an arbitrary function (minimization of variance over K datapoints here), with $L1$ error norm. Additionally, using a random number generator for profiles across 1,000 parallel SMP (Origin 2000) processors at LANL, we construct 1,000 subsets, with $K = 2,000$ and $r = 0.006$, for separate likelihood regression analysis, averaging κ, λ, γ, and ξ by weighting the inverse variance.

For recreational diving, both estimators are roughly equivalent, because little dissolved gas has separated into free phases (bubbles). Analysis shows this true for all cases examined, in that estimated risks for both overlap at the 95% confidence level. The only case where dissolved gas and phase estimators differ (slightly here) is within repetitive diving profiles. The dissolved gas estimator cues on gas buildup in the slow tissue compartments (staircasing for repets within an hour or two), while the phase estimator cues on bubble gas diffusion in the fast compartments (dropping rapidly over hour time spans). This holding true within all recreational diving distributions, we proceed to the risk analysis.

Nonstop limits (NDLs), denoted t_n as before, from the US Navy, PADI, and NAUI Tables, and those employed by the Oceanic decometer provide a set for comparison of relative DCI risk. Listed below in Table 42 are the NDLs and corresponding risks (in parentheses) for the profile, assuming ascent and descent rates of 60 fsw/min (no safety stops). Haldane and RGBM estimates vary little for these cases, and only the phase estimates are included.

Table 42. Risk Estimates For Various NDLs

d (fsw)	USN t_n (*min*)	PADI t_n (*min*)	NAUI t_n (*min*)	Oceanic t_n (*min*)
35	310 (4.3%)	205 (2.0%)		181 (1.3%)
40	200 (3.1%)	140 (1.5%)	130 (1.4%)	137 (1.5%)
50	100 (2.1%)	80 (1.1%)	80 (1.1%)	80 (1.1%)
60	60 (1.7%)	55 (1.4%)	55 (1.4%)	57 (1.5%)
70	50 (2.0%)	40 (1.2%)	45 (1.3%)	40 (1.2%)
80	40 (2.1%)	30 (1.3%)	35 (1.5%)	30 (1.3%)
90	30 (2.1%)	25 (1.5%)	25 (1.5%)	24 (1.4%)
100	25 (2.1%)	20 (1.3%)	22 (1.4%)	19 (1.2%)
110	20 (2.2%)	13 (1.1%)	15 (1.2%)	16 (1.3%)
120	15 (2.0%)	13 (1.3%)	12 (1.2%)	13 (1.3%)
130	10 (1.7%)	10 (1.7%)	8 (1.3%)	10 (1.7%)

Risks are internally consistent across NDLs at each depth, and agree with the US Navy assessments in Table 41. Greatest underlying and binomial risks occur in the USN shallow exposures. The PADI, NAUI, and Oceanic risks are all less than 2% for this set, thus binomial risks for single DCI incidence are less than 0.02%. PADI and NAUI have reported that field risks (p) across all exposures are less than 0.001%, so considering their enviable track record of diving safety, our estimates are liberal. Oceanic risk estimates track as the PADI and NAUI risks, again, very safely.

Next, the analysis is extended to profiles with varying ascent and descent rates, safety stops, and repetitive sequence. Table 43 lists nominal profiles (recreational) for various depths, exposure and travel times, and safety stops at 5 msw. Mean DCI estimates, r, are tabulated for both dissolved gas supersaturation ratio (ZHL) and bubble number excess (RGBM) risk functions, with, employing maximum variance, $r_\pm = r \pm .004$.

Table 43. Dissolved And Separated Phase Risk Estimates For Nominal Profiles.

Profile (depth/time)	Descent rate (msw/min)	Ascent rate (msw/min)	Safety stop (depth/time)	Risk r_{RGBM}	risk r_{ZHL}
14 msw/38 min	18	9	5 msw/3 min	.0034	.0062
19 msw/38 min	18	9	5 msw/3 min	.0095	.0110
28 msw/32 min	18	9		.0200	.0213
37 msw/17 min	18	9	5 msw/3 min	.0165	.0151
18 msw/31 min	18	9	5 msw/3 min	.0063	.0072
	18	9		.0088	.0084
	18	18		.0101	.0135
	18	18	5 msw/3 min	.0069	.0084
17 msw/32 min SI 176 min	18	9	5 msw/3 min		
13 msw/37 min SI 174 min	18	9	5 msw/3 min		
23 msw/17 min	18	18	5 msw/3 min	.0127	.0232

The ZHL (Buhlmann) NDLs and staging regimens are widespread across decompression meters presently, and are good representation for Haldane risk analysis. The RGBM is newer and more modern (and more physically correct), and is coming online in decometers and associated software. For recreational exposures, the RGBM collapses to a Haldane dissolved gas algorithm. This is reflected in the risk estimates above, where estimates for both models differ little.

Simple comments hold for the analyzed profile risks. The maximum relative risk is 0.0232 for the 3 dive repetitive sequence according to the Haldane dissolved risk estimator. This translates to 0.2% binomial risk, which is comparable to the maximum NDL risk for the PADI, NAUI, and Oceanic NDLs. Again, this type of dive profile is common, practiced daily on liveaboards, and benign. According to Gilliam, the absolute incidence rate for this type of diving is less than 0.02%. Again, our analyses overestimate risk.

Effects of slower ascent rates and safety stops are noticeable at the 0.25% to 0.5% level in relative surfacing risk. Safety stops at 5 *m* for 3 *min* lower relative risk an average of 0.3%, while reducing the ascent rate from 18 msw/min to 9 msw/min reduces relative risk an average of 0.35%.

Staging, NDLs, and contraints imposed by decometer algorithms are consistent with acceptable and safe recreational diving protocols. Estimated absolute risk associated across all ZHL NDLs and staging regimens analyzed herein is less than 0.232%, probably much less in actual practice. That is, we use $p = 0.006$, and much evidence suggests $p < 0.0001$, some ten times safer.

Implicit in such formulations of risk tables are assumptions that given decompression stress is more likely to produce symptoms if it is sustained in time, and that large numbers of separate events may culminate in the same probability after time integration. Though individual schedule segments may not be replicated enough to offer total statistical validation, categories of predicted safety can always be grouped within subsets of corroborating data. Since the method is general, any model parameter or meaningful index, properly normalized, can be applied to decompression data, and the full power of statistical methods employed to quantify overall risk. While powerful, such statistical methods are neither deterministic nor mechanistic, and cannot predict on first principles. But as a means to table fabrication with quoted risk, such approaches offer attractive pathways for analysis.

Validation procedures for schedules and tables can be quantified by a set of procedures based on statistical decompression analysis:

- select or construct a measure of decompression risk, or a probabilistic model;
- evaluate as many dives as possible, and especially those dives similar in exposure time, depth, and environmental factors;
- conduct limited testing if no data is available;
- apply the model to the data using maximum likelihood;
- construct appropriate schedules or tables using whatever incidence of decompression sickness is acceptable;
- release and then collect profile statistics for final validation and tuning.

Questions of what risk is acceptable to the diver vary. Sport and research divers would probably opt for very small risk (0.01% or less), while military and commercial divers might live with higher risk (1%), considering the nearness of medical attention in general. Many factors influence these two populations, but fitness and acclimatization levels would probably differ considerably across them. While such factors are difficult to fold into any table exercise or analysis, the simple fact that human subjects in dive experiments exhibit higher incidences during testing phases certainly helps to lower the actual incidence rate in the field, noted by Bennett and Lanphier.

Keyed Exercises

- *What is the probability, $P(3)$, for 3 DCI cases in 100 dives, given an underlying incidence rate of 5%?*

$$P(n) = \frac{N!}{n!\,m!} p^n q^m, \quad N = 100, \quad n = 3, \quad m = 97$$

$$p = .05, \quad q = .95$$

$$P(3) = \left[\frac{100!}{3!\,97!}\right] \times (.05)^3 \times (.95)^{97} = \left[\frac{100 \times 99 \times 98}{1 \times 2 \times 3}\right] \times (.0001) \times (.0069) = .111$$

What is the probability, $Q(97)$, for 97 cases no DCI in the same sample?

$$Q(97) = P(3) = .111$$

- *What is the probability, $P(1)$, for one hit (DCI) in 20 dives with underlying incidence, $p = .01$?*

$$P(1) = .16$$

What is the probability, $P_>(2)$, for two or more hits in 20 dives for the same underlying incidence?

$$P_>(2) = .02$$

- *What is the survivor fraction, $1 - \chi$, for decompression of saturated air divers across, $G = 35\ fsw$?*

$$1 - \chi = exp\ \left[-\frac{G - 14.3}{25.1} \right]^{4.73}$$

$$1 - \chi = exp\ \left[-\frac{21.7}{25.1} \right]^{4.73} = exp\ (-.46) = .63$$

What is the cumulative DCI incidence rate, χ?

$$\chi = 1 - .63 = .37$$

- *What can you say about the DCI relative incidence, p, for a nonstop exposure at 80 fsw for 40 min?*

$$0.01\ <\ p\ <\ 0.05$$

What can you say about the (old) USN nonstop limit of 200 min at 40 fsw?

$$p\ >\ 0.05$$

- *A table modeler wants to use maximum likelihood in fitting the data to a DCI risk function, ϕ, of the temporal form, $\phi = exp\ (-qt)$, for 1000 trial dives with some 200 cases of DCI. What are the risk forms, ρ and σ (probabilities)?*

$$\rho(t) = 1 - exp\ \left[-\int_0^t \phi(t')dt' \right] = 1 - exp\ [-(exp\ (-qt) - 1)/q]$$

$$\sigma(t) = exp\ \left[-\int_0^t \phi(t')dt' \right] = exp\ [-(exp\ (-qt) - 1)/q]$$

What are the asymptotic limits, $\rho(\infty)$ and $\sigma(\infty)$?

$$\rho(\infty) \rightarrow 1 - exp\ (-1/q)$$

$$\sigma(\infty) \rightarrow exp\ (-1/q)$$

What is the value of q for the asymptotic forms?

$$\Psi = 200\ln\ [1 - exp\ (-1/q)] + 800\ln\ [exp\ (-1/q)]$$

$$\frac{\partial \Psi}{\partial q} = \left[\frac{-200}{1 - exp\ (-1/q)} \right] \left[\frac{exp\ (-1/q)}{q^2} \right] + \left[\frac{800}{exp\ (-1/q)} \right] \left[\frac{exp\ (-1/q)}{q^2} \right] = 0$$

$$exp\left(-1/q\right) = .800, \quad -\left[\frac{1}{q}\right] = \ln .8$$

$$q = -\left[\frac{1}{\ln .8}\right] = 4.48$$

Data Banks and Model Correlation

Profile Data Banks are extended collections of dive profiles with conditions and outcomes. To validate tables, meters, and software within any computational model, profiles and outcomes are necessarily matched to model parameters with statistical (fit) rigor. Profile-outcome information is termed a Data Bank (DB) these days, and there are a couple of them worth discussing. Others will surely develop along similar lines. Their importance is growing rapidly in technical and recreational sectors not only for the information they house, but also for application to diving risk analysis and model tuning.

One well known DB is the DAN Project Dive Exploration (PDE) collection. The PDE collection focuses on recreational air and nitrox diving up to now, but is extending to technical, mixed gas, and decompression diving. Approximately 87,000 profiles reside on PDE computers with some 97 cases of DCS across the air and nitrox recreational diving. PDE came online in the 1995, under the guidance of Dick Vann and Petar Denoble. DAN Europe, under Alessandro Marroni, joined forces with DAN USA in the 2000s extending PDE. Their effort in Europe is termed Dive Safe Lab (DSL). DSL has approximately 50,000 profiles with 8 cases of DCS. For simplicity following, we group PDE and DSL together as one DB, as information is easily exchanged across their computers. In combo, PDE and DSL house some 137,000 profiles with 105 cases of DCS. The incidence rate is 0.0008 roughly. This is a massive and important collection.

Another more recent DB focused on technical, mixed gas, decompression diving is the Data Bank at Los Alamos National Laboratory (LANL DB). Therein some 2,879 profiles with 20 cases of DCS reside. The Author is mainly responsible for bringing the LANL DB online in the early 2000s. Much of the LANL DB rests on data extracted from C&C Dive Team operations over the past 20 years or so. In LANL DB, the actual incidence rate is 0.0069, roughly 10 times greater than PDE and SDL. Such might be expected as LANL DB houses mixed gas, decompression profiles, a likely riskier diving activity with more unknowns.

In both cases, data collection is an ongoing effort, and profile information can be narrowed down to its simplest form, most of it coming from dive computer downloads tagging information across variable time intervals (3–5 *seconds*) which is then processed into a more manageable format for future statistical analysis:

- bottom mix/p_{O_2}, depth, and time;
- ascent and descent rates;
- stage and decompression mix/p_{O_2}, depths, and times;
- surface intervals;

- time to fly;
- diver age, weight, sex, and health complications;
- outcome rated 1–5 in order of bad to good;
- environmental factors (temperature, current, visibility, equipment).

Different DBs will use variations on reported data, but the above covers most of the bases.

Staging is properly a single most concern in diving. Depths, exposure times, gas mixes and switches, ascent and descent rates, open circuit (OC)and rebreather (RB) systems, shallow or deep stops are a few of many choices facing divers. Within that set, there are an infinity of possibilities to bring a diver to the surface, but not all safe.

The question of diving data then becomes important. Many feel that the matching of models and data requires data across a spectrum of diving activities, with the more the better, rather than just directed clinical but scattered tests. While manned tests of single profiles are certainly important, it is usually difficult to extrapolate results to all *other* cases because of the multiplicity of possible events for differing depths, gas mixtures, ascent rates, level stagings, and combinations of all. In other words, isolated tests are hard to kluge together, and, therefore, the widest possible spectrum of diving profile-outcomes is preferrable. Besides, there is likely not enough money nor time to test all pertinent mixed gas, decompression profiles of interest across all diving sectors. In that same vein, the focus of Data Banks is operational diving, and not clinical tests.

Another concern is deep stop data across OC and RB diving. The shallow stop paradigm of Haldane has persisted for almost a century and most data taken over the years reflects shallow stop staging as the focus for testing and dive planning. While it can be shown that both deep stop and shallow stop diving can be effected within the same relative risk levels, deep stop diving is more efficient timewise (shorter) than shallow stop diving. To fill the gap in deep stop data, Data Banks need engage in collecting profile-outcomes for deep stop (bubble) models for correlation of bubble models with both deep stop and shallow stop data. Recall that bubble models generally require deeper decompression staging than dissolved (Haldane) gas models, and collapse to dissolve gas models in the limit of little, or no, bubble excitation and growth. The real task is deep stop decompression data correlations, as it has been shown that bubble models recover shallow stop staging as the failsafe option. In fairness to Haldane, we need note that he tested deep stops 100 years ago, but they never made it into his tables, nor other dissolved gas tables later. Reasons are sundry and various.

Both DBs are storing important dive information as summarized. Specific profile entry points span recreational to technical, OC to RB, air to mixed gas, and shallow to deep diving. That's a lot of territory. PDE and DSL are focused on no decompression diving, while LANL DB is focused on decompression diving. Of course, overlaps exist. Consider both DBs in more detail.

PDE plus DSL houses some 137,000 profiles with 105 cases of DCS. The underlying incidence rate is roughly $p = 105/137,000 = 0.0008$, well below 1%. Both gather data on dives, conditions, and outcomes to assess DCS and risk factors.

One interesting study contrasted risk in 3 dive groups, namely, warm water divers, cold water divers, and USN chamber (wet pod) divers. Outcomes are tabulated in Table 44. The main purpose of including USN chamber dives is one of calibration of model to data across all 3 cases. USN divers were also immersed and exercising too.

Table 44. Three Group Population Sample

Dive group	Dives	DCS hits	Incidence
warm water	51497	8	0.0002
cold water	6527	18	0.0028
USN chamber	2252	70	0.0311

The highest overall hit rate occurs in USN chamber divers, and lowest in warm water divers. But there is more info in this 3 class sample, as extensive statistical analysis shows.

While USN chamber dive risks are absolutely and relatively higher, a further breakdown of cold water versus (just) Scapa Flow risk shows that Scapa Flow risks are also inherently smaller by comparison to other cold water risks. Scapa Flow is located off the northern coast of Scotland in the Orkney Islands and is the historical cemetary for wrecks dating back to the Vikings. During WW1 and WW2, Scapa Flow was home to the Royal Navy. It is plausible to speculate that long, decompression dives put USN divers at higher risk than short, no decompression, warm water dives due to thermal stresses (temperature). And more particularly, the lower risks for Scapa Flow divers are thought to result from extensive use of drysuits to offset heat loss as a thermal stress. Recall also that low risk dives require many more trials than high risk dives to extract credible statistical info.

An important spinoff of the DSL collection is Doppler data collected off recreational air divers making 1/2 deep stops for 2–3 *min* after no decompression exposures. Bennett and Marroni clocked Doppler (bubble count) minima in divers performing 1/2 deep stops after exposures close to the old USN NDLs for various depths. Parallel analyses using profiles from the LANL DB exhibit risk minimization in the same time frames for the 1/2 deep stop within bubble models, but not supersaturation models. This is seen in Table 45. Supersaturation risk increases

Table 45. Doppler and Bubble Risk Minimization

depth/time (fsw/min)		bubble risk			supersaturation risk		
	no stop	1 *min*	2.5 *min*	4 *min*	1 *min*	2.5 *min*	4 *min*
80/40	0.0210	0.0193	0.0190	0.0191	0.0212	0.0218	0.0226
90/30	0.0210	0.0187	0.0183	0.0184	0.0213	0.0220	0.0229
100/25	0.0210	0.0174	0.0171	0.0172	0.0215	0.0223	0.0234
110/20	0.0220	0.0165	0.0161	0.0162	0.0224	0.0232	0.0241
120/15	0.0200	0.0150	0.0146	0.0147	0.0210	0.0220	0.0238
130/10	0.0170	0.0129	0.0125	0.0126	0.0178	0.0191	0.0213

monotonically with deep stop time. Though relatively small, bubble risk reaches a minima somewhere in the 2–3 *min* 1/2 deep stop following dives to the air NDLs. Such represents a useful symbiosis between DSL and LANL DBs.

In all cases, supersaturation risk tracks higher than bubble risk, but all are relatively small. This comes as no surprise as USN NDLs have been used safely and successfully with and without deep safety stops for many years. Having just said that, however, Doppler scores are certainly a modern concern for all divers, and most would likely prefer to dive regimens that minimize Doppler counts.

Some 2,879 profiles now reside in the LANL DB. There are 20 cases of DCS in the data file. The underlying DCS incidence rate is, $p = 20/2879 = 0.0069$, below but near 1%. Stored profiles range from 150 fsw down to 840 fsw, with the majority above 350 fsw. All data enters through the author, that is, divers, profiles, and outcomes are filtered.

A summary breakdown of DCS hit (bends) data consists of the following:

- OC deep nitrox reverse profiles – 5 hits (3 DCS I, 2 DCS II)
- OC deep nitrox – 3 hits (2 DCS I, 1 DCS II)
- OC deep trimix reverse profiles – 2 hits (1 DCS II, 1 DCS III)
- OC deep trimix – 2 hits (1 DCS I, 1 DCS III)
- OC deep heliox – 2 hits (2 DCS II)
- RB deep nitrox – 2 hits (1 DCS I, 1 DCS II)
- RB deep trimix – 2 hits (1 DCS I, 1 DCS III)
- RB deep heliox – 2 hits (1 DCS I, 1 DCS II)

DCS I means limb bends, DCS II implies central nervous system (CNS) bends, and DCS III denotes inner ear bends (occurring mainly on helium mixtures). Both DCS II and DCS III are fairly serious afflictions, while DCS I is less traumatic. Deep nitrox means a range beyond 150 fsw, deep trimix means a range beyond 200 fsw, and deep heliox means a range beyond 250 fsw as a rough categorization. The abbreviation OC denotes open circuit, while RB denotes rebreather. Reverse profiles are any sequence of dives in which the present dive is deeper than the previous dive. Nitrox means an oxygen enriched nitrogen mixture (including air), trimix denotes a breathing mixture of nitrogen, helium, oxygen, and heliox is a breathing mixture of helium and oxygen. None of the trimix nor heliox cases involved oxygen enriched mixtures on OC, and RB hits did not involve elevated oxygen partial pressures above 1.4 *atm*. Nitrogen-to-helium (*heavy-to-light*) gas switches occurred in 4 cases, violating contemporary ICD (isobaric counterdiffusion) protocols . Isobaric counterdiffusion refers to two inert gases (usually nitrogen and helium) moving in opposite directions in tissues and blood. When summed, total gas tensions (partial pressures) can lead to increased supersaturation and bubble formation probability.

None of the set exhibited full body nor CNS (central nervous system) oxygen toxicity (*oxtox*). The 20 cases come after the fact, that is diver distress with hyperbaric chamber treatment following distress. Profiles originate with seasoned divers as well as from broader field testing reported to us, coming from divers using wrist slate decompression tables with computer backups. Most profiles reach us directly as computer downloads, which we translate to a requisite format. Approximately 88% of LANL DB entries emanate from computer downloads.

The data is relatively coarse grained, making compact statistics difficult. The incidence rate across the whole set is small, on the order of 1% and smaller. Fine graining into depths is not meaningful yet, so we breakout data into gas categories (nitrox, heliox, trimix), as tabulated earlier. Table 46 indicates the breakdown.

Table 46. Profile Gas-DCS Summary

Mix	Total profiles	DCS hits	Incidence
OC nitrox	344	8	0.0232
RB nitrox	550	2	0.0017
all nitrox	894	10	0.0112
OC trimix	656	4	0.0061
RB trimix	754	2	0.0027
all trimix	1410	6	0.0042
OC heliox	116	2	0.0172
RB heliox	459	2	0.0044
all heliox	575	4	0.0070
total	2879	20	0.0069

The DCS hit rate with nitrox is higher, but not statistically meaningful across this sparse set. The last entry is all mixes, as noted previously. In the above set, there are 35 *marginals*, that is, DCS was not diagnosed, but the diver surfaced feeling badly. In such cases, many do not weight the dive as a DCS hit.

It is also interesting to break mixed gas profiles into 100 fsw increments, though we do not do depth dependent statistics on these profiles. It is obvious that 500 fsw or so is the limit statistically to the data set. It is for that reason that we limit applications of the LANL algorithm to 540 fsw.

Table 47. Profile Gas-Depth Summary

	100 to 199 fsw	200 to 299 fsw	300 to 399 fsw	400 to 499 fsw	500 to 599 fsw	600+ fsw	total
OC nitrox	268	76					344
RB nitrox	213	246	91				550
OC trimix	10	388	226	26	4	2	656
RB trimix	22	358	266	108			754
OC heliox		42	49	25			116
RB heliox	12	195	143	107	2		459
total	525	1305	775	266	6	2	2879

The corresponding DCS hit summary for Table 47 is given in Table 48.

Table 48. DCS Gas-Depth Summary

	100 to 199 *fsw*	200 to 299 *fsw*	300 to 399 *fsw*	400 to 499 *fsw*	500 to 599 *fsw*	600+ *fsw*	total
OC nitrox	5	3					8
RB nitrox		1	1				2
OC trimix		2		1		1	4
RB trimix			1	1			2
OC heliox			2				2
RB heliox			1	1			2
total	5	6	5	3		1	20

Profiles come from technical diving selectively, essentially mixed gas, extended range, decompression, and extreme diving. Profiles from the recreational community are not included, unless they involve extreme exposures on air or nitrox (many repetitve dives, deeper than 150 *fsw*, altitude exposures, etc.). This low rate makes statistical analysis difficult, and we use a global approach to defining risk after we fit the model to the data using maximum likelihood. The maximum likelihood fit links directly to the binomial probability structure of DCS incidence in divers and aviators. Just a few comments here hopefully suffice to outline the complex mathematical process applied to model and data in what is termed maximum likelihood. The approach is used extensively across diving data. Exact details are presented in the next section for profile and risk analyses.

To analyze risk, a risk estimator must be used and fitted to the data. Two are very popular, that is, the supersaturation and bubble growth risk functions. These are explained qualitatively as follows:

- supersaturation (ratio) risk estimator—uses the difference between total inert gas tension and ambient pressure divided by ambient pressure as a measure of risk;
- bubble (ratio) risk estimator—uses the bubble growth rate divided by the initial volume of bubbles excited by compression-decompression as a measure of risk.

Mathematical expressions, and arbitrary parameters contained therein, are then fitted to the data in the process of maximum likelihood, that is, a probability function of all dive profiles and outcomes across the DB is matched in parameter and outcome space as best possible. Very high speed computers and sophisticated mathematical software are necessary in matching parameters to outcomes. Here at LANL, the world's largest and fastest supercomputers in parallel processing mode make short work of the fitting process.

In many studies, the supersaturation risk function does not correlate deep stop data well, while the bubble risk function fits both deep stop and shallow stop data. The bubble risk function we employ derives from the LANL bubble model (RGBM), of course, having enjoyed safe utility across many diving sectors in diverse application.

But it is no stretch to note that many modern bubble models would suggest much the same, generically, compared to dissolved gas models. Broadband analyses of PDE and SDL data suggests:

- models do not always extrapolate outside their calibration (data) points;
- probabilistic techniques coupled to real models are useful vehicles for diver risk estimation;
- dive conditions (environmental stresses) may significantly affect risk;
- the body mass index (BMI) often correlates with DCS risk, particularly for older and overweight divers;
- human characteristics such as age, sex, and certification level affect the likelihood of diving morbidity and fatality;
- leading causes of morbidity and mortality in diving are drowning, near drowning, barotrauma during ascension, and DCS;
- only 2% of recreational divers use tables for dive planning, with the rest relying on dive computers;
- nitrox diving is exploding in the recreational sector.

LANL DB profile analysis of dissolved gas staging versus bubble staging and related metrics, suggests broadly:

- deep stop data is intrinsically different from data collected in the past for diving validation, in that previous data is mainly based on shallow stop diver staging, a possible bias in dive planning;
- deep stop data and shallow stop data yield the same risk estimates for nominal, shallow, and nonstop diving because bubble models and dissolved gas models converge in the limit of very small phase separation;
- if shallow stop data is only employed in analyses, dissolved gas risk estimates will be usually higher than those computed with deep stop data;
- pure O_2 or $EAN80$ are standard OC switch gases in the 20 fsw zone;
- deep stops are standard across mixed gas diving, and DCS spikes are nonexistent;
- deep switches to nitrogen mixes off helium mixes are avoided by technical divers, instead oxygen fraction is increased by decrease in helium fraction;
- deep stop dive computers serve mostly as backup or bailout, with tables and dive planning software the choice for deep stop diving;
- DCS spikes across mixed gas, decompression, and deep stop diving are non existent using deep stop tables, meters, and software;
- DCS incidence rates are higher for technical diving versus recreational diving, but still small;
- RB usage is increasing across diving sectors;
- wrist dive computers possess chip speeds that allow full resolution of even the most extensive bubble models;
- technical diving data is most important for correlating models and data;

- technical divers do not dive air, particularly deep air, with trimix and heliox the choices for deep excursions;
- released deep stop tables, software, and meters enjoy extensive and safe utility among professional divers;
- technical diving is growing in leaps and bounds, with corresponding data accessible off computers and bottom timers;

Comparative Profiles and Risk

To perform risk analysis with the LANL Data Bank, an estimator need be selected. For diving, dissolved gas and phase estimators are useful. Two, detailed earlier, are extended here. First is the dissolved gas supersaturation ratio, historically coupled to Haldane models, ρ, written in modified ratio form,

$$\rho(\kappa,\lambda,t) = \kappa \left[\frac{\Pi(t) - P(t)}{P(t)} \right] - \kappa \, exp \, (-\lambda t)$$

and second, ψ, is the separated bubble volume, invoked by dual phase models,

$$\psi(\gamma,\mu,t) = \gamma \left[\frac{\phi(t)}{\phi_i(t)} \right] - \gamma \, exp \, (-\mu t)$$

with $\phi(t)$ the bubble volume due to excitation, diffusion, and Boyle expansion-contraction and ϕ_i the initial bubble excitation volume. The exponential terms in both risk functions merely insure data smoothing for short dives, that is, as $t \to 0$, then $r \to 0$, too. For long dives, $t \to \infty$, the exponential terms vanish. Physically, the exponential terms also link to bubble extinction, not discussed herein. Both risk functions vary in time, exposure, and staging. For simplicity, the asymptotic exposure limit is used in the likelihood integrals for both risk functions, r, across all compartments, τ,

$$1 - r(\kappa,\lambda) = exp \left[- \int_0^\infty \rho(\kappa,\lambda,t)dt \right]$$

$$1 - r(\gamma,\mu) = exp \left[- \int_0^\infty \psi(\gamma,\mu,t)dt \right]$$

with *hit* $-$ *no hit*, likelihood function, Ω, of form,

$$\Omega = \prod_{k=1}^{K} \Omega_k$$

$$\Omega_k = r_k^{\delta_k} (1 - r_k)^{1-\delta_k}$$

and logarithmic reduction, Ψ,

$$\Psi = ln \, \Omega$$

where, $\delta_k = 0$ if DCS does not occur in profile, k, or, $\delta_k = 1$ if DCS does occur in profile, k. To estimate κ, λ, γ, and μ in maximum likelihood, a modified Levenberg-Marquardt algorithm is employed (*SNLSE*, Common Los Alamos Applied Mathematical Software Library), a nonlinear least squares data fit (NLLS) to an arbitrary logarithmic function (minimization of variance over K data points with $L2$ error norm). The same technique was applied to estimating separated phase volume and inert gas densities. The mathematical approach is well known. To estimate a function Φ, using a fit set, Υ, that is,

$$\Phi = \frac{1}{2} \sum_{m=1}^{M} [\Upsilon_m(x_m)]^2$$

or, in vector notation,

$$\mid \Phi \mid = \frac{1}{2} \Upsilon(x) \cdot \Upsilon(x)$$

a solution vector, **p**, is found satisfying,

$$[\mathbf{J}^\dagger \mathbf{J} + \chi \mathbf{I}] \, \mathbf{p} = -\mathbf{J}^\dagger \mathbf{f}$$

with **J** the Jacobian (derivative determinant) of Υ,

$$\mathbf{J} = \frac{\partial \Upsilon}{\partial \mathbf{x}}$$

$\mathbf{J}^\dagger$ the hermitian inverse (transpose) of **J**, and **I** the identity operator. The χ are positive constants, and **p** is the approximation to Φ. Numerically, all Jacobian derivatives are estimated and used in the minimization fit. Functions are generally nonlinear in form and behavior, and the error is $L2$ (variance in fit to exact values). The process is iterative, with each update, **q**, of **p**, obtained from the Jacobian differential expansion,

$$\Upsilon(\mathbf{p}+\mathbf{q}) = \Upsilon(\mathbf{p}) + \mathbf{J}\mathbf{q}$$

The likelihood maximization technique amounts to numerically determining κ, γ, λ, and μ according to,

$$\frac{\partial \Psi}{\partial r} = \frac{\partial \Psi}{\partial \kappa}\frac{\partial \kappa}{\partial r} + \frac{\partial \Psi}{\partial \lambda}\frac{\partial \lambda}{\partial r} = 0$$

for the dissolved gas gradient ratio estimator, ρ, and,

$$\frac{\partial \Psi}{\partial r} = \frac{\partial \Psi}{\partial \gamma}\frac{\partial \gamma}{\partial r} + \frac{\partial \Psi}{\partial \mu}\frac{\partial \mu}{\partial r} = 0$$

for the phase estimator, ψ.

We assign numerical tasks to processors on the LANL Blue Mountain Machine, a massively parallel processor (MPP) with 2,000 nodes according to:

• each tissue compartment, τ, then, within each compartment;
• only nitrox data points;
• only trimix data points;
• only heliox data points;

- both nitrox and trimix data points;
- both nitrox and helium data points;
- both heliox and trimix data points;
- all heliox, nitrox, and trimix data points.

estimating κ, λ, γ, and μ across all domains. The last case, all data, is the full set employed in risk analysis, but there wasn't much difference in the estimators, seen in mean error estimates across the partitioned data structures. For 11 tissue compartments, and 7 data sets, 77 risk estimates emerge. Only maximum tissue risks are finally averaged and variance computed. In diver staging, certain tissue compartments control the exposure, This is true within dissolved gas algorithms, as well as bubble algorithms. Finally, we find across the partitioned data structures, 2–8 above:

$$\kappa = 0.91 \pm 0.14 \ min^{-1}$$

$$\lambda = 0.28 \pm 0.11 \ min^{-1}.$$

and, similarly.

$$\gamma = 0.09 \pm 0.07 \ min^{-1}$$

$$\mu = 0.88 \pm 0.46 \ min^{-1}$$

For notational shorthand, we abbreviate supersaturation and bubble risk functions,

$$\sigma = r(\kappa, \lambda)$$

$$\beta = r(\gamma, \mu)$$

The data is relatively coarse grained, making compact statistics difficult. The incidence rate across the whole set is small, on the order of 1% and smaller. Fine graining into depths is not meaningful yet, so we breakout data into gas categories (nitrox, heliox, trimix), as tabulated earlier. Table 49 indicates the breakdown.

Table 49. Profile Data

Mix	Total profiles	DCS hits	Incidence
OC nitrox	344	8	0.0232
RB nitrox	550	2	0.0017
all nitrox	894	10	0.0112
OC trimix	656	4	0.0061
RB trimx	754	2	0.0027
all trimix	1410	6	0.0042
OC heliox	116	2	0.0172
RB heliox	459	2	0.0044
all heliox	575	4	0.0070
all	2879	20	0.0069

The DCS hit rate with nitrox is higher, but not statistically meaningful across this sparse set. The last entry is all mixes, as noted previously.

The logarithmic likelihood (LL), Ψ, is a rough metric for fits to bubble and supersaturation risk estimators. The canonical value, Ψ_6, is the LL for the 6 RB/OC control data set. No fit value, Ψ, will better the canonical value, Ψ_6, that is,

$$\Psi_6 = -112.9$$

$$\Psi \leq \Psi_6$$

meaning all fits will be more negative (smaller LL). Results are tabulated as follow in Table 50.

Table 50. Logarithmic Likelihood And Logarithmic Likelihood Ratio

estimator	LL	parameters	LLR	α
6 step set	$\Psi_6 = -112.9$	$p = 0.0232, 0.0061, 0.0172,$ $0.0036, 0.0027, 0.0044$		
3 step set	$\Psi_3 = -118.4$	$p = 0.0112, 0.0042, 0.0079$	$\Gamma_3 = 11.0$	0.013
full set	$\Psi_{full} = -119.2$	$p = 0.0069$	$\Gamma_{full} = 12.6$	0.033
σ	$\Psi_{sat} = -210.6$	$\kappa = 0.91 \pm 0.14 \ min^{-1}$ $\lambda = 0.28 \pm 0.11 \ min^{-1}$	$\Gamma_{sat} = 92.2$	0.001
β	$\Psi_{bub} = -113.3$	$\gamma = 0.09 \pm 0.07 \ min^{-1}$ $\mu = 0.88 \pm 0.46 \ min^{-1}$	$\Gamma_{bub} = 0.8$	0.933

The logarithmic likelihood ratio (LLR), denoted Γ, tests two models, and is χ^2 distributed,

$$\Gamma = 2(\Psi_6 - \Psi)$$

for Ψ the bubble and supersaturation estimators in Table 50. The percentage point, α, is the area under the χ^2 curve, from $\chi^2_{\alpha,v} = \Gamma$ to ∞,

$$\int_{\chi^2_{\alpha,v}}^{\infty} \chi^2(x,v)dx = \alpha$$

for v the degrees of freedom (6 - the number of bubble, supersaturation, 3 step, or full fit degrees of freedom). The *hit − no hit* criteria for the bubble estimator is the phase volume, Φ, while standard USN M-values are the criteria for the supersaturation estimator. Deep stops clobber M-values.

Clearly, the supersaturation risk function does not correlate well, compared to the bubble risk function. It does not work here in the deep decompression arena, but others have shown it correlates in the nonstop and light decompression limits. In those limits, bubble models and supersaturation models tend to converge, simply because phase growth is minimal.

This analysis suggests that deep stops are both safe and compact statistically for the LANL model and set. Coupled gas transport analysis suggests that deep stops and shallow stops can both be staged safely, but deep stops are more efficient in controlling bubble growth and are usually shorter in overall dive time duration. The deep stop approach to staging via the RGBM is the regimen encoded into a host of modern dive computers, including the EXPLORER from HydroSpace, the COBALT from Atomic Aquatics, the XEO from Liquivision, the VYPER, VYTEC, D9, and HelO2 from Suunto, the M1, NEMO, and PUCK from Mares, the UDI from UTC, the LEONARDO from Cressi, and others to name a few. All rely on the LANL Data Bank for statistical surety across both recreational and technical diving.

Nonstop limits (NDLs), denoted t_{nn}, from the US Navy, PADI, NAUI, and ZHL (Buhlmann) Tables provide a set for comparison of relative DCS risk. Listed in Table 51 are the NDLs and corresponding risks for the nonstop excursion, assuming ascent and descent rates of 60 fsw/min (no safety nor deep stops). Dissolved gas and phase risk estimates vary little for cases, and only the phase estimates are included. Surface intervals (SIs) between dives are time spent at the surface.

Table 51. Risk Estimates For Standard Air NDLs.

d (fsw)	USN NDL t_n (min)	risk β	PADI NDL t_n (min)	risk β	NAUI NDL t_n (min)	risk β	ZHL NDL t_n (min)	risk β
35	310	4.3%	205	2.0%			181	1.3%
40	200	3.1%	140	1.5%	130	1.4%	137	1.5%
50	100	2.1%	80	1.1%	80	1.1%	80	1.1%
60	60	1.7%	55	1.4%	55	1.4%	57	1.5%
70	50	2.0%	40	1.2%	45	1.3%	40	1.2%
80	40	2.1%	30	1.3%	35	1.5%	30	1.3%
90	30	2.1%	25	1.5%	25	1.5%	24	1.4%
100	25	2.1%	20	1.3%	22	1.4%	19	1.2%
110	20	2.2%	13	1.1%	15	1.2%	16	1.3%
120	15	2.0%	13	1.3%	12	1.2%	13	1.3%
130	10	1.7%	10	1.7%	8	1.3%	10	1.7%

Risks are internally consistent across NDLs at each depth, and agree with the US Navy assessments in Table 42. Greatest underlying risks occur in the USN shallow exposures. The PADI, NAUI, and ZHL risks are all less than 2% for this set, and risks for single DCS incidence are less than 0.02. PADI and NAUI have reported that incidence rates (p) across all exposures are less than 0.001%, so considering their enviable track record of diving safety, our estimates are liberal. ZHL risk estimates track as the PADI and NAUI risks, again, very safely. Estimates were corroborated within data sets at Duke both in Table 51 and Table 52.

Next, the analysis is extended to profiles with varying ascent and descent rates, safety stops, and repetitive sequence. Table 52 lists nominal profiles (recreational) for various depths, exposure and travel times, and safety stops at 5 *msw*. Mean DCS estimates, r, are tabulated for both dissolved gas supersaturation ratio and excited bubble volume risk functions, with nominal variance, $r_{\pm} = r \pm 0,004$, across all profiles.

Table 52. Dissolved And Separated Phase Risk Estimates For Nominal Profiles.

Profile (*depth/time*)	Descent rate (*msw/min*)	Ascent rate (*msw/min*)	Safety stop (*depth/time*)	Risk β	risk σ
14 *msw*/38 *min*	18	9	5 *msw*/3 *min*	0.0034	0.0062
19 *msw*/38 *min*	18	9	5 *msw*/3 *min*	0.0095	0.0110
28 *msw*/32 *min*	18	9		0.0200	0.0213
37 *msw*/17 *min*	18	9	5 *msw*/3 *min*	0.0165	0.0151
18 *msw*/31 *min*	18	9	5 *msw*/3 *min*	0.0063	0.0072
	18	9		0.0088	0.0084
	18	18		0.0101	0.0135
	18	18	5 *msw*/3 *min*	0.0069	0.0084
17 *msw*/32 *min* SI 176 *min*	18	9	5 *msw*/3 *min*		
13 *msw*/37 *min* SI 174 *min*	18	9	5 *msw*/3 *min*		
23 *msw*/17 *min*	18	18	5 *msw*/3 *min*	0.0127	0.0232

The ZHL (Buhlmann) NDLs and staging regimens are widespread across decompression meters presently, and are good representations for dissolved gas risk analysis. The RGBM is newer, more modern, and is coming online in decometers and associated software. For recreational exposures, the RGBM collapses to a dissolved gas algorithm. This is reflected in the risk estimates above, where estimates for both models differ little.

Simple comments hold for the analyzed profile risks. The maximum relative risk is 0.0232 for the 3 dive repetitive sequence according to the dissolved risk estimator. This translates to 2% profile risk, which is comparable to the maximum NDL risk for the PADI, NAUI, and ZHL NDLs. This type of dive profile is common, practiced daily on liveaboards, and benign. According to Gilliam, the absolute incidence rate for this type of diving is less than 0.02%. Again, our analyses overestimate risk. Effects of slower ascent rates and safety stops are seen only at the 0.25% to 0.5% level in relative surfacing risk. Safety stops at 5 *msw* for 3 *min* lower relative risk an average of 0.3%, while reducing the ascent rate from 18 *msw/min* to 9 *msw/min* reduces relative risk an average of 0.35%. Staging, NDLs, and constraints imposed by decometer algorithms are consistent with acceptable and safe recreational diving protocols. Estimated absolute risk associated across all ZHL NDLs and staging regimens analyzed herein is less than 2.32%, probably much less in actual practice. That is, we use $p = 0.0069$, and much evidence suggests $p < 0.0001$, some ten times safer.

Implicit in such formulations of risk tables are assumptions that given decompression stress is more likely to produce symptoms if it is sustained in time, and that large numbers of separate events may culminate in the same probability after time integration. Though individual schedule segments may not be replicated enough to offer total statistical validation, categories of predicted safety might be grouped within subsets of corroborating data. For instance, risks on air dives might be estimated from just nitrox data, risks on trimix from just trimix data, risks on heliox just from heliox data, etc. Since the method is general, any model parameter or meaningful index, properly defined, can be applied to decompression data, and the full power of statistical methods employed to quantify overall risk. While powerful, such statistical methods are neither deterministic nor mechanistic, and cannot predict on first principles. But as a means to table fabrication with quoted risk, such approaches offer attractive pathways for analysis.

Questions of what risk is acceptable to the diver vary. Sport and research divers would probably opt for small risk (1% or less), while military and commercial divers might live with higher risk (5%), considering the nearness of medical attention in general. Many factors influence these two populations, but fitness and acclimatization would probably play strategically.

Recent Doppler and wet tests are interesting, including our recorded CCR 16 dive sequence to 450 fsw. Gas transport analysis of these applications follows, along with bubble risk estimates.

- Bennett and Maronni 2.5 Minute Recreational Deep Stop
  Deep stops are already mainliners in some training agency protocols for no and light decompression diving on air and nitrox. The prescription is to make a deep stop at half depth for 1–3 min, followed by a shallow stop in the 15 fsw zone for 1–2 min. In Table 53, we cite bubble surfacing risks for a deep stop at half depth for 1 min, 2.5 min, and 4 min, the middle case suggested by Bennett and Maronni from Doppler scoring, followed by direct ascent to the surface. Surfacing supersaturation risks are tabulated in Table 54 for comparison. Dives are carried out to the (old) US Navy NDLs for easy reference. Deep stops for less than 2.5 min reduce recreational risk out to the Navy NDLs in all cases. Bubble risks decrease for short deep stops and then increase as stop times increase. As stop times continue to increase, the dives will require decompression. In other words, with increasing deep stop time, the dives become multilevel decompression dives. Obviously, the playoff of deep stop time against bottom time is a minimax problem. This is traced to bubble behavior with increased gas tensions for increasing deep stop time. In all cases, stop time in the shallow zone was 1 min. Longer stop times in the shallow zone

had little effect on surfacing risks. Shallow stops in training regimens probably serve better to teach buoyancy control to neophytes.

Table 53. Comparative Bubble Risks For Recreational Deep Stops

depth (*fsw*)	time (*min*)	no stop β	1 *min* stop β	2.5 *min* stop β	4 *min* stop β
80	40	2.10%	1.93%	1.90%	1.91%
90	30	2.10%	1.87%	1.83%	1.84%
100	25	2.10%	1.74%	1.71%	1.72%
110	20	2.20%	1.65%	1.61%	1.62%
120	15	2.00%	1.50%	1.46%	1.47%
130	10	1.70%	1.29%	1.25%	1.26%

Ascent and descent rates were standard in the analysis, that is, 30 fsw/min and 60 fsw/min respectively. The small risk spread for 1–4 *min* accommodates recreational deep stop training regimens, that is, 1–3 *min* deep half stop for many agencies.
Corresponding supersaturation risks in Table 54 are seen to increase montonically with length of deep stop. This is to be expected in dissolved gas models, with exposures at increasing depths for increasing times cascading tissue tensions, oblivious to any bubble-dissolved gas interactions tracked in Table 53.

Table 54. Comparative Supersaturation Risks For Recreational Deep Stops

Depth (*fsw*)	Time (*min*)	No stop σ	1 *min* Stop σ	2.5 *min* Stop σ	4 *min* Stop σ
80	40	2.10%	2.12%	2.18%	2.26%
90	30	2.10%	2.13%	2.20%	2.29%
100	25	2.10%	2.15%	2.23%	2.34%
110	20	2.20%	2.24%	2.32%	2.41%
120	15	2.00%	2.10%	2.20%	2.38%
130	10	1.70%	1.78%	1.91%	2.13%

- C & C Team 450/20 Multiple RB Dive Sequence At 1.4 *atm*

  Details of a 16 dive sequence by members of the C & C Team to 450 *fsw* for 20 *min* at 1.4 *atm* follow. Dives were successfully completed in tandem without DCS problems, and are included in the LANL Data Bank. All dives follow the same schedule, as given in Table 55. Oxtox (both CNS and full body) metrics are included. Diver Tags and Outcomes are tabulated, according to the LANL Data Bank profile schema described previously. Diver Tag 1 is the author (BRW). Risk estimates (both bubble and supersaturation) are noted along with binomial probabilities for 16 tandem dives within a LANL Data Bank underlying incidence rate of 0.69%. Four additional dives in the same sequence were also performed without mishap, but are not included because of larger fluctuations about 450 *fsw*. Bottom fluctuations in the 16 dive sequence were ± 5 *fsw* maximum for longer than a minute.

  Diluent is 10/80 trimix with a pp_{O_2} setpoint of 1.4 *atm*. The cumulative CNS clock fractions exceed a (traditional) limit of 1.0, while OTU uptake remains below a (traditional) limit of 650 *min*. There is likely greater variability in oxtox limit points than decompression limit points. Descent and ascent rates are standard, except in the 30 *fsw* zone where the ascent rate is 1 *fsw/min*. The binomial probability of no hits is $P(0)$, while the probability of 1 hit is $P(1)$. The probability of 2 or more hits is vanishingly small for underlying incidence of 0.69%.

These are very interesting dives for a number of reasons:

- dives were very deep;
- oxtox clock, like many technical dives, was exceeded;
- divers surfaced feeling tired, but not sick;
- ascent rate of 1 *fsw/min* in the 30 *fsw* zone has been practiced by WKPP divers out of a habitat at 30 *fsw* with success;
- dive was a relatively controlled exposure and provides good metrics for the LANL Data Bank;
- age span of divers was 25–68 yrs at the time (2008);
- setpoint of 1.4 *atm* was high compared to common RB usage, and offers another good set of data points.

The use of RBs for technical, exploration, scientific, and military diving is both on the rise and important. High oxygen fractions with helium and/or nitrogen diluents for deep exposures is an area fertile for model and data correlation. Such activity, outside the military, is a recent development, like the past 10–15 years, or so. Users of RB systems also rely heavily on dive planning software for decompression and deep diving. Some pertinent diveware is detailed in the Part 7.

Table 55. RB 16 Dive Sequence At 1.4 *atm.*

Dive Tags = 2042–2058
Diver Tags = 3,20,5,**1**,9,6,10,2,14,4,15,7,8,11,16,12
Diver Outcomes = 3,4,3,**3**,4,3,4,3,4,3,3,3,4,3,4,3
Underlying Incidence = 20/2879

Depth (*fsw*)	Time (*min*)	CNS clock (*fraction*)	OTU uptake (*min*)
450	20	.17	32.6
360	0.5	.01	0.8
350	0.5	.01	0.8
340	0.5	.01	0.8
330	0.5	.01	0.8
320	0.5	.01	0.8
310	0.5	.01	0.8
300	1.0	.02	1.6
290	1.0	.02	1.6
280	1.0	.02	1.6
270	1.0	.02	1.6
260	1.0	.02	1.6
250	1.0	.02	1.6
240	1.0	.02	1.6
230	1.5	.03	1.8
220	1.5	.03	1.8
210	2.0	.03	4.1
200	2.0	.03	4.1
190	2.0	.03	4.1
180	2.0	.03	4.0
170	2.0	.02	4.0
160	2.5	.02	4.0
150	2.5	.02	3.9
140	3.5	.03	5.7
130	5.0	.05	9.0
120	5.0	.04	8.5
110	5.0	.04	8.4
100	5.5	.04	9.0
90	6.0	.05	9.8
80	8.0	.07	13.0
70	8.0	.07	12.5
60	9.5	.08	15.5
50	11.0	.10	17.9
40	12.0	.10	19.5
30	8.5	.07	13.8
20	10.5	.09	17.1
10	17.0	.11	25.2
	211.5	1.38	262.2

$$\beta = 4.27\%, \quad \sigma = 12.67\%$$
$$P(0) = 89.4\%, \quad P(1) = 10.4\%$$

Computed bubble risk, β, is below the binomial probability, $P(1)$.

- NEDU Deep Stop Air Tests

The Navy Experimental Diving Unit recently tested their version of air deep stops with a moderate DCS rate. Profiles tested are given in Table 56, along with a suggested LANL deep stop profile. Profile NEDU 1 incurred a 5.5% DCS hit rate, while NEDU 2 incurred a lower 1.5% DCS hit rate.

Table 56. Comparative NEDU Air Deep Stop Schedules

depth $fsw)$	NEDU 1 time (min)	NEDU 2 time (min)	LANL time (min)
170	30	30	30
120			0.5
110			1.5
100			2.5
90			3.5
80			4.5
70			5.0
70	12		5.0
60	17		7.0
50	15		11.0
40	18	9	14.5
30	23	23	22.0
20	17	52	28.5
10	72	93	59.9
	206	207	195
σ	5.6%	2.4%	3.4%
β	10.6%	3.2%	2.6%

Bubble risk is higher in both NEDU 1 and NEDU 2, but large in NEDU 1. NEDU 1 is a multilevel decompression dive with inadequate treatment in the shallow zone. Initial deep stops in NEDU 1 did not control bubble growth, and the length of the stay in 70, 60, and 50 fsw builds up dissolved gas in the middle range tissues, which then diffuses into bubbles causing them to grow. NEDU 2 is classic with no deep stops, and very long times in the shallow zone to effect decompression. The LANL schedule has deeper stops, shorter midzone times, and then shorter times in the shallow zone compared to both NEDU 1 and NEDU 2. One important factor here is the shape of the decompression schedule, that is the LANL profile is shorter overall, with NEDU 1 and NEDU 2 profiles exhibiting supersaturation staging with shallow belly and tail, while the LANL profile is steeper exhibiting bubble staging with deeper stops and steeper ascent rate. Both NEDU profiles are not of the genre typically dived by users of modern deep stop tables, software, and meters.

Gas transport analyses on both NEDU schedules suggests that NEDU 1 produces 15%–30% larger bubble volumes on surfacing, due to the longer stay in the mid zone, while NEDU 2 produces surfacing bubble volumes 3% - 5%

larger than surfacing bubble volumes in the LANL profile. Surfacing bubble volumes in the LANL profile were close to the staging limit point.

- French Navy Deep Stop Schedules
  The French Navy also tested deep stop air schedules. Three protocols on deep air were employed and none exhibited Grade 4 Doppler bubbles. Analysis centered on just Grade 3 bubbles. For purposes of deep stop analysis, Protocol 1, a dive similar to NEDU 1, is interesting. Protocol 1 is a deep air dive to 200 fsw for 20 *min*, with ascent staging according to Table 57. Contrasting staging strategies are denoted MN90, the standard French Navy dissolved gas regimen, and LANL. Outside of World Navies, few diving sectors today even contemplate air decompression diving to 200 fsw. Risks in air dives beyond 150 fsw are known to increase by factors of 10 over similar dives at shallower depth. This is, of course, one major reason why trimix and heliox become mixtures of choice for deep and decompression diving worldwide, across commercial, scientific, exploration, and research sectors.

Table 57. French Navy Air Deep Stop Schedules At 200 fsw

	Protocol 1	MN90	LANL
ascent rate fsw/min			
starting at 90 fsw	10	20	30
depth	time	time	time
(fsw)	(*min*)	(*min*)	(*min*)
200	20	20	20
130			0.5
120			0.5
110			1.0
100			1.0
90			1.0
80	1		1.5
70	1		2.0
60	2		2.0
50	2		2.5
40	4		3.0
30	6	3	6.0
20	9	8	7.0
10	22	32	8.0
	78	68	65
β	3.9%	2.2%	2.1%

By contrast, LANL staging starts deeper, is shorter overall, and has smaller bubble risk than Protocol 1. Protocol 1, however, tracks more closely with LANL than NEDU 1, and exhibits lower risk than NEDU 1. However, run time for Protocol 1 versus MN90 is longer, unlike conventional bubble model run times. Estimated bubble risks, β, are tabulated at the bottom of Table 57.

With regard to the preceding dives and schedules, a couple of points are interesting. These follow from a closer look at dissolved and bubble gas phases across the profiles, using LANL tools and selected way points on the dives. These comments also apply to deep and decompression staging using traditional dissolved gas models and tables. Remember these comments are made within the LANL model framework and attendant data correlation:

- bubble growth in the deep zone of decompression profiles NEDU 1 and Protocol 1 is not constrained in their version of deep stop air tests;
- deep stops are not deep enough in NEDU 1 and Protocol 1, nor are follow stops;
- critical phase volume limit points are exceeded in NEDU 1 and Protocol 1 even before the diver exits, in other words, along the decompression glide path underwater;
- the recreational 2.5 *minute* stop at 1/2 depth within the NDLs of even the old USN Tables maintains the phase volumes below limit points;
- the LANL 450/20 profiles also surface below the phase volume limit point, no surprise because profiles were designed to meet that constraint;
- supersaturation profiles MN90 and NEDU 2 also do not control bubble growth in the deeper zones, but the separated phase volume is below model limit points, with pressure in the shallow zone sufficient to constrain bubble growth and maintain adequate dissolution, but time consuming because bubbles are now larger in the shallow zone.

Much the same can be said of supersaturation versus bubble staging strategies in general.

To finish up analysis, consider other applications across tables, meters, and software, focusing on shallow stop versus deep stop profiles, risk, and data. The time span of these applications is the past 3–5 *yrs*, and they represent real mixed gas diving across many venues.

- UW Seafood Diver Air Tables

  As another application of the LANL Data Bank to table construction and analysis, we detail a set of tables of interest to the University of Wisconsin (UW), along with estimated risk for various nonstop limits gleaned from the data. These Tables have no groups, and simple rules. Released mixed gas RGBM Tables resulted from similar analyses across both the technical and recreational segments. Such Tables are certainly useful for a broad spectrum of diving, and are easy to use.

  Table 58 lists the maximum NDLs for any series of dives (up to 3) with 60 *min* SIs between dives. Divers need make a deep stop at half the maximum bottom pressure for 1 *min*, plus a shallow safety stop in the 15 *fsw* zone for 2 *min*. Descent rate is 60 *fsw/min*, and ascent rate is 30 *fsw/min*. The NDLs are listed for maximum risk after 3 repetitive dives to the (same) depth indicated, or to a lesser depth.

Table 58. RGBM Repetitive Risks For Air Dives

depth (*fsw*)	β 5.14% maximum time (*min*)	β 3.29% maximum time (*min*)	β 1.37% maximum time (*min*)	
100	24	20	14	deep stop 60/1 shallow stop 15/2
80	38	32	24	deep stop 50/1 shallow stop 15/2
60	50	42	32	deep stop 40/1 shallow stop 15/2
40	130	120	100	deep stop 30/1 shallow stop 15/2

Tables like these are of interest to Puerto Rican diving fishermen, and fishing sport divers. NAUI uses a variant, detailed next, for training. Technical Training Agencies also employ mixed gas tables for decompression diving, as well as dive planning software, all based on the RGBM algorithm. Some risk estimates of profiles in these RGBM Technical Tables also follow.

- NAUI Air and Nitrox Recreational Tables (sea level - 10,000 *ft*)
For comparison, consider similar RGBM Tables 59–61 employed by NAUI for air and nitrox diver training, sea level up to 10,000 *ft*. They are basically the same as the Puerto Rican seafood diver tables above, except that successive dives must always be shallower than the previous. Descent and ascent rates are 75 *fsw/min* and 30 *fsw/min*, and SIs are 60 *min*. At sea level to 2,000 *ft* elevation, three dives may be made in a day on air or nitrox. At elevations above 2,000 *ft*, only two dives are sanctioned. There are 9 RGBM Tables in all, 3 for air, 3 for EAN32, and 3 for EAN36, ranging in altitude, 0–2,000 *ft*, 2,000–6,000 *ft*, and 9,000–10,000 *ft*. In Tables 59-61, risks are tabulated at the end of the 3 or 2 dive sequence, for just 3 Tables (air at 6,000–10,000 *ft*, EAN32 at 2,000 - 6,000 *ft*, and EAN36 at 0- 2,000 *ft*). Risks decrease at any elevation as the oxygen fraction increases, while elevation increases risk for any mixture of nitrogen and oxygen. Moving from left to right (first dive through last permitted dive) successive decrements in permissible depths are seen. Safety stops at half the bottom depth are required for 1–2 *min*, plus a shallow stop in the 15 *fsw* zone for 2 *min*. The shallow stop mostly serves to control ascent speed. Maximum risk is seen in the air tables at 10,000 *ft* elevation, and minimum risk in the EAN36 tables at sea level.

Table 59. NAUI RGBM Air Tables (6,000 - 10,000 ft)
Maximum Risk After Dive 2, $\beta = 2.36\%$

Dive 1		Dive 2	
depth	*time*	*depth*	*time*
(fsw)	*(min)*	*(fsw)*	*(min)*
90	11	60	28
80	15	55	28
70	21	50	40
60	28	45	40
50	40	40	64
40	64	35	64
30	103	30	103

Table 60. NAUI RGBM EAN32 Tables (2,000–6,000 ft)
Maximum Risk After Dive 2, $\beta = 1.65\%$

Dive 1		Dive 2	
depth	*time*	*depth*	*time*
(fsw)	*(min)*	*(fsw)*	*(min)*
100	20	65	43
90	26	60	57
80	33	55	57
70	43	50	84
60	57	45	84
50	84	40	120
40	120	35	120
30	150	30	150

Table 61. NAUI RGBM EAN36 Tables (0–2,000 ft)
Maximum Risk After Dive 3, $\beta = 1.12\%$

Dive 1		Dive 2		Dive 3	
depth	*time*	*depth*	*time*	*depth*	*time*
(fsw)	*(min)*	*(fsw)*	*(min)*	*(fsw)*	*(min)*
110	31	80	60	50	150
100	35	75	60	50	150
90	46	70	85	50	150
80	60	65	85	50	150
70	85	60	115	50	150
60	115	55	115	50	150
50	150	50	150	50	150

These air and nitrox tables have been backbones in NAUI training regimes. They are simple to use, and easy to teach, avoiding USN Group tags.

- Helitrox Nonstop Limits (NDLs)
  Helitrox is enriched trimix, that is, the oxygen fraction is above 21% in the breathing mixture. Helitrox is gaining in popularity over nitrox when helium is available for gas mixing. Diving agencies often use helitrox in the beginning

sequence of technical diver training. Listed below in Table 62 are nonstop time limits and corresponding risks, β, for exposures at that depth-time. The mixture is helitrox (enriched 26/17 trimix), sometimes called triox.

Table 62. Helitrox NDLs And Risk

depth $d\ (fsw)$	time $t_n\ (min)$	risk β
70	35	1.4%
80	25	1.4%
90	20	1.4%
100	15	1.4%
110	10	1.5%
120	8	1.5%
130	6	1.4%
140	5	1.5%
150	4	1.6%

These NDL triox risks track closely with NDL risks for air and nitrox.

• Comparative Helium and Nitrogen Staging and Risk
Consider a deep trimix dive with multiple switches on the way up. This is a risky technical dive, performed by seasoned professionals. Table 63 contrasts stop times for two gas choices at the 100 fsw switch. The dive is a short 10 min at 400 fsw on 10/65/25 trimix, with switches at 235 fsw, 100 fsw, and 30 fsw. Descent and ascent rates are 75 fsw/min and 25 fsw/min. Obviously, there are many other choices for switch depths, mixtures, and strategies. In this comparison, the oxygen fractions were the same in all mixes, at all switches. Differences between a nitrogen or a helium based decompression strategy, even for this short exposure, are nominal. Such usually is the case when oxygen fraction is held constant in helium or nitrogen mixes at the switch.
Comparative profile reports suggest that riding helium to the 70 fsw level with a switch to EAN50 is good strategy, one that couples the benefits of well being on helium with minimal decompression time and stress following isobaric switch to nitrogen. Shallower switches to enriched air also work, with only a nominal increase in overall decompression time, but with deeper switches off helium to nitrox a source of isobaric counterdiffusion (ICD) issues that might best be avoided. Note the risk, β, for the helium strategy, 40/20/40 trimix at 100 fsw, is slightly safer than the nitrogen strategy, EAN40 at 100 fsw, but in either case, the risk is high.

Table 63. Comparative Helium And Nitrogen Gas Switches

depth (fsw)	$\beta = 6.42\%$ time (*min*) 10/65 trimix	$\beta = 6.97\%$ time (*min*) 10/65 trimix
400	10.0	10.0
260	1.5	1.5
250	1.0	1.0
240	1.0	1.0
	18/50 trimix	18/50 trimix
230	0.5	0.5
220	0.5	0.5
210	0.5	0.5
200	0.5	0.5
190	1.0	1.0
180	1.5	1.5
170	1.5	1.0
160	1.5	1.5
150	1.5	2.0
140	2.0	1.5
130	2.0	2.5
120	4.0	4.0
110	4.5	4.0
	40/20 trimix	EAN40
100	2.5	2.0
90	2.5	2.0
80	2.5	2.0
70	5.0	4.0
60	6.5	5.5
50	8.0	6.5
40	9.5	7.5
	EAN80	EAN80
30	10.5	10.5
20	14.0	14.0
10	21.0	20.5
	123.0	116.0

The logistics of such deep dives on OC are formidable for both diver and surface support crew if any. The number of stage bottles (decompression tanks) is forbidding for a single diver, of course, but surface support teams, themselves at high risk for placing bottles on a line at depth, can effect such a dive. These surface support teams are often called "push teams" and are vested with immense responsibility for diver safety. With that in mind, the following WKPP and record OC trimix dives are mind boggling.

- WKPP Extreme Exploration Dives
The Woodville Karst Plain Project (WKPP) has reported a number of 300 fsw dives with OC and RB systems on trimix for many hours bottom time, and some 8 hrs of decompression. Pure oxygen is employed in the 30 fsw zone with the help of an underwater habitat. Successful regimens systematically

roll back the helium fraction and increase the oxygen fraction in roughly the same proportions, thus maintaining nitrogen fractions low and fairly constant. Diving starts in the cave systems of Wakulla Springs in Florida. Table 64 summarizes the ascent and decompression profile. The risk is high, but WKPP professionals continue to attempt and complete such extreme exposures, pushing the exploration envelope. These dives served as calibration points for the RGBM algorithm on whole.

Table 64. WKPP Extreme Trimix Dives
Surfacing Risk, $\beta = 13.67\%$

Depth (fsw)	Time (min)	Trimix (fsw)	Depth (min)	Time	Trimix
270	360	11/50	140	5	
260	1		130	6	
250	1		120	7	35/25
240	1	18/40	110	8	
230	2		100	9	
220	2		90	10	
210	2		80	12	
200	3		70	16	50/16
190	3		60	34	
180	3	21/35	50	41	
170	4		40	49	
160	4		30	60	pure O_2
150	5		20	90	

- Record OC Trimix Dive
  Consider risk after an OC dive to 1040 fsw on trimix, with matched ICD switches maintaining the relative fraction of nitrogen constant as helium is reduced in the same measure as oxygen is increased. Dives without this rather well known strategy ended in some serious hyperbaric chamber time for treatment of vestibular DCS. Reports hint this dive was attempted, maybe accomplished, but contradictions abound. We merely treat it as academic exercise for risk prediction. One attempt ended in the Phuket hyperbaric chamber, as reported by a hyperbaric specialist and support team. Earlier dives to 540 fsw using RGBM schedules are recounted in trade magazines and at Internet sites. Dives like these with deep stops are becoming more common these days, both on OC and CCR systems.
  Table 65 roughly summarizes the RGBM profile and ascent protocol. Stops range from 740 fsw to 10 fsw for times ranging 0.5 min to 31.0 min. Descent rate is assumed to be 60 fsw/min, and ascent rate between stages is assumed to be 30 fsw/min. Mixes and switch depths are indicated, as in Table 64. Stops are made in 10 fsw increments all the way to the surface.

Table 65. Trimix Dive To 1040 *fsw* And Risk
Surfacing Risk, $\beta = 26.13\%$

Depth (*fsw*)	Time (*min*)	Trimix	Depth (*fsw*)	Time (*min*)	Trimix
1049	0.5	5/67	380	3.0	
750	0.5		370	3.0	
740	0.5		360	3.0	
730	0.5		350	3.0	
720	0.5		340	3.5	
710	0.5		330	3.5	
700	0.5		320	3.5	
690	0.5		310	3.5	
680	0.5		300	3.5	
670	0.5		290	2.5	14/56
660	0.5		280	3.0	
650	0.5		270	3.5	
640	0.5		260	3.5	
630	0.5		250	3.5	
620	0.5		240	3.5	
610	0.5		230	4.0	
600	0.5		220	4.0	
590	0.5		210	5.0	
580	0.5		200	6.0	
570	1.0		190	6.5	
560	1.0		180	6.5	
550	1.0		170	6.5	
540	1.0		160	7.5	
530	1.0		150	9.0	
520	1.5		140	9.5	
510	1.5		130	8.0	27/56
500	1.5		120	8.5	
490	1.5		110	9.0	
480	1.5		100	13.0	
470	1.5		90	13.5	
460	1.5		80	14.0	
450	1.5		70	15.5	
440	2.0		60	16.0	
430	2.0		50	17.5	
420	2.5		40	21.0	
410	2.5		30	22.0	EAN80
400	2.5		20	24.5	
390	3.0		10	31.0	pure O_2

The computed risk for this dive is very high, near 30%. Total decompression time is near 415 *min*. Logistics for stage cylinders are beyond formidable, and the risk for deep support divers is also high.

- HydroSpace EXPLORER Extreme RB Profile
Table 66 is a deep RB dive downloaded off the HydroSpace EXPLORER computer. From a number of corners, reports of 400 *fsw* dives on rebreather

systems are becoming commonplace. Consider this one to 444 *fsw* for 15 *min*. Diluent is 10/85 trimix, and ppo_2 setpoint is 1.1 *atm*. From a decompression standpoint, rebreather systems are the quickest and most efficient systems for underwater activities. The higher the ppo_2, the shorter the overall decompression time. That advantage, however, needs to be played off against increasing risks of oxygen toxicity as oxygen partial pressures increase, especially above 1.4 *atm*. The higher percentage of oxygen and lower percentage of inert gases in higher ppo_2 setpoints of closed circuit rebreathers (CCRs) results in reduced risks, simply because gas loadings and bubble couplings are less in magnitude and importance. This shows up in any set of comparative ppo_2 RB calculations, as well as in OC versus RB risk estimates.

Table 66. Extreme RB Dive And Risk
Surfacing Risk $\beta = 5.79\%$

Depth (*fsw*)	Time (*min*)	Depth (*fsw*)	Time (*min*)
444	15.	150	2.0
290	0.5	140	2.0
280	0.5	130	2.0
270	0.5	120	2.5
260	0.5	110	3.0
250	0.5	100	3.5
240	0.5	90	4.0
230	1.0	80	4.5
220	1.0	70	5.0
210	1.0	60	7.0
200	1.0	50	7.5
190	1.5	40	8.0
180	1.5	30	12.5
170	1.5	20	14.0
160	1.5	10	15.5

Risk associated with this 444 *fsw* dive is less than a similar dive on trimix to roughly the same depth for a shorter period of time, that is, Table 14.

- USS Perry Deep RB Wreck Dives
  A team of divers uncovered the wreck of the USS Perry in approximately 250 *fsw* off Anguar, and explored it for a week on RBs. Diving in extremely hazardous and changing currents, their repetitive decompression profile appears in Table 67. Profiles and risk for the two dives, separated by 4 *hrs* SI, are nominal, with no accounting of exertion effort in current implied. Diluent is 10/50 trimix, with a ppo_2 setpoint of 1.3 *atm*.
  The repetitive decompression dive sequence here is noteworthy. First dive is 260/40 with 270 *min* SI, followed by a second dive with profile 210/20. Repetitive decompression dives are not common and the team effort provides a valuable data point for the profiles in the RGBM DB. Profile risks for both

dives are in the 5% range. Run time for dissolved gas staging here is about 30% longer.

Table 67. USS Perry RB Repetitive Decompression Dives And Risk
Surfacing Risk After Dive 1, $\beta = 5.32\%$
Surfacing Risk After Dive 2, $\beta = 5.89\%$

Depth (fsw)	Time (min)	Depth (fsw)	Time (min)
260	40	40	5
170	1	30	6
160	1	20	9
150	1	10	12
140	1	0	270
130	1	210	20
120	1	90	1
100	2	80	1
90	2	70	1
80	2	60	1
70	3	50	2
60	3	40	2
50	4	30	9

Keyed Exercises

- *Profile data collection items include*
  ( ) tank rating
  ( ) diver certification
  (x) age, weight, and gender

- *Data Banks focus on*
  (x) operational diving
  ( ) clinical testing
  ( ) only DCS profiles

- *Bubble models generally require*
  ( ) shallower staging
  ( ) no decompression stops
  (x) deeper decompression stops

- *LANL DB profiles span*
  ( ) OC and RB shallow diving
  ( ) just computer downloads
  (x) 2879 exposures across all deep diving

- *DAN PDE and DSL house*
  (x) around 137,000 dive profiles
  ( ) mostly decompression profiles
  ( ) only oxtox profiles

- *DCS I hits affect*
  (x) the limbs
  ( ) the brain
  ( ) the lungs

- *DCS II hits affect*
  ( ) the vestibular organs
  (x) the central nervous system
  ( ) the hands

- *DCS III hits affect*
  (x) the inner ear
  ( ) the outer ear
  ( ) the eyes

- *The supersaturation risk estimator*
  ( ) uses the partial nitrogen gas tension
  (x) uses total gas tension minus ambient pressure
  ( ) counts VGE

- *The bubble risk estimator*
  ( ) counts helium bubbles
  ( ) tracks only supersaturation
  (x) employs the bubble growth rate

- *In the LANL DB, the underlying incidence is*
  ( ) 0.56
  (x) 20/2879
  ( ) indeterminate

- *Data from the DAN PDE and SDL suggests*
  (x) only 2% of recreational divers use tables
  ( ) trimix diving is decreasing
  ( ) models correlate outside data limit points

- *Data from the LANL DB suggests*
  ( ) dissolved gas and bubble models give the same decompression schedules
  (x) deep stop DCS spikes are not seen in the data
  ( ) pure oxygen switches are prevalent at 55 fsw

- *The mathematical technique for correlating data and models is called*
  ( ) Monte Carlo
  ( ) least squares
  (x) maximum likelihood

- *Match the entries in the first column with the best single the entry in the second column.*

(f) Recreational deep stops	(a) 1040 fsw on constant N_2 fractions
(c) Multiple 450/20 RB dives	(b) Enriched trimix
(j) NEDU deep stop air tests	(c) CNS clock greater than 1.0
(g) French Navy deep stop profile	(d) Roughly same decompression times
(i) UW Seafood Diver tables	(e) Hazardous currents
(l) NAUI air and nitrox tables	(f) Reduced bubble counts
(b) Helitrox NDLs	(g) High risk air dives
(d) Comparative He and N_2 staging	(h) Computer downloaded dives
(k) WKPP exploration dives	(i) Tables from LANL DB
(a) Record OC trimix dive	(j) Too long in mid zone
(h) EXPLORER extreme RB dives	(k) Calibration of RGBM
(e) USS Perry deep RB dives	(l) No group dive tables

Maladies

Diving has its own brand of medical complications, linked to ambient pressure changes. For brief consideration, a few of the common medical problems associated with compression-decompression and diving follow. The bubble problem has been long discussed, but we can start off by summarizing a few concensus opinions concerning decompression sickness. A cursory discussion of some drugs then follows.

But to start off, a few clinical observations are listed, not to scare the reader, but rather to point out that diving, like all other environmentally changing activities, has its own set of risk factors. Risk, obviously here, relates to pressure changes and exposure times:

- in 1976, Palmer and Blakemore reported that 81% of goats with CNS bends and 33% with limb bends exhibited permanent spinal cord damage on autopsy;
- in 1978, the same investigators reported that clinically bent, but cured, goats, also exhibited brain damage on autopsy;
- in 1979, a Workshop in Luxemborg reported that even asymptomatic dives may cause permanent brain and spinal impairment;
- in 1982, Idicula reported CT scans of the brains of veteran divers showed characteristics similar to punch drunk divers;

- in 1984, Edmonds conducted physchological and psychometric studies on abalone divers in Australia and reported strong evidence for dementia;
- in 1985, Hoiberg reported the USN divers who once suffered the bends had a higher rate of headaches, vascular diseases, and hospitalizations than a matched sample who had never been bent;
- in 1986, Morris reported that English divers with more than 8 years experience has significantly poorer short term memory;
- in the 1980s and 1990s, Workshops repeatedly voiced concern about the long term effects of transient hematological changes in divers, such as sedimentation, red cell configuration, alteration of lipoprotein, platelet reduction, and vascular stress;
- in 1984, Brubakk noted ultrasonically detected bubbles (VGE) in animals for as long as a month after hyperbaric exposure;
- now, Calder examines the spinal cord of every diver in the United Kingdom who dies of any cause;
- in 1985, Dick reported that mild (self) neurological complaints are common after diving and go untreated, and that many serious cases never violated the USN Tables.

Of course, it comes as no surprise that the medical community continues to push for shorter and shallower exposures, ultra conservatism in tables and meters, and all other risk ameliorating avenues. Enough said here, the above list points out some concerns for all of us. Conservative approaches, coupled to the most modern and correlated biophysical.

Bends

Clinical manifestations of decompression sickness, or decompression illness (DCI), can be categorized as pulmonary, neurological, joint, and skin DCI, as summarized by the diving medical community. All are linked to bubbles upon pressure reduction, with embolism also included in the categorization. Pulmonary DCI manifests itself as a sore throat with paroxysmal cough upon deep inspiration, followed by severe chest pain, and difficult respiration, a condition collectively called the *chokes*. Chokes is seen often in severe high altitude exposures. Neurological DCI affects the heart, brain, and spinal cord, through arterial gas emboli, venous gas emboli, shunted venous gas emboli (VGE that pass through the pulmonary circulation and enter the arterial circulation), and stationary, extravascular (*autochthonous*) bubbles. Joint DCI is a common form of mild bends, affecting the nervous (*neurogenic*), bone marrow (*medullar*), and joint (*articular*) assemblies. Neurogenic pain is localized at remote limb sites, usually without apparent cerebral or spinal involvment. Bubbles in the bone have been proposed as the cause of both dull aching pain and bone death. Expanding extravascular bubbles have been implicated in the mechanical distortion of sensory nerve endings. Skin DCI manifests itself as itching, rash, and a sense of localized heat. Skin DCI is not considered serious enough for hyperbaric treatment, but local pain can persist for a few days. Blotchy purple patching of the skin has been noted to precede serious DCI, especially the chokes.

Most believe that bends symptoms follow formation of bubbles, or the gas phase, after decompression. Yet, the biophysical evolution of the gas phase is incompletely understood. Doppler bubble and other detection technologies suggest that:

- moving and stationary bubbles do occur following decompression;
- the risk of decompression sickness increases with the magnitude of detected bubbles and emboli;
- symptomless, or *silent*, bubbles are also common following decompression;
- the variability in gas phase formation is likely less than the variability in symptom generation.

Gas phase formation is the single most important element in understanding decompression sickness, and is also a crucial element in preventative analysis.

Treatment of decompression sickness is an involved process, requiring a recompression chamber and various hyperbaric treatment schedules depending on the severity of the symptoms, location, and initiating circumstance. Recompression is usually performed in a double lock hyperbaric chamber, with the patient taken to a series of levels to mitigate pain, first, and then possibly as deep as 165 fsw for treatment. Depending on the depth of the treatment schedule, oxygen may, or may not, be administered to washout inert gas and facilitate breathing. Treatment of air embolism follows similar schedules.

High Pressure Nervous Syndrome

Hydrostatic pressure changes, particularly in the several hundred atm range, are capable of affecting, though usually reversibly, central nervous system activity. Rapidly compressed divers, say 120 fsw/min to 600 fsw, breathing helium, experience coarse tremors and other neurological disorders termed *high pressure nervous syndrome* (HPNS). At greater depths, near 800 fsw, cramps, dizziness, nausea, and vomiting often accompany the tremor. Although HPNS can be avoided by slowing the compression rate, the rate needs to be substantially reduced for compressions below 1,100 fsw.

While the underlying mechanisms of HPNS are not well understood, like so many other pressure related afflictions, the use of pharmacological agents, some nitrogen in the breathing mixture, staged compressions, alcohol, and warming have been useful in ameliorating HPNS in operational deep diving.

Gas induced osmosis has been implicated as partially causative in high pressure nervous syndrome. Water, the major constituent of the body, shifting between different tissue compartments, can cause a number of disorders. Mechanical disruption, plasma loss, hemoconcentration, and bubbles are some. Under rapid pressure changes, gas concentrations across blood and tissue interfaces may not have sufficient time to equilibrate, inducing balancing, but counter, fluid pressure gradients (osmotic gradients). The strength of the osmotic gradient is proportional to the absolute pressure change, temperature, and gas solubility.

Inert Gas Narcosis

It is well known that men and animals exposed to hyperbaric environments exhibit symptoms of intoxication, simply called *narcosis*. The narcosis was first noticed in subjects breathing compressed air as early as 1835. The effect, however, is not isolated to air mixtures (nitrogen and oxygen). Both helium and hydrogen, as well as the noble (rare) gases such as xenon, krypton, argon, and neon, cause the same signs and symptoms, though varying in their potency and threshold hyperbaric pressures. The signs and symptoms of inert gas narcosis have manifest similarity with alcohol, hypoxia (low oxygen tension), and anesthesia. Exposure to depths greater than 300 *fsw* may result in loss of consciousness, and at sufficiently great pressure, air has been used as an anesthetic. Individual susceptibility to narcosis varies widely from individual to individual. Other factors besides pressure potentiate symptoms, such as alcohol, work level, apprehension, and carbon dioxide levels. Frequent exposure to depth with a breathing mixture, as with DCS, affords some level of adaptation.

Many factors are thought contributory to narcosis. Combinations of elevated pressure, high oxygen tensions, high inert gas tensions, carbon dioxide retention, anesthetically blocked ion exchange at the cellular interface, reduced alveolar function, and reduced hemoglobin capacity have all been indicted as culprits. But, still today, the actual mechanism and underlying sequence is unknown.

The anesthetic aspects of narcosis are unquestioned in most medical circles. Anesthesia can be induced by a wide variety of chemically passive substances, ranging from inert gases to chloroform and ether. These substances depress central nervous system activity in a manner altogether different from centrally active drugs. Anesthetics have no real chemical structure associated with their potency, and act on all neural pathways, like a bulk phase. Physicochemical theories of anesthetics divide in two. One hypothesis envisions anesthetics interacting with hydrophobic surfaces and interfaces of lipid tissue. The other postulates anesthetic action in the aqueous phases of the central nervous system. The potency and latency of both relate to the stability of gas hydrates composing most anesthetics. The biochemistry of anesthetics and narcosis in divers has not, obviously, been unraveled.

Hyperoxia and Hypoxia

Elevated oxygen tensions (*hyperoxia*), similar to elevated inert gas tensions, can have a deleterious effect on divers, aviators, and those undergoing hyperbaric oxygen treatment. The condition is known as oxygen toxicity, and was first observed, in two forms, in the final quarter of the 1800s. Low pressure oxygen toxicity (Lorraine Smith effect) occurs when roughly a 50% oxygen mixture is breathed for many hours near 1 *atm*, producing lung irritation and inflammation. At higher partial pressures, convulsions develop in high pressure oxygen toxicity (Bert effect), with latency time inversely proportional to pressure above 1 *atm*. Factors contributing to the onset of symptoms are degree of exertion, amount of carbon dioxide retained and inspired, and individual susceptibility. Early symptoms of oxygen poisioning include muscular twitching (face and lips), nausea, tunnel vision, difficulty hearing and ringing, difficulty breathing and taking deep breaths, confusion, fatigue, and coordination problems. Convulsions are the most serious manifestation of oxygen poisioning, followed ultimately by unconsciousness. Oxygen toxicity is not a problem whenever oxygen partial pressures drop below 0.5 *atm*.

Oxygen toxicity portends another very complex biochemical condition. Elevated oxygen levels interfere with the enzyme chemistry linked to cell metabolism, especially in the central nervous system. Reduced metabolic and electrolytic transport across neuronal membranes has been implicated as a causative mechanism. The role of carbon dioxide, while contributory to the chain of reactions according to measurements, is not understood, just as with inert gas narcosis. On the other hand, it has been noted that only small increases in brain carbon dioxide correlate with severe symptoms of oxygen toxicity. Carbon dioxide seems to play an important, though subtle, part in almost all compression-decompression afflictions.

Breathing air at atmospheric pressure after the onset of oxygen toxicity symptoms can restore balance, depending on severity of symptoms. Deep breathing and hyperventilation can also forestall convulsions if initiated at the earliest sign of symptoms.

When the tissues fail to receive enough oxygen, a tissue debt (*hypoxia*) develops, with varying impact and latency time on body tissue types. Hypoxia can result with any interruption of oxygen transport to the tissues. Although the nervous system itself represents less than 3% of body weight, it consumes some 20% of the oxygen inspired. When oxygen supply is cut, consciousness can be lost in 30 *seconds* or less, respiratory failure follows in about a *minute*, and irreparable damage to the brain and higher centers usually occurs in about 4 *minutes*. Obviously, the brain is impacted the most. The victim of hypoxia may be unaware of the problem, while euphoria, drowsiness, weakness, and unconsciousness progress. Blueness of the lips and skin results, as blood is unable to absorp enough oxygen to maintain its red color. When oxygen partial pressures drop below 0.10 *atm*, unconsciousness is extremely rapid.

Hypoxia is a severe, life threatening condition. However, if fresh air is breathed, recovery is equally as rapid, providing breathing has not stopped. If breathing has stopped, but cardiac function continues, artificial respiration can stimulate the breathing control centers to functionality. Cardiopulmonary resuscitation can be equally successful when both breathing and heart action have ceased.

Hypercapnia and Hypocapnia

Tissue carbon dioxide excess (*hypercapnia*) can result from inadequate ventilation, excess in the breathing mixtures, or altered diver metabolic function. All tissues are affected by high levels of carbon dioxide, but the brain, again, is the most susceptible. The air we breathed contains only some 0.03% carbon dioxide. As partial pressures of carbon dioxide approach 0.10 *atm*, symptoms of hypercapnia become severe, starting with confusion and drowsiness, followed by muscle spasms, rigidity, and unconsciousness. Carbon dioxide at 0.02 *atm* pressure will increase breathing rate, and carbon dioxide at 0.05 *atm* pressure induces an uncomfortable sensation of shortness of breath. Factors which increase the likelihood and severity of hypercapnia include corresponding high partial pressure of oxygen, high gas densities, breathing dead spaces, and high breathing resistance.

Any process which lowers carbon dioxide levels in the body below normal (*hypocapnia*), can produce weakness, faintness, headache, blurring of vision, and, in the extreme case, unconsciousness. Hypocapnia often results from hyperventilation. The respiratory system monitors both carbon dioxide and oxygen levels to stimulate breathing. Rising carbon dioxide tensions and falling oxygen tensions trigger the breathing response mechanism. Hyperventilation (rapid and deep breathing) lowers the carbon dioxide levels, leading to hypocapnia.

Extended breathholding after hyperventilation can lead to a condition known as shallow water blackout. Following hyperventilation and during a longer breathholding dive, oxygen tensions can fall to a very low level before a diver returns to the surface and resumes breathing. Oxygen levels are lowered because exertion causes oxygen to be used up faster, but also the sensitivity to carbon dioxide drops as oxygen tension drops, permitting oxygen levels to drop even further. Upon ascension, the drop in the partial pressure of oxygen in the lungs may be sufficient to stop the uptake of oxygen completely, and, with the commensurate drop in carbon dioxide tension, the urge to breathe may also be suppressed.

While the short term effects of both hypercapnia and hypocapnia can be disastrous in the water, drowning if consciousness is lost, the long term effects following revival are inconsequential. Treatment in both cases is breathing standard air normally. Residual effects are minor, such as headache, dizziness, nausea, and sore chest muscles.

Carbon dioxide seems to be a factor in nearly every other compression-decompression malady, including decompression sickness, narcosis, hyperoxia, and hypoxia. It is a direct product of metabolic processes, with about 1 l of carbon dioxide produced for every 1 l of oxygen consumed. Carbon dioxide affects the metabolic rate, and many other associated biochemical reactions. The physical chemistry of carbon dioxide uptake and elimination is much more complex than that of inert gases, such as nitrogen and helium. Transfer of inert gases follows simple laws of solubility (Henry's law) in relation to partial pressures. Carbon dioxide transport depends on three factors, namely, gas solubility, chemical combination with alkaline buffers, and diffusion between the cellular and plasma systems. Only relatively small changes in partial pressures of carbon dioxide can induce chain reactions in the three mechanisms, and larger scale biological impact on gas exchange and related chemistry.

Barotrauma

With pressure decrease, air contained in body cavities expands. Usually, this expanding air vents freely and naturally, and there are no problems. If obstructions to air passage exist, or the expanding air is retained, overexpansion problems, collectively called barotrauma, can occur. One very serious overexpansion problem occurs in the lungs. The lungs can accommodate overexpansion to just a certain point, after which continued overpressurization produces progressive distention and then rupture of the alveoli (air exchange sacs). Problems with lung overexpansion can occur with pressure differentials as small as 5 fsw. This distention can be exacerbated by breathholding on ascent or inadequate ventilation, and partial obstruction of the bronchial passageways.

The most serious affliction of pulmonary overpressure is the dispersion of air from the alveoli into the pulmonary venous circulation (arterial embolism), thence, into the heart, systemic circulation, and possibly lodging in the coronary and cerebral arterioles. Continuing to expand with further decrease in pressure, these emboli (bubbles) can block blood flow to vital areas. Clinical features of arterial gas embolism develop rapidly, including dizziness, headache, and anxiety first, followed by unconsciousness, cyanosis, shock, and convulsions. Death can result from coronary or cerebral occlusion, inducing cardiac arrhythmia, shock, and circulatory and respiratory failure. The only treatment for air embolism is recompression in a hyperbaric chamber, with the intent of shrinking emboli in size, and driving the air out of the emboli into solution.

Gas from ruptured alveoli may pass into the membrane lining the chest, the parietal pleura, and also rupture the lining (*pneumothorax*). Trapped in the intrapleural lining, the gas may further expand on ascent, and push against the heart, lungs, and other organs. Often the lungs collapse under the pressure. Symptoms of pneumothorax include sudden chest pain, breathing difficulty, and coughing of frothy blood. Recompression is the indicated treatment for a concomitant condition, along with thoracentesis.

Gas trapped in the tissues about the heart and blood vessels, and the trachea (*mediastinal emphysema*), can adversely impact the circulation, particularly, the venous flow. Symptoms include pain in the sternum, shortness of breath, and sometimes fainting. The condition is exacerbated on ascent as gas trapped in tissues expands. In severe cases, hyperbaric treatment is utilized.

If the bubbles migrate to the tissues beneath the skin (*subcutaneous emphysema*), often a case accompanying mediastinal emphysema, their presence causes a swelling of neck tissue and enhanced local pressure. Feeling of fullness, and change of voice are associated with subcutaneous emphysema. Treatment consists of oxygen breathing, which accelerates tissue absorption of the air trapped in the neck region.

Pressure increases and decreases can be tolerated by the body when they are distributed uniformly, that is, no local pressure differentials exist. When pressure differentials exist, outside pressure greater than inside pressure locally, and vice versa, distortion of the shape of the local site supporting the pressure difference is the outcome. Burst alveoli are one serious manifestation of the problem. Other areas may suffer similar damage, for instance, the ears, sinuses, teeth, confined skin under a wetsuit, and the intestines. Though such complications can be very painful, they are usually not life threatening. When local pressure differentials develop because of inside and outside pressure imbalances, blood vessels will rupture in attempt to equalize pressure. The amount of rupture and degree of bleeding is directly proportional to the pressure imbalance.

Pressures in ear spaces in the sinuses, middle ear, and teeth fillings are often imbalanced during compression-decompression. To accommodate equalization when diving, air must have free access into and out of these spaces during descent and ascent. Failure to accommodate equalization on descent is termed a squeeze, with outside pressure greater than inside (air space) pressure, while failure to accommodate equalization on ascent is called a reverse block, with inside pressure (air space) greater than ambient pressure. In the case of the ear, it is the eustachian tube which does not permit air passage from the throat to the middle ear. The sinuses have very small openings which close under congestive circumstance, inhibiting air exchange. Similarly, small openings in and around teeth fillings complicate equalization of the air space under the filling (usually a bad filling). In all cases, slow descents and ascents are beneficial in ameliorating squeeze and reverse block problems.

Altitude Sickness

At altitudes greater than some 7,000 *ft*, decreased partial pressures of oxygen can cause arterial hypoxemia. Under hypoxic stimulation (low oxygen tension), hyperventilation occurs with secondary lowering of arterial carbon dioxide and production of alkalosis. Newcomers to high altitude typically experience dyspnea (shortness of breath), rapid heart rate, headache, insomnia, and malaise. Symptoms disappear within a week, and general graded exercise may hasten acclimatization.

Acclimatization is usually lost within a week at lower altitudes. Although increased oxygen at depth may be beneficial, the surface malaise often precludes diving until acclimatization. In itself, altitude sickness is not life threatening.

Pulmonary Edema

Pulmonary edema (fluid buildup in the lungs) can affect nonacclimatized individuals who travel within a day or two to elevations near, or above, 10,000 *ft*. Symptoms usually appear within 18 *hr* after arrival, consisting of rasping cough, dyspnea, and possible pain in the chest. Treatment requires immediate removal to lower altitude, hospitalization with rest, oxygen, and diuretic therapy. Prevention includes adequate acclimatization and reduced levels of exertion. A month of graded exercise may be requisite. Again, increased oxygen partial pressures at depth are helpful, but diving rigors can precipitate pulmonary edema. Symptoms might resemble the chokes (decompression sickness).

Pulmonary edema can be a serious, even fatal, affliction, as noted by its yearly toll on mountain climbers. At altitude, evidence of cough, shortness of breath, or tightness serves as a warning. Rapid treatment, including lower altitude, hospitalization, and appropriate therapy, is recommended.

Hypothermia and Hyperthermia

Exposure to cold results in heat loss, called *hypothermia*, with the rate dependent upon body area, temperature difference, body fat, insulation properties of wet or dry suit, and physical activity. Exercise always increases heat loss. As core temperatures drop, symptoms progress from shivering, to weakness, to muscle rigidity, to coma, and then death. Rewarming at the earliest signs of hypothermia is prudent. While more of a cold water problem, hypothermia can also occur in relatively warm and even tropical waters. Severe hypothermia is a life threatening condition. Shivering and a feeling of being very cold are first symptoms of hypothermia, and the situation gets worse fast. Rewarming in dry clothing is standard and obvious treatment, as well as ingestion of balanced electrolytes. Exercise, caffeine, and alcohol are to be avoided. Care in the choice of protective suit to conserve body heat, attention to feelings of cold, and good physical condition help to minimize hypothermia.

Inadequate ventilation and body heat loss, called *hyperthermia*, usually in the presence of high environmental temperatures and low body fluid levels, lead to a progressive raising of temperatures in vital organs. As temperatures rise, symptoms progress from profuse sweating, to cramps, to heat exhaustion, to heat stroke, to coma, and then death. Dehydration is a contributing factor. Replacement of body fluids and reduction of body temperature are necessary in effective treatment of hyperthermia. Cool water immersion is employed in severe cases, but the usual treatment consists of fluids, salt, and full body ventilation. Like hypothermia, severe hyperthermia is life threatening.

Hyperthermia can be avoided by proper attention to water intake and protection from environmental heat. Environmental temperatures above body temperature are potentially hazardous, especially with increasing levels of physical exertion.

Dysbaric Osteonecrosis

Bone rot (*dysbaric osteonecrosis*) is an insidious disease of the long bones associated with repeated high pressure and saturation exposures. Deep and saturation diving portend problems with temperature control in environmental suits, habitats, respiration and surface monitoring, compression and decompression, inert gas reactivity, communication, oxygen levels, and many others, all falling into an operational control category, that is, problems which can be ameliorated through suitable application of sets of established diving protocols. But aseptic bone necrosis is a chronic complication about which we know little.

Affecting the long bones as secondary arthritis or collapsed surface joints, lesions, detected as altered bone density upon radiography, are the suspected cause. Statistics compiled in the early 1980s by the US Navy, Royal Navy, Medical Research Council, and commercial diving industry suggest that some 8% of all divers exposed to pressures in the 300 *fsw* range exhibited bone damage, some 357 out of 4,463 examined divers. No lesions were seen in divers whose exposures were limited to 100 *fsw*. Some feel that very high partial pressures of oxygen for prolonged periods is the ultimate culprit for bone lesions, leading to fat cell enlargement in more closed regions of the bone core, a condition that reduces blood flow rate and probably increases local vulnerability to bubble growth. The facts, however, are still not clear. And commercial divers continue to be at higher risk of osteonecrosis.

Drugs

Very few studies have systematized the overall effects of drugs underwater. Drug utilization by divers is connected with medication used to ameliorate diving problems, medication used to treat illness, and recreational drugs.   Recent studies suggest that drug effects are compounded at increasing depth, having been described as potentiating, antagonizing, and unpredictable as far as altered behavior with increasing pressure.   Side effects can be subtle and also variable, possibly exacerbated by other risk factors such as cold water, oxygen, or nitrogen concentrations. Many different types of drugs are utilized.

Among the more common drugs used by divers are decongestants, taken for ear and sinus relief. These drug products are typically antihistamines, providing relief by constricting blood vessels, reducing tissue swelling, and opening passages between sinuses and middle ear for air exchange. Antihistamines often produce drowsiness and decreased mental acuity. Another decongestant, with trade name terfenadine, has no sedative effects. Drugs addressing motion sickness may lead to functional motor impairment. Antihistamines, particularly *meclizine* and *dimenhydrate* are often employed for motion sickness, additionally causing sedation. The skin patch drug, *scopolamine*, also possesses sedative properties, with some additional side effects of blurred vision and dry mouth. Individual reactions vary widely.

Sedative and pain agents also alter mental function. Anti-anxiety drugs, such as *valium, halcion,* and *dalmane,* are strong agents, producing significant changes in mental outlook. Muscle relaxants, such as *flexiril* and *robaxin,* induce drowsiness. Analgesics containing *propoxyphene, codein, oxycodone,* or *hydrocodone* reduce mental and physical exercise capacity. Agents used in the treatment of depression or psychosis cause sedation, and have been noted to induce cardiac dysfunction. Tradename drugs in this category, *elavil, haldol,* and *sinequan,* impair cognitive abilities.

Hypertension drugs can limit diving performance.   Diuretics, like *lasix* and *hydrochlorothiazide,* cause fluid loss, possibly compounding dehydration and electrolytic imbalance. Agents affecting heart rate and peripheral vasculature may cause drowsiness and reduce blood flow capacity. These drugs include *metoprolol, hytrin, tenex,* and others. Bronchodilators, used in the treatment of asthma, include *theophylline* and *steroids.*   In the former category, tradename drugs, such as *theodur, uniphyl, metaprel,* and *ventolin* can cause cardiac dysrhythmias and CNS impairment. Gastrointestinal drugs containing histamines can also affect the central nervous system, causing drowsiness and headache. Antacids seem to have no noted adverse effects on divers.

According to the diving medical community at large, the bottom line on drugs underwater is caution, since little is known about many, particularly newer ones. Narcotics and hallucinogens, alcohol, and heavy doses of caffeine have been linked to reduced mental and physical acuity, sedation, vasodilatation, diuresis, and dehydration on the mild side, and extreme neurological, respiratory, and cardiovascular stress on the more severe side.

Keyed Exercises

• *For the following set of conditions and/or symptoms, identify some possible diving maladies:*

Partial oxygen tension of 1.85 *atm?*

Hyperoxia

Partial carbon dioxide tension of .10 *atm, with muscle spasms?*

Hypercapnia (*Severe*)

Rasping cough at an elevation of 13,000 *ft?*

Pulmonary Edema

Intense shivering in a dry suit?

Hypothermia

Light-headedness on an air dive to 145 *fsw?*

Nitrogen Narcosis

Weakness and headache following a hyperventilated skin dive?

Hypocapnia

Pain in the sternum and coughing of blood?

Pneumothorax

Shortness of breath at 6,555 *ft elevation?*

Altitude Sickness

Lesions and cracks in the long bones of the leg?

Dysbaric Osteonecrosis

Paralysis of the lower legs?

DCI (*Neurological*)

Partial oxygen tension of .09 *atm?*

Hypoxia (*Moderate*)

Chest pain and swelling of the neck?

> *Subcutaneous Emphysema*

Profuse sweating and muscle cramps?

> *Hyperthermia*

Dull aching pain in the joints?

> *DCI (Articular)*

• *Match some of the following side effects to drugs possibly avoided when diving?*
Drowsiness?

> *Scopolamine, Flexiril, Robaxin, Elavil, Haldol, Sinequan*

Motor impairment?

> *Meclizine, Dimenhydrate, Propoxyphene, Codein, Oxycodone, Hydrocodone*

Reduced blood flow capacity?

> *Metoprolol, Hytrin, Tenex, Theophylline*

Cardiac dysrhythmias?

> *Theodur, Metaprel, Uniphyl, Ventolin*

Blurred vision?
> *Scopolamine*

Reduced cognitive functionality?

> *Valium, Halcion, Dalmane, Elavil, Haldol, Sinequan*

Appendix A

FUNDAMENTAL CONCEPTS AND RELATIONSHIPS

Matter

Matter has definite mass and volume, can change form and phase, and consists of tiny atoms and molecules. A gram molecular weight ($gmole$) of substance, that is, an amount of substance in grams equal to its atomic weight, A, possesses Avogadro's number, N_0, of atoms or molecules, some 6.025×10^{23} constituents. Molecules of a gas are in constant motion. Liquid molecules are free to move and slide over each other, while loosely bound. Molecules in a solid are relatively fixed, but can oscillate about their lattice points.

Matter cannot be created nor destroyed, but it can be transformed by chemical and nuclear reactions. In the most general sense, matter and energy are equivalent. For instance, the nuclear and chemical binding energies of molecules and atoms result from very small mass reductions in constituent particles (mass defect) when in bound states. The postulate of conservation of mass-energy is fundamental, and cannot be derived from any other principle. Stated simply, mass-energy can neither be created nor destroyed. All of observable science is based on this premise.

The concepts of mass and corresponding occupied volume are fundamental perceptions. The mass, m, in unit volume, V, is the mass density,

$$\rho = \frac{m}{V},$$

and gases are usually the least dense, followed by fluids, and then solids. Weight density is the weight per unit volume. Specific density, η, is the ratio of material density to density of water. States of matter usually have much different densities. Matter interactions are generically termed mechanics.

Mechanics

Mechanics is concerned with the effects of forces to produce or retard motion (kinetic energy), change position, induce material deformation, or cause chemical and nuclear reactions (potential energy). Forces may be gravitational, nuclear, or electromagnetic in origin. Mechanical properties describe the change in shape of matter when external forces are applied. Examples include the simple bending of a beam, the propagation of sound waves, the permanent deformation of metals into useful shapes, and the flow of liquids and gases around obstacles. For matter in the gaseous state, the usual force is the hydrostatic pressure, and deformation is a change in volume. For matter in the solid state, both tensile and shearing forces come into play to produce deformations.

Time rate of change distance is velocity, v, or, using vector notation,

$$\mathbf{v} = \frac{d\mathbf{s}}{dt}$$

with $d\mathbf{s}$ the inifinitesimal change in position over change in time, dt. Time rate of change of velocity is acceleration, $\mathbf{a}$,

$$d\mathbf{a} = \frac{d\mathbf{v}}{dt}$$

The above set of equations are cast in vector notation, and Figures 69 and 70 review the addition, subtraction, velocity and particle displacement (Figure 62), velocity and particle displacement in a curved trajectory, and acceleration (Figure 63) in terms of vector diagrams.

Force is a push or a pull. Newton's first law states that a body in motion tends to stay in motion unless acted upon by an unbalanced force. Forces, $\mathbf{F}$, acting upon bodies of mass, m, produce accelerations, $\mathbf{a}$, linked by Newton's second law,

$$\mathbf{F} = m\mathbf{a}.$$

with t the time, the most general form of the force law is,

$$\mathbf{F} = \frac{d\mathbf{p}}{dt},$$

with $\mathbf{p}$ the momentum, defined in terms of mass, m, and velocity, $\mathbf{v}$,

$$\mathbf{p} = m\mathbf{v},$$

allowing for changes in mass to generate force. Such situation obviously presents itself in the relativistic case, where mass depends on velocity. Another case where force depends on rate of mass loss occurs with fuel burnup in rocket propulsion systems. Newton's third law states that for every action, there is an equal and opposite reaction. Stated another way, for every applied force, there is an equal and opposite reaction force, a stipulation requiring the conservation of momentum in all reactions.

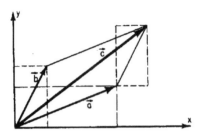

The addition of vectors.

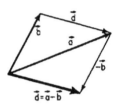

The subtraction of vectors.

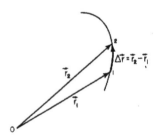

The displacement of a
particle in a short time interval $\Delta t =$
$t_2 - t_1$.

Figure 62. Addition And Subtraction Of Vectors

To add vectors, place them tip to tail, preserving their magnitudes and directions, and draw the resultant from the tail of the first to the tip of the second vector. Or to subtract vectors, reverse the direction of the subtracted vector, and place it on the tip of the first vector. Then proceed as with vector addition.

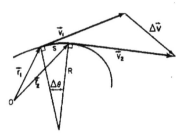

A curved trajectory.

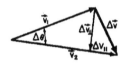

**Diagram for calculating
the acceleration.**

Figure 63. Velocity And Particle Displacement In A Curved Trajectory

*In vectors terms, velocity, **v**, and acceleration, **a**, are rates of change in position, **r**, and velocity, **v**, as shown below.*

The rectilinear equations above generalize for the curvilinear case. Angular momentum, **L**, about some fixed point a distance, **r**, away, is defined as,

$$\mathbf{L} = \mathbf{r} \times \mathbf{p}$$

and the corresponding torque, **N**, is then,

$$\mathbf{N} = \frac{d\mathbf{L}}{dt}$$

Obviously, in terms of the force, **F**,

$$\mathbf{N} = \mathbf{r} \times \mathbf{F}$$

A force applied to an element of surface area, at angle, θ, to the surface element normal, generates a pressure, P, given by,

$$P = \cos\theta \frac{dF}{dA},$$

with dF and dA scalar elements of force and area. Pressure at a point is equal in all directions, and thus is not a specifically directed (vector) quantity.

Energy in simplest terms is the ability to do work. Or equivalently, the ability to do work requires an interchange of energy between a system and its surroundings. Energy takes two main forms, kinetic and potential. Kinetic energy is the energy associated with motion. Potential energy is the energy associated with position in a force field. Binding energy is the energy associated with changes in both kinetic and potential energies in bound composite systems, undergoing chemical, nuclear, or molecular interactions. Electromagnetic and acoustical energies are kinetic and potential energies associated with light and pressure waves. Heat energy can be kinetic energy associated with random molecular translations, vibrations, and rotations, or potential energy of frictional surface distortions and stress fatigue, nuclear and chemical reactions, and phase transformations. In all processes known to man, mass-energy is conserved, which is to say that mass can be converted to energy, and vice versa.

In the most general (relativistic) sense, mass and energy are equivalent, as mentioned, which follows as a consequence of the constancy of the speed of light in any inertial frame. An inertial frame is a frame of reference moving with constant velocity (no acceleration). Einstein postulated that the laws of physics are identical for two observers moving with constant velocity with respect to each other (first law of relativity), and that the speed of light, c, is constant independent of relative motion between reference frames (second law of relativity). This requires that the mass, m, of a body moving with speed, v, increases over its resting value, m_0, according to the relativistic equation,

$$m = \frac{m_0}{(1 - v^2/c^2)^{1/2}}$$

for c the speed of light. The corresponding total energy, E, becomes,

$$E = mc^2$$

and the momentum, $\mathbf{p}$, satisfies,

$$\mathbf{p} = m\mathbf{v}$$

as before, but employing the relativistic mass. In the low energy limit, that is, the classical realm,

$$\lim_{v/c \to 0} \frac{m_0 c^2}{(1 - v^2/c^2)^{1/2}} \approx m_0 c^2 + \frac{1}{2} m_0 v^2$$

so we write the total energy as the sum of rest mass energy, E_0, plus kinetic energy K,

$$E = m_0 c^2 + \frac{1}{2} m_0 v^2 = E_0 + K$$

with

$$E_0 = m_0 c^2$$

$$K = \frac{1}{2} m_0 v^2$$

in the usual (nonrelativistic) sense.

Force, **F**, acting along a pathlength, **ds**, does work, dW,

$$dW = \mathbf{F} \cdot \mathbf{ds},$$

or, in terms of pressure, P, effecting a volume change, dV,

$$dW = P\,dV,$$

imparting, or taking, energy to, or from, a system. If there are zero net forces on a system, total energy, $H = K + U$, remains constant, with K kinetic energy and U potential energy. Various forms of the system energy can change, but the total, H, cannot change. If net forces do work on a system and if, when the processes are reversed, the system returns to its initial value of energy, H, the forces are said to be conservative, and the energy of the system is independent of how the work was done. One nonconservative force is friction, since the amount of energy lost to friction by a moving body depends on the distance over which the body slides, and not just on initial and final states. Conservative forces are said to derive from potentials, U, so that we write,

$$\mathbf{F} = -\nabla U,$$

in which case, the total energy, $H = K + U$, is a constant of motion. In a conservative force field, the change in energy associated with initial and final states depends only on initial and final state energies, and is independent of the path chosen between points. Then two (energy) states, i and f, for a conservative transition, are linked according to,

$$H_i = K_i + U_i = H_f = K_f + U_f$$

Potential, U, will depend on position in force fields (gravitation, electromagnetism, strong and weak interactions, and combinations). In the gravitational field of the Earth, we reference the geopotential with respect to position, h,

$$U = mgh$$

with m the mass, g the local acceleration of gravity, and h measured from any convenient Earth reference point in the vertical direction (center, surface, satellite orbit).

Power, J, is the rate of doing work,

$$J = \frac{dW}{dt},$$

for corresponding small changes in energy and time, dW and dt.

The interactions of matter and energy are sometimes broken down into light, heat, and sound. Macroscopically, this is a classical division, suitably splitting mechanics into major observable categories, but with understanding that each is a detailed science by itself.

Light

Light is energy in the form of radiation, equivalently regarded as photons (particles) or electromagnetic packets (waves). Light, regarded as photons in the energy range, 2.5 up to 5.2×10^{-19} *joule*, or electromagnetic waves in the wavelength range, 380 *nm* up to 800 *nm*, causes sensation of vision. Solar radiation reaching the Earth's surface is peaked in this same spectral range, a range where humans and animals possess sensitive receptors. Light forms a small part of the continuous spectrum of electromagnetic radiation, which encompasses radio waves and infrared radiation at wavelengths longer than light, and ultraviolet, x-ray, gamma ray, and cosmic ray radiation at progressively shorter wavelenghts. As a wave, light is characterized by crossed electric and magnetic field vectors, **E** and **B**.

Electromagnetic waves are transverse, that is, **E** and **B** oscillate in a plane perpendicular to the direction of travel, unlike acoustical waves which are longitudinal and oscillate in the direction of travel. In terms of frequency, f, and wavelength, λ, electromagnetic waves propagating in a vacuum satisfy, $\lambda f = c$, and, treating as photons, light possess particle energy, $\varepsilon = hf$, for h Planck's constant $(6.625 \times 10^{-34}$ *joule sec*). In a vacuum, light (waves or photons) travels at constant speed, c, but in a material medium, however, photons are absorbed and emitted by molecules, slowing down the speed of propagation in the medium.

Refractive index, n, is really a function of wavelength, so that two light beams of different color (wavelength) propagate through materials at different speeds. Across the visible spectrum, differences in refractive indices are small. In glass, 0.009 is the difference between blue and red light indices of refraction. Table 68 lists refractive indices of a few materials.

Table 68. Refractive Indices.

media	Refractive index n	Media speed of light c/n (*m/sec*)
vacuum	1.0000	2.99 x 10^8
air	1.0003	2.98 x 10^8
glass	1.4832	2.02 x 10^8
quartz	1.4564	2.05 x 10^8
steam	1.3178	2.27 x 10^8
salt water	1.3340	2.24 x 10^8
pure water	1.3321	2.24 x 10^8

When light passes from one dielectric medium to another, it is refracted and reflected according to the refractive indices of the media. Figure 64 depicts the relationships between angles of incidence, ϕ, refraction, ϕ', reflection, ϕ, and the indices of refraction, n and n', assuming $n' > n$. Quantitatively, the relationship is called Snell's law,

$$n' \sin \phi' = n \sin \phi$$

At the interface of denser media, there exists a critical angle, ϕ_c, such that for all larger angles of incidence in that media, all light is reflected (grazing incidence),

$$\sin \phi_c = \frac{n}{n'}$$

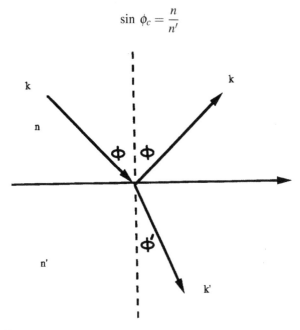

Figure 64. Incidence, Reflection, and Refraction Of Light

Plane electromagnetic waves, such as light, striking the interface between two transmitting media, with permittivities, ε and ε', and permeabilities, μ and μ', experience reflection and refraction according to Snell's law,

$$n' \sin \phi' = n \sin \phi$$

for,

$$n = \left[\frac{\varepsilon\mu}{\varepsilon_0\mu_0}\right]^{1/2} \quad n' = \left[\frac{\varepsilon'\mu'}{\varepsilon_0\mu_0}\right]^{1/2}$$

with ε_0 and μ_0 vacuum permittivity and permeability. The case is drawn for $n' > n$.

Water is transparent to light. Although a glass of water seems to allow all the light to pass through, it is obvious that as one goes deeper underwater, it gets darker. In the ocean, with so much water available, the amount of light energy absorbed becomes important. Water clarity and lack of turbidity are also primary factors in determining light penetration in different regions, or layers. Thus, it is difficult to determine at what depth water becomes dark. Some indication of light penetration is the depth at which microscopic plants exist underwater, because marine plants, like land plants, require light for photosynthesis. The vertical region in the ocean where light exists is called the euphotic zone, existing from the surface down to where only 1% of the light remains. The lower limit varies from 45 fsw along the coasts, down to as much as 500 fsw in the clear tropical zones. As one descends, white sunlight is selectively absorbed, starting with the red part of the spectrum, and then continuing to the green and blue parts. Colors, such as red, perceived in fish and other creatures underwater, do not come from surface light. Pigments in these creatures absorb the remaining blue-green light, and then remit the light as red. At a depth of 33 fsw, little or no color distinction is possible. There are no shadows, and light seems to be coming from all around. At 330 fsw, visibility is limited to a few feet. At 950 fsw, all is quite dark.

Unlike sound waves encountering density interfaces, light transmission through opaque dielectric interfaces is slightly attenuated, with energy passing easily from one media to the other. Because of refraction, however, perceived images of source objects differ across the media interface. Such refractive phenomena change image size and relative position, the study of which is called optics.

Optics

Optics deals with ray phenomena that are not dependent in any way on the wave or quantum behavior of light. In geometrical optics, light travels along straight lines, or rays, in homogeneous media, which are bent at the interfaces separating media, or curved in media with variable refractive indices. At any point along a fan of rays emitted by an object point source of light, there is a surface everywhere perpendicular to the rays, called the wave front. The wave front is the locus of points reached by light after a given time along all possible ray paths. If the wave front emerging from a lens or other optical interface is a true sphere, a perfect image will be formed. Any departure from a true sphere represents the presence of optical aberrations, or, more simply, image distortions. An optical system consists of an assembly of mirrors, lenses, prisms, and apertures, usually with spherical surfaces to facilitate precise image formation. The human eye is an optical system consisting of lenses, apertures, and image forming planes.

Each ray from an object point, after passing through an optical system (such as the eye), strikes a specified image plane at a single point, with all such points for all possible rays passing through the system constituting the geometrical image of the source as formed by the optical system. While the number of rays are infinite, only a few rays, strategically chosen with regard to the optical system, are actually traced in an image assembly called a spot diagram. The spot diagram represents an outline picture of the image produced by the optical system, but lacking fine structure caused by light wave interference and diffraction. In spite of microstructural limitations, the simple ray tracing technique can quantify gross relationships between source and image sizes, distances, focal lengths, and refractive indices of optical media.

Refraction of paraxial rays (very nearly normally incident), as shown in Figure 65, is a good example of the power of simple ray tracing techniques in optical applications. The ratio of image to object distance, σ, is termed shortening, while the ratio of image to object height, μ, is the lateral magnification. For paraxial bundles of rays, the dispersion is small and the bundle is clustered at near normal incidence. Always, $\sigma\mu = 1$. Objects underwater, viewed at the surface, appear larger and closer than their actual size and position. The shortening is 3/4, while the lateral magnification is 4/3, taking $n = 4/3$ for water, and $n' = 1$ for air. The opposite occurs underwater, when viewing an object above the surface. Underwater viewing of surface objects is also limited by the critical angle, ϕ_c. Outside the viewing cone, limited by ϕ_c underwater, no surface images can be transmitted through the water to the eyes.

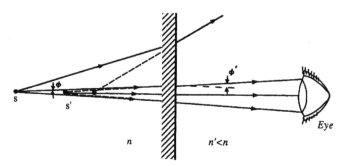

Figure 65. Virtual Images And Refraction At Plane Surfaces

When observing through a plane surface of a refracting medium, objects are seen clearly, but not necessarily in their true position. As virtual images, they appear closer, or farther away, depending on the ratio of refractive indices of both media. The actual distance, s, in medium, n, and the apparent distance, s', in medium, n', are related through the paraxial approximation (almost normal incidence),

$$s' = \frac{n'}{n}s$$

When looking into water from air, objects underwater are foreshortened by a factor of 3/4, the ratio of air to water refractive indices. Objects are also magnified in size by the reciprocal of the foreshortening and thus, for water, the magnification is 4/3.

The eyes focus using paraxial rays. The ability to accommodate angular spread in the paraxial bundle is called peripheral vision. The greater the ability to accommodate angular dispersion in rays striking the eye, the greater is the corresponding peripheral vision. Cutting off the most widely dispersed rays in the bundle reaching the eyes, for instance, with a mask underwater, causes tunnel vision, or the perception of a brightly illuminated foreground, and dark peripheral background.

The refraction and focusing of overhead sunlight by wave motion produces the pattern of light ripples often seen on sandy bottoms below shallow, clear water. Wave crests act like converging lenses, focusing light rays into spatial regions of higher intensity, while the troughs act like diverging lenses, defocusing light rays into spatial regions of lesser intensity.

Sound

Any change in stress or pressure leading to a local change in density, or displacement from equilibrium, in an elastic medium can generate an acoustical wave. Acoustics is concerned with fluctuations in mechanical properties characterizing the state of matter, such as pressure, temperature, density, stress, and displacement. Primary acoustical measurements determine the magnitude and wave structure of one of these mechanical properties, whereas secondary measurements characterize the propagation speed and the rate of dissipation of acoustical energy.

The time averaged energy density, I, of an acoustical wave is a sum of kinetic and potential (strain) contributions, and can be written, $I = 2\pi^2 f^2 U^2 \rho u$, for u sound speed, ρ material density, f frequency, and U wave amplitude. At an interface, energy is both transmitted and reflected. The transmitted wave amplitude, TU, and reflected wave amplitude, RU, depend on the density and acoustical speed in both media. Across dissimilar interfaces, very little energy, emanating as an acoustical signal in either water or air, is transmitted. For an air-water interface, we have

$$T = 0.0081,$$

$$R = 0.9919,$$

in approximately both cases (air-water, or water-air propagation), using nominal values of water and air densities, and acoustical speeds. Corresponding ratios of transmitted to incident intensity, and reflected to incident intensity, measures of the acoustical energy transmitted and reflected across the boundary, are given by

$$\frac{I_T}{I} = T^2 = 0.0092,$$

$$\frac{I_R}{I} = R^2 = 0.9839,$$

These results parallel electromagnetic wave propagation across a metallic-dielectric (conducting-nonconducting) interface.

Sound propagation is but one aspect of acoustics. When we speak, we utter sound. Someone nearby hears the sound. In studying the production and reception of sound and transmission through media, acoustics is a discipline of physics, but speech and hearing obviously invoke biological elements and processes. When speaking, a slight disturbance is produced in the air in front of the mouth, a compression resulting in a change in air pressure near 1 $dyne/cm^2$. Since air is an elastic medium, it does not stay compressed and expands again passing on the disturbance to its neighbor. That neighbor in turn passes the disturbance on to its next neighbor, and so on, resulting in a pressure fluctuation that moves through the air column in the form of a sound (acoustical) wave. Reaching the ear of an observer, the disturbance moves the eardrum, which in turn displaces the little bones in the middle ear, communicating motion to the hair cells in the cochlea, with the ultimate biophysical interpretation of the hearing of the sound by the brain.

A great bulk of data gathered about the ocean bottom, and other underwater objects, uses sound navigation and ranging (sonar). Sonar may be active or passive. Passive sonar equipment listens to noises underwater, and can determine presence and relative direction of sound sources. Active sonar, or echo sounding, acts like radar, sending out an acoustical signal which is reflected back to a receiver. If sounding from the bottom, the depth is equal to 1/2 the time for the signal to leave and return, multiplied by the speed of sound in water, about 4,950 ft/sec. Ships tracing out prescribed paths can continuously map the bottom with sonar, is sinusoidal, as with light waves. Sound speeds in various media are tabulated in Table 69, at 0 ^oC and 1 atm.

Table 69. Sound Speeds at Standard Temperature and Pressure.

media	sound speed $u\ (m/sec)$
vacuum	0
air	333
steel	5302
copper	3292
parafin	1395
wood	2984
salt water	1452
pure water	1461

Heat

In thermodynamics, heat denotes the quantity of energy exchanged by thermal interaction of any system with its environment. For example, if a flame is applied to a cool metal plate, the energy content of the plate increases, as evidenced by its temperature increase, and we say that heat has passed from the flame to the plate. If energy losses to the surrounding air can be ignored, the heat transferred from the flame is equal to the energy gain of the plate. In more complex processes, involving mechanical as well as thermal interactions, the heat transferred is more difficult to identify. Thermodynamics focuses on the controlled and slow evolution of heat, energy, and entropy, and the distinctions between them in mechanical systems. While heat is a tenuous concept, linked to observables such as internal energy change and external work, we often deal with systems at different temperatures, exchanging heat in the absence of mechanical interactions, or external forces. Specific heat, c, measures change in heat capacity, dQ, for corresponding change in temperature, dT, per unit mass, m, of substance. At constant pressure, the specific heat is denoted, c_P,

$$c_P = \frac{1}{m}\left[\frac{dQ}{dT}\right]_P$$

while at constant volume, the specific heat, c_V, is similarly written,

$$c_V = \frac{1}{m} \left[\frac{dQ}{dT} \right]_V$$

Generally, it is c_P that concerns us as divers and underwater. The molal specific heat is the heat capacity per unit mole (n replaces m). Heat, then, is the energy exchanged between parts of mechanical systems at different temperatures. Three fundamental and well known mechanisms include convection, conduction, and radiation. In practical situations, near standard temperatures and pressures, heat exchange usually involves the first two, conduction and convection. Radiative transfer underscores fairly high temperatures.

Heat conduction is the exchange of heat from one body at a given temperature to another body at a lower temperature with which it is in contact. Transfer of molecular kinetic energy occurs directly by molecular impacts or collisions. Heat conduction is governed by Fourier's law,

$$\phi = -K \nabla T,$$

with, ϕ, heat flux, K, conductivity, and, T, temperature.

Heat convection is a special case of conduction that occurs when a fluid or gas flows past the outer boundary of a system. Then the determination of K involves solving the fluid equations of a viscous, heat conducting fluid or gas, coupled to the heat flow equations in the system. Table 70 summarizes specific heats, conductivities, and corresponding densities for a cross section of materials.

Radiative transfer is a different mechanism completely from conduction and convection. The mechanism is electromagnetic wave emission from a heated surface, with the spectrum of wavelengths a complex function of surface temperature. For a point (idealized) source at temperature, T, the radial (isotropic) heat flux, ϕ, is given by the Stefan-Boltzmann relationship,

$$\phi = \sigma T^4,$$

for T the temperature, and σ the radiation constant ($5.67 \times 10^{-8} watt/m^2 \ {}^oK^4$. The most complex heat transfer phenomena are those in which extended physical systems interact by combinations of the above, in addition to phase transformations such as boiling, condensation, or solidification.

Table 70. Specific Heats, Conductivities, And Densities.

material	Specific heat c_P $(cal/g\,^oC)$	Conductivity K $(cal/sec\;cm\,^oC)$	Density ρ (g/cm^3)
air	.242	.0001	.00024
iron	.121	.0858	16.623
aluminum	.207	.5375	2.721
polyethylene	.912	.6939	.925
neoprene	.381	.0004	.189
glass	.135	.0025	2.312
salt water	.949	.0013	1.025
pure water	1.000	.0014	1.000
alcohol	.653	.0010	.791

Radiation is absorbed in passing through matter, and the fraction absorbed is characteristic of the material. The ratio of absorbed to incident radiation at a certain wavelength is called the absorptivity, α, and depends on the wavelength. A body with absorptivity equal to one is called a *black* body. Perfect black bodies do not exist in nature, but there are many approximate black bodies, especially in the infrared, or long wavelength, region. Of the incident radiation that is not absorbed, part is reflected and part is transmitted. The ratio of reflected to incident radiation is called the reflectivity, ρ, and the ratio of transmitted to incident radiation is called the transmissivity, τ. Obviously, the three quantities are related by,

$$\alpha + \rho + \tau = 1.$$

For a black body, $\rho = \tau = 0$, and $\alpha = 1$. A molecule which absorbs radiation at a particular wavelength is also able to emit radiation at the same wavelength. The emissivity, ε, is defined to be the ratio of emitted radiation to the maximum possible at a given temperature, and by Kirchhoff's law,

$$\varepsilon = \alpha.$$

Equation of State

The relationship between pressure, volume, and temperature for any substance is called the equation of state (EOS). In the case of solids and liquids, equations of state are typically quite complicated, mainly because molecular interactions in solids and liquids are extended (long range). Gases, however, present a simpler situation. Interactions of gas molecules are localized (short range), compared to solids and liquids, and the corresponding equation of state reflects the point nature of interactions.

Long before kinetic theory and statistical mechanics provided the molecular basis for gas laws, chemists (and probably alchemists) deduced that, under pressure, P, volume, V, and temperature, T, changes, to good order of the day,

$$\lim_{P \to 0} \frac{PV}{nT} = R,$$

for n the number of moles of the gas, with R a constant, and temperature, T, measured on an absolute (^oK) scale. Obviously, their range of investigation was limited in phase space, but it is still interesting to note that all gas laws reduce to the simple form in the limit of low pressure, for any temperature.

With this subset of definitions, the relationship between pressure, volume, temperature, and number of moles of gas is ideal gas law, and R the universal gas constant $(8.317 \ joule/gmole \ ^oK)$. If temperature is kept constant, pressure increases linearly with inverse volume. If pressure is kept constant, the volume varies linearly with temperature, or, if the volume is kept constant, the pressure increases linearly with temperature. The fact that real gases approximate this behavior has been known for centuries, in fact, the quantifications are often called the laws of Boyle, Charles and Gay-Lussac, after the Eighteenth century investigating chemists.

Rheology

Rheology is the interdisciplinary study of the deformation and flow of material under internal and external forces. Rheology tries to correlate macroscopic response and flow of solids, liquids, and gases with constitutive equations spanning atomic, molecular, intermolecular, and broader domain scales. Irreversible processes, such as macroscopic flow, heat generated by internal friction, mechanical aging, fatigue, solid deformation, shearing, and stressing can be collectively quantized through constitutive equations. The mechanical relationships, describing the change in shape or flow of matter under internal and external forces, are also called the *material properties*.

Deformation

A solid is elastic if the amount of deformation is directly proportional to the applied force, implying that the deformation process is reversible and independent of the way the force is applied. A solid is inelastic if the displacement depends on the rate, or direction, of the applied force. Interest in the elastic and inelastic properties of matter date back to Galileo.

For most metals and ceramics, the rate dependent effects are small, but play an important role in the dissipation of oscillational energy, causing damping of vibrations in machines and oscillating mechanical systems. In plastics and rubbers, inelastic contributions to deformations are large, and these types of materials are termed viscoelastic. The categorization, plastic solid, or plastic deformation, is appropriate for materials in which deformation is a nonlinear, irreversible function of the applied force. Examples include the permanent deformation of metals by large forces, the response of organic polymers, and glass at high temperature. For perfectly elastic solids, stress and strain are completely reversible, so that the energy stored in the solid under stress is returned when the stress is removed. In such case, a stressed solid will vibrate and oscillate between deformed and relaxed state indefinitely.

Friction and viscosity are certainly dissipative forces, tending to convert kinetic energy into mostly heat and potential energy that is not recoverable. Frictional and viscous forces impart irreversibility to physical processes, contributing to overall increase in entropy. Perpetual motion machines, indefinite oscillations, and perfect multidirectionality of physical phenomena are precluded because of dissipative mechanisms. Yet, without frictional and viscous forces, we could not walk on the Earth, drive cars, nor swim underwater with fins.

Friction and Tribology

Friction is the tangential force necessary to overcome resistance in sliding contacting surfaces against each other, under a normal force pressing the surfaces together. Friction is mainly a surface phenomenon, depending primarily on conditions at the interfacial surfaces. By definition, friction is the ratio of the magnitudes of the required moving force, F, to the normal (load) force, N, and takes the form,

$$\mu = \frac{F}{N},$$

with the coefficient of friction, μ, ranging from small to large values. For lubricated surfaces, μ ranges from 0.001 to 0.2, for dry surfaces, μ, varies between 0.1 and 2.0, while for ultraclean surfaces, μ becomes very large. For ultrasmooth surfaces, μ is large because of large cohesive forces, while for very rough surfaces, μ is large because of high asperity interlocking.

The maximum value of frictional force required to start sliding is known as *static* friction, while the amount of frictional force necessary to maintain sliding is known as *kinetic* friction. Static friction is always slightly greater than kinetic friction. Some static coefficients of friction for metals are listed in Table 71 below. Kinetic coefficients are no more than 5% to 10% less.

Table 71. Coefficients Of Static Friction

metal	against itself	against steel
aluminum	1.3	0.6
brass	1.4	0.5
bronze	1.2	0.4
copper	1.3	0.8
iron	0.4	0.4

Contact between surfaces that are dry, and ordinarily rough, usually involves the tips of tall asperities. Thus, total contact area is only a small fraction of the entire interfacial area. Tips adhere to opposing surfaces, and must be sheared if motion is to occur. Total force requisite to shear these junctions is roughly the product of the shear strength of the materials times the area of all junctions at the onset of sliding. Wear (tribology), concerned with the loss or transfer of material in contact, results from many interactive frictional forces, including adhesion, abrasion, corrosion, fatigue, and worse, combinations of all. The volume of wear (material lost), w, is proportional to the applied normal load, N, distance moved or slid, x, and inversely proportional to the material hardness, β, so that,

$$w = \frac{kNx}{\beta},$$

with k the proportionality constant, obviously a function of many variables. Lubrication attempts to mitigate wear by imposing films of foreign substances between contacting bodies, with films solid (graphite), fluid (oil), or chemically active substances. Elastohydrodynamic lubrication occurs in highly loaded assemblies with changes in fluid viscosities under high pressure and temperature, seen, for instance, in multiple viscosity oil for car engines and compressors.

Viscosity

Fluid flow is invariably accompanied by drag, that is, mechanical work is expended to keep the fluid in motion, and is then converted into heat. The effect is linked to viscosity, or internal fluid friction as it is termed in analogy to material properties. Viscosity arises in fluids and gases as a result of momentum transfer between adjacent layers of molecules, simply, shear forces resulting from velocity differences between molecules in interacting layers. Velocity differences can arise through applied forces, temperature differences, boundary effects, or local turbulence and mixing. Like friction, viscosity is dissipative, tending to resist motion, or changes in motion.

In gases, viscosity is proportional to the square root of absolute temperature, and is essentially independent of pressure. For actual gases, viscosity is indeed constant over a wide range of pressures, somewhere in the range of 0.01 *atm* up to 10 *atm* In liquids, on the other hand, viscosity falls off rapidly with increasing temperature Additionally, viscosity in liquids has a short range, intermolecular force component

Measurement of viscosity is simple, conceptually. Two plates of cross sectiona area, A, separated by a distance, Δx, are placed in a fluid. The force, F, requirec to drag one plate with velocity, Δv, with respect to the other, in parallel direction defines the viscosity, X, through the relationship,

$$F = \frac{XA\Delta v}{\Delta x}.$$

The statement above assumes that the shear process does not alter the gas or flui structure. Certainly for gases this poses no problems, but for fluids, this may no always be true. For instance, within polymers, the shearing and flow result in partia alignment of elongated molecules.

Shocks

Shocks are wave disturbances propagating at supersonic speeds in materials, characterized by rapid rise in local pressure, density, and temperature in frontal regions. Shock waves are generated by the sudden release of large amounts of energy in a small region, for instance, detonations in high explosives, passage of supersonic aircraft in the atmosphere, or discharges of lightning bolts in a narrow air channel. Shock waves, not sustained in propagation, lose energy through viscous dissipation, reducing to ordinary sound (acoustical) waves.

Detonation waves are special types of self-sustaining shock waves, in which exothermal reactions move with supersonic speed into the undetonated material, compressing, heating, and igniting chemical reactions that sustain shock propagation. The detonation process usually requires a shock wave to initiate reactions. Deflagrations, or flames, differ from shocks and detonation waves because deflagrations propagate at subsonic speeds.

A unique feature of shock wave propagation in gases is the high shock temperatures attainable, near 15,000 ^{o}K. Such high temperatures are very useful for the study and application of shock tubes to measurements of reaction rate processes in science and aeronautics. Measurements of chemical reaction, vibrational relaxation, dissociation, and ionization rates have been effected with shock tubes, over large temperature ranges. Modified shock tubes can be used as short duration wind tunnels, so to speak, producing high Mach number ($\mu = 16$), high temperature ($T = 6,000$ ^{o}K) environments replicating the gas dynamics encountered by missiles and reentry vehicles (RVs). Conventional wind tunnels are constrained by Mach numbers approximately half shock tube Mach numbers.

The shock equation of state, simply the relationship between pressure and volume for given shock speed, has been established for many materials, and up to pressures of 10 *Mbar*. Pressures and densities attained in shock compressed geologic material are comparable to those found in the Earth, and have provided valuable data for geophysical analysis. Volcanism, plate faulting, and marine disturbances generate geological shocks of enormous potential destructive force, and an accurate assessment of their propagation characteristics in the Earth is an important component of seismology and geophysics. Thermodynamics, like rheology, deals with macroscopic properties of extended matter, such as density and pressure, where temperature is a significant variable. Thermodynamics provides a complete description of these properties under conditions of equilibrium, and offers a starting point for investigation of nonequilibrium phenomena such as hydrodynamics, transport, and chemical reactions. Collectively, thermodynamics relates mechanics to heat and temperature changes, assigns directionality to physical processes, and serves as the basis for descriptions of macroscopic interactions. Thermodynamics grew naturally out of early studies of temperature.

Thermometry

While thermometry is concerned with heat measurements and fixed calibration points for instruments, some indicated in Table 72 below, what thermometers measure is the average kinetic energy, $\bar{e}$, of the molecular ensemble, the essence of temperature. Typically, thermometers employ linear or logarithmic scales, most often using two (sometimes three) calibration points. In the 1,000 to 5,000 ^oK temperature range, at 1 *atm* pressure, all condensed phases (solid and liquid) are unstable against the gaseous phase. There are no known stable solids above 4,200 ^oK, the approximate melting point of a mixture of tantalum carbide and hafnium carbide. Stable liquids do exist over the entire range, although not extensively studied. The normal boiling point of tungsten, for example, is about 6,200 ^oK. Although intermolecular forces responsible for the stability of solids and liquids begin to weaken as temperature is increased from 1,000 to 5,000 ^oK, chemical valence binding is still of considerable importance in the gas phase. Molecular species that are unstable at room temperatures are sometimes found in conditions of equilibrium in high temperature vapors. In the 5,000 to 10,000 ^oK range, no stable molecules can exist in the gas phase. At temperatures near 10,000 ^oK, atoms and ions can exist together, while above 10,000 ^oK appreciable numbers of free electrons are present. At 50,000 ^oK, mostly electrons and bare nuclei persist. In the 100,000,000 ^oK region, like charged ions in a plasma possess sufficiently high collisional energy to overcome mutual Coulomb repulsion, supporting, in the case of deuterium and tritium, fusion.

Table 72. Temperature Calibration Points.

calibration point	Kelvin (^oK)	Fahrenheit (^oF)	Centigrade (^oC)
absolute zero	0	-460	-273
hydrogen triple	14	-434	-259
neon boiling	27	-410	-246
oxygen boiling	90	-297	-183
water triple	273	32	0
water boiling	373	212	100
sulfur boiling	717	831	444
gold freezing	1336	1945	1063

When reference points, such as freezing and boiling, are known, it is simple to construct thermometers, devices which interpolate and extrapolate over ranges near the reference points. Both linear and logarithmic forms are employed. Denoting the freezing point calibration, X_i, at temperature, T_i, and then boiling point calibration, X_s, at temperature, T_s, linear and logarithmic temperature scales are given by,

$$\frac{T - T_i}{T_s - T_i} = \frac{X - X_i}{X_s - X_i}$$

and,

$$\frac{T - T_i}{T_s - T_i} = \frac{\ln\left(X - X_i\right)}{\ln\left(X_s - X_i\right)}$$

with T the temperature for reading X. Not unexpectedly, standard Kelvin, Centigrade (Celsius), Rankine, and Fahrenheit temperatures are defined on linear scales,

$$^{o}F = \frac{9^{o}}{5} C + 32,$$

$$^{o}K = ^{o} C + 273,$$

$$^{o}R = ^{o} F + 460.$$

Thermodynamics

The first law of thermodynamics is really a statement of conservation of energy in any system. Denoting the internal energy of the system, U, the net heat flow into the system, Q, and the work, W, done on the system, the first law requires that infinitesimal changes dQ, dU, and dW satisfy the balance,

$$dU = dQ - dW,$$

The second law requires an ordering variable, S, called entropy, so that for any process, the heat transferred, dQ, takes the form,

$$dQ = T dS,$$

with $dS \geq 0$. The requirement that the entropy change, dS, associated with the process must be greater than or equal to zero imparts directionality to the process. Combining first and second laws, considering only mechanical work, $dW = PdV$, we see that,

$$dU = T dS - PdV.$$

In mechanics, energy and momentum are usually introduced as derived concepts. Advanced treatments introduce energy and momentum as fundamental quantities. Similarly, in thermodynamics, internal energy and entropy may be introduced as fundamental quantities, instead of pressure, volume, and temperature.

Phase Transformations

Every substance obeys an equation of state, some fundamental relationship between pressure, temperature, and volume. That of ideal gases is a simple example. Real substances can exist in the gas phase only at sufficiently high temperatures. At low temperature and high pressures, transitions occur to the liquid and solid phases. Figure 66 depicts the phase diagram for a substance like carbon dioxide that contracts on freezing. Inspection of the figure shows that there exist regions in which the substance can exist only in a single phase, regions labeled solid, liquid, vapor, and gas. A vapor is just the gas phase in equilibrium with its liquid phase. In other regions, labelled solid-vapor, solid-liquid, and liquid-vapor, both phases exist simultaneously. Along a line called the triple line, all three phases coexist.

The Clausius-Clapeyron equation relates pressure, temperature, volume, and heat of transformation along the solid-liquid, solid-vapor, and liquid-vapor equilibration lines, according to,

$$\frac{dP}{dT} = \frac{l}{T\Delta v},$$

with l the appropriate heat of transformation, and Δv the difference in the specific phase volumes at temperature, T. The equation describes the reversible processes of condensation-vaporization, freezing-melting, and accretion-sublimation, that is, processes proceeding in either direction with the same latent heats of transformation. At the triple point, the latent heats of transformation are additive, specifically, the heat of sublimation equals the sum of the heats of vaporization and melting. For water, the heat of melting is 80 cal/g at 0 ^oC, while the heat of vaporization is 540 cal/g at 100 ^oC and standard pressure (1 atm).

Vapor Pressure

Liquids tend to evaporate, or vaporize, by releasing molecules into the space above their free surfaces. If this is a confined space, the partial pressure exerted by released molecules increases until the rate at which molecules return to the liquid equals the rate at which they leave the liquid surface. At this equilibrium point, the vapor pressure is known as the saturation pressure.

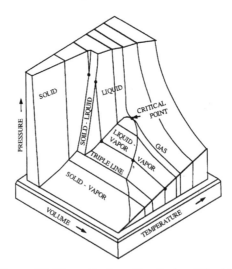

Figure 66. Phase Surfaces For Carbon Dioxide

The equation of state (EOS) is a relationship between pressure, temperature, and volume for any substance. All possible states lie on a surface, as portrayed below for carbon dioxide. In certain regimes, only the gas, solid, or liquid phases are possible. In other regions two phases, solid-liquid, solid-vapor, or liquid-vapor, are possible. A vapor is a gas in equilibrium with its liquid phase. Along the triple point, all three phases coexist.

Molecular evaporation increases with increasing temperature, hence the saturation pressure increases with temperature. At any one temperature, the pressure on the liquid surface may be higher than this value, but it cannot be lower. Any slight reduction below saturation pressure induces the very rapid rate of evaporation called boiling.

Saturation vapor pressures of known liquids vary widely. Table 73 lists saturation vapor pressures for a number of liquids. At 70 ^oF, vapor pressures of mercury and gasoline are seen to differ by a factor of 10^5 approximately.

Table 73. Saturated Vapor Pressures.

liquid	temperature (^oF)	vapor pressure (lbs/in^2)
mercury	70	0.000025
mercury	320	0.081
water	200	7.510
water	70	0.363
water	32	0.089
kerosene	70	0.492
alcohol	70	1.965
gasoline	70	4.439
ammonia	200	794.778
ammonia	50	89.190
ammonia	-100	1.238

Electrodynamics

Electrodynamics is the study of charged particles and their associated electrical and magnetic field interactions. The word was coined by Ampere in 1850 to describe all electromagnetic phenomena. The comprehensive description of all electromagnetic phenomena, embodied in Maxwell's equations, is another crowning achievement in science.

The coupling of thermodynamics and electrodynamics is the basis of plasma physics, the study of high temperature matter composed of charged particles. Stellar and interstellar matter is mostly in the plasma state, as is matter in the upper atmosphere (magnetosphere, ionosphere), flames, chemical and nuclear explosions, and electrical discharges. Matter in a controlled thermonuclear reactor would also be in a plasma state, and the study of fusion as a source of energy and power has led to extensive knowledge and advances in plasma physics. In terms of gross properties, plasmas differ from nonionized gases because of their high electrical and thermal conductivity, unusual dielectric and refractive properties, their emission of electromagnetic radiation, collective, long range particle interactions due to the Coulomb force, and very high temperatures.

Electrodynamics is specifically a study of charges in motion, the associated electric and magnetic fields produced, and their interaction with, and in, matter.

The fundamental entity is electrical charge, and only electrical charge, since corresponding magnetic poles have not been found to date. Electrodynamics describes moving charges and time varying fields, while electrostatics and magnetostatics are concerned with stationary charges and constant fields in time, obviously a subcase. Electrical charge is a property of matter, first observed in ancient Greece in materials we now call dielectrics. Centuries ago, it was noted that amber, upon being rubbed, attracts bits of straw and lighter objects. The Greek word for amber is electron. That electrified bodies attract and repel was noted by Cabeo in the early 1700s, while du Fay and Franklin denoted these two types of electricities, positive and negative, a convention still holding today, and established the notion that charge can be neither created nor destroyed (conservation of charge in physical processes).

Two charges, q and Q, attract (or repel) each other with force, $\mathbf{F}$, given by the Coulomb law,

$$\mathbf{F} = -\kappa_0 \frac{qQ}{r^3} \mathbf{r}$$

for r the distance, κ_0 the Coulomb constant $(8.91 \times 10^9 \ m/f)$, and $\mathbf{r}$ the separation vector. A charge, q, moving with velocity, $\mathbf{v}$, through electric and magnetic fields, $\mathbf{E}$ and $\mathbf{B}$, experiences a Lorentz force, $\mathbf{F}$, from both fields,

$$\mathbf{F} = q(\mathbf{E} + \mathbf{v} \times \mathbf{B}).$$

Maxwell's equations are four partial differential equations relating electric field, $\mathbf{E}$, magnetic field, $\mathbf{B}$, current density, $\mathbf{J}$, and charge density, ρ. Defining the displacement, $\mathbf{D}$, and magnetic intensity, $\mathbf{H}$,

$$\mathbf{H} = \frac{\mathbf{B}}{\mu},$$

$$\mathbf{D} = \varepsilon \mathbf{E},$$

with ε and μ the material permittivity and permeability, we can write Maxwell's equations,

$$\nabla \cdot \mathbf{D} = \rho,$$

$$\nabla \times \mathbf{E} = -\frac{\partial \mathbf{B}}{\partial t},$$

$$\nabla \cdot \mathbf{B} = 0,$$

$$\nabla \times \mathbf{H} = \mathbf{J} + \frac{\partial \mathbf{D}}{\partial t}.$$

The relationship between $\mathbf{H}$ and $\mathbf{B}$ is analogous to the relationship between $\mathbf{D}$ and $\mathbf{H}$ that is, $\mathbf{H}$ and $\mathbf{D}$ depend only on the source of the fields, while $\mathbf{B}$ and $\mathbf{E}$ also depend on the local material properties. Thus, $\mathbf{B}$ and $\mathbf{E}$ are fundamental, but $\mathbf{H}$ and $\mathbf{D}$ can be easier to employ in applications.

In a conductor, with conductivity, σ, permeability, μ, and permittivity, ε, current density, $\mathbf{J}$, is linearly coupled to the electric field, $\mathbf{E}$, by Ohm's law,

$$\mathbf{J} = \sigma \mathbf{E},$$

serving as a corollary to Maxwell's equations. The current driving potential, V, in the conductor also satisfies the electromotive generalization of Ohm's law,

$$V = iR,$$

with R the electrical resistance, and i the current. Similarly, an electrostatic potential, V, is generated when a conductor cuts through magnetic field lines, that is, the magnitude of the electromotive force is given by,

$$V = \frac{\partial \phi}{\partial t},$$

with,

$$\phi = \int \mathbf{B} \cdot d\mathbf{A},$$

and $d\mathbf{A}$ the area swept out by the conductor in cutting magnetic field lines.

Conservation of charge demands that the charge density, ρ, and current density, $\mathbf{J}$, are related by a continuity equation,

$$\frac{\partial \rho}{\partial t} + \nabla \cdot \mathbf{J} = 0,$$

which is just a simple statement that any increase, or decrease, in charge in a small volume must correspond to a flow of charge into, or out of, the same volume element. Electrostatics is defined by the condition,

$$\frac{\partial \rho}{\partial t} = 0,$$

while magnetostatics similarly requires,

$$\nabla \cdot \mathbf{J} = 0,$$

Magnetic materials have traditionally been considered as elements, alloys, or compounds permitting ordered arrangements, or correlations, among electron magnetic moments or spins. Net magnetic polarization can be ferromagnetic, in which all spins are aligned parallel, antiferromagnetic, in which neighboring spins are aligned antiparallel, or ferrimagnetic, in which spins of two dissimilar atoms are aligned antiparallel. Metals such as iron, cobalt, and nickel are ferromagnetic, while manganese and chromium are antiferromagnetic. The temperature necessary to induce a phase transition from an unordered magnetic state to a magnetically ordered state is the Curie temperature, whether ferrromagnetic or antiferromagnetic in the final state. The permanent properties of such materials are useful in magnetic devices, such as computers and transformers.

An essential difference between electric and magnetic interactions appears in the direction of the force. The electrical force acts in the direction of motion, while the magnetic force acts normal to the direction of motion. Hence the magnetic force can only change direction of the moving charge, but cannot do work on it. Interestingly, both the Coulomb and Ampere laws exhibit an inverse square dependence on the separation of source and field point.

Plasmas

Plasma physics is the physics of ionized gases, and is a relatively new science. Not until development of the electrical power industry were controlled experiments on ionized gases possible, so plasma physics is some $100\ yr$ old. Studies at the turn of the century of gas discharges and radio propagation off the ionosphere, along with impetus for controlled thermonuclear reaction programs in the 1950s, fueled study of the complex mechanisms attending plasma interactions. The discovery of the solar wind and Van Allen radiation belts in the 1960s provided much data for integration of plasma theory and experiment. Plasmas are complex, exhibiting fluid turbulence and collective motion, linear and nonlinear behavior, and wave and particle motions.

Plasmas exhibit a state of matter in which a significant number, if not all, of the electrons are free, not bound to an atom or molecule. Practically speaking, matter is in the plasma state if there are enough free electrons to provide a significant electrical conductivity, σ. Usually, only a small fraction of electrons need be free to meet this criterion. Collisional ionization, caused by energetic thermal motions of atoms at high temperature, is the source of large numbers of free electrons in matter. Large densities of free electrons are also found in metals at solid densities, independent of the temperature, accounting for the electrical conductivity of metals at room temperatures and lower. Most terrestrial plasmas, excepting metals which are not plasmas, are very hot and not very dense. The plasma state is the highest temperature state of matter, occurring certainly at much higher temperatures than the gaseous state. Plasmas are hot, ionized gases. Plasmas in discharge tubes, for instance, have subatmospheric densities on the whole. On the cosmological scale, most of the matter in the Universe is thought to reside in stellar interiors, where the density is so high that it is called a stellar plasma independent of its temperature. Of course, the temperature is also so high that only the plasma phase could exist.

In the laboratory, much research interest centers on economical means to exploit plasmas for energy production. Borrowing from what we already know of energy production in solar and stellar plasmas, one focus is fusion energy production in thermonuclear fuels, such as deuterium and tritium.

Fusion Energy

Fusion processes in the solar plasma are responsible for energy radiated to the Earth. For the past four decades, scientists have pursued the dream of controlled thermonuclear fusion. The attraction of this pursuit is the enormous energy potentially available in fusion fuels, and the widely held view of fusion as a safe and clean energy source. The fusion reaction with the highest cross section as a reaction process,

$$D+T \rightarrow n+He,$$

releases some $17.6\,MeV$ of energy, denoting deuterium, D, tritium, T, neutron, n, and helium, He. To produce fusion reactions in a deuterium-tritium plasma, very high collisional temperatures are necessary to overcome the Coulomb repulsion between interacting nuclei, and the plasma must be confined for long time scales so that many fusion collision reactions can take place to make the process economically feasible. Temperatures near $3\,keV$ ($3.47 \times 10^7\,{}^oK$) are necessary for plasma ignition and sustained thermonuclear burn.

Development of an economically viable fusion reactor would literally give us the energy equivalent of oceans of oil. Because seawater contains about 40 g of deuterium and 0.1 g of lithium per ton, every barrel of seawater contains the energy equivalent of almost 30 barrels of oil in deuterium fuel, and about 1/5 barrel of oil in tritium fuel (with tritium produced, or *bred*, from neutron capture on lithium). A volume of seawater equal to the top meter of the oceans would yield enough fuel to power electrical generators for thousands of years at the present consumption rate.

Two methods for producing controlled fusion are popular today, certainly areas of investigation, called magnetic confinement fusion (MCF) and inertial confinement fusion (ICF). Magnetic fusion uses very intense magnetic fields to squeeze a DT plasma to high enough temperatures and densities to ignite and sustain fusion burn. Inertial fusion attempts the same by imploding small pellets, containing DT, with high energy light, ion, or electron beams focused across the pellet. Both are tough problems technologically. With DT fuel, both processes require fuel temperatures in excess of $10^8\,{}^oK$, and fuel particle densities, n, and confinement times, τ, such that, $n\tau \geq 10^{15}\,sec/cm^3$. Magnetic fusion operates in a regime, $\tau \approx 1\,sec$, and therefore, $n \approx 10^{15}\,cm^{-3}$. For magnetic confinement fusion, the density is limited by the maximum magnetic field strength that can be generated, often determined by the material strength of the confining vessel. Inertial fusion relies on the mass of the imploding target to provide confinement. For inertial fusion, $\tau \approx 10^{-10}\,sec$, so that, $n \approx 10^{25}\,cm^{-3}$. Again, these are tough technological constraints in the Earth laboratory, but minor operational limitations in the interior furnace of the Sun, which keeps bathing the Earth with direct solar energy from fusion processes, some $2\,cal/min\,cm^2$.

Stellar Evolution

The Sun is a star with nuclear furnace, like countless others in the Universe. The evolution of nominal stars is detailed by four continuity equations in space and time, much like the equations of hydrodynamics. Star birth occurs following a gravitational instability in interstellar dust clouds, actually a dynamical contraction phase due to gravity against a counteracting pressure gradient. At sufficiently high densities and temperatures in the keV range, thermonuclear reactions occur, with the release of large amounts of energy. In such simplified approach, the star is assumed to be a gaseous sphere, subjected to its own gravity while maintaining spherical symmetry throughout its evolution, from a contracting protostar in interstellar dust, to a very hot, and dense, radiating plasma, to a fuel depleted, dying core. External forces, magnetic fields, and stellar rotation are not included. The hydrostatic equation, balancing gravity against pressure, takes the form,

$$\frac{\partial P}{\partial m} = -\frac{G_0 m}{4\pi r^4}$$

with P pressure, m the mass inside a stellar sphere at radius, r, and G_0 the gravitational constant. The radial distribution of mass is written,

$$\frac{\partial r}{\partial m} = \frac{1}{4\pi\rho r^2}$$

with ρ the mass density. Conservation of energy requires that the variation in heat content per unit mass be the difference between fusion energy production, ε, and the radiative energy loss, δ,

$$\frac{\partial L}{\partial m} = \varepsilon - \delta$$

with L the stellar luminosity (Hertzsprung-Russell) at distance, r. The temperature gradient, using the radiative Stefan-Boltzmann law, takes the form,

$$\frac{\partial T}{\partial m} = 3\omega L \sigma 16\pi^2 r^4 T^3$$

with T the temperature, ω the photon opacity, and σ the Stefan-Boltzmann constant. These four equations close upon themselves in the same manner as the hydrodynamic equations of particle, momentum, and energy conservation, and the equation of state. The Hertzprung-Russell luminosity is a photometric measurement of stellar radiative output. The Hertsprung-Russell diagram, as it is called, depicts luminosities as a function of temperature. Variations in Hertzsprung-Russell diagrams for different clusters of stars have aided theories of stellar evolution.

Most stars follow four steps of evolution, namely, gravitational contraction until thermonuclear ignition, expansion due to fusion burn of light elements (hydrogen), lesser expansion due to fusion burn of heavier elements (helium), and final contraction (death) into a white dwarf, neutron star, or black hole (depending on stellar mass) as thermonuclear fuel is depleted, or sometimes enormous explosion (nova). Lightweight stars, with masses less than 4 times the solar mass, usually die as white dwarfs (including the Sun). Middleweight stars, up to about 8 solar masses, because they are thought to burn carbon later in their evolution, may die as white dwarfs, or possibly explode as nova and supernova. Heavyweight stars, beyond 8 solar masses, may also explode, but can degenerate (burn) into cold neutron stars or black holes. Neutron stars are very dense objects, essentially compressed neutrons, supported against gravitational collapse by neutron degeneracy (quantum exclusion limit) pressure, while black holes are collapsed gravitational fields, so strong that light emerging from within is completely trapped by gravity, acccording to general relativity. Matter densities in such stellar objects are enormous, on the order of ton/cm^3.

Elementary Particle Interactions

Stellar interactions of enormous proportions are driven mainly by gravity. While such interactions on the cosmological scale are beyond imagination, there exist interactions that are up to 10^{36} stronger than the gravitational forces compressing massive stellar objects, the so called strong, weak, and electromagnetic forces. Elementary particle physics deals with all four at a fundamental level, but a modern focus has been the latter three, namely, strong, weak, and electromagnetic interactions.

The past 40 years have witnessed an explosion of experimental particle data, gathered from high energy accelerators and outer space. Information has been integrated in a consistent picture of elementary particle interactions. Particles are classified in distinct categories. Particles of spin 1/2, with weak and electromagnetic interactions, are called leptons. Leptons include electrons, muons, neutrinos, and their antiparticles. Masses typically range from .511 *MeV* (electron) possibly up to 1,800 *MeV* (τ lepton). Neutrinos are massless. Particles with strong interactions, including weak and electromagnetic, are called hadrons. Integer spin hadrons are mesons, while half integer spin hadrons are baryons. Masses of hadrons range from 135 *MeV* (pion) up to as high as 10,200 *Mev* (short lived resonances). Baryon numbers are conserved in all interactions. Meson numbers are not. Hadrons include protons, neutrons, pions, kaons, short lived resonances, and their antiparticles.

The long range forces of gravity and electromagnetism account for large scale macroscopic phenomena, like planetary attraction and charged particle scattering. The short range strong and weak forces account for microscopic phenomena, such as nucleon binding, radioactive nuclear transmutation, and hadron decay into leptons and photons. Strengths of the fundamental forces inversely as their ranges, in order, strong, weak, electromagnetic, and gravitational, and roughly in the ratio, $10^{36} : 10^{22} : 10^{10} : 1$.

One very interesting aspect of elementary particle interactions is matter-antimatter annihilation, and particularly proton-antiproton annihilation. Antiprotons are negatively charged protons, with the same mass and spin. Proton-antiproton annihilation in matter is one of the most energetic reactions observed routinely in high energy physics, some 1.88 *GeV* per annihilation. Antiprotons, as negatively charged protons, continuously slow down in matter until they are stopped and captured on the surface of a nucleus by a proton, in which case, both proton and antiproton annihilate into gammas, pions, and other shortlived particles. When an antiproton annihilates at rest on the surface of an actinide nucleus (such as uranium and plutonium) many fragments and neutrons are also produced, following direct reaction, nuclear evaporation, and fission processes, along with production of high energy gammas and pions. Collectively, these processes have been termed antiproton fission, for simplicity, because many neutrons are produced as the end result of all reactions. Recent experiments suggest that as many as 15 to 20 neutrons are emitted following antiproton annihilation on U^{238}, that their distribution is peaked near 5 *Mev* in energy, and that a sizeable fraction (45%–75%) of the annihilation energy (1.88 *GeV* per annihilation) is deposited locally in the U^{238}. Using hybrid fission-fusion capsules in a pulsed power propulsion engine, it has been estimated theoretically that 8 *mg* of antiprotons could drive a 10 ton rocket payload to Mars, and back, in 3 months. While technology for producing 8 *mg* of antiprotons is nonexistent today, the energy densities of antiproton fuels are more than fascinating, and the possibilities more than imagination.

Potential schemes for employing antiproton-proton annihilation as a driver for space propulsion, power generation, condensed matter physics experiments, biomedical treatment, and others, enter the realm of possibility with the advent of portable storage traps (Penning) and related proof-of-principle storage experiments at the European Center For Nuclear Research (CERN) Low Energy Antiproton Ring (LEAR). As many as 10^6 antiprotons have been trapped in Penning traps, and an upper theoretical limit is near 10^{12} antiprotons. Such technology is growing and will port to other interesting systems and experiments, and many new applications are developing.

Keyed Exercises

• *What does a wrist thermometer of mass, m = 10 g, weigh, w?*

$$w = mg$$

$$w = 10 \times 980 \, dynes = 9.8 \times 10^3 \, dynes$$

• *What does a 1.5 lb abalone iron weigh, w?*

$$w = 1.5 \, lb$$

• *What is the density of fresh water, ρ, of weight, w = 31.2 lbs, occupying .5 ft³?*

$$\rho = \frac{w}{V} = \frac{31.2}{.5} \, lb/ft^3 = 62.4 \, lb/ft^3$$

• *What is the density of salt water, ρ, of mass, m = 2050 kg, occupying 2.0 m³?*

$$\rho = \frac{m}{V} = \frac{2050.}{2.0} \, kg/m^3 = 1025 \, kg/m^3$$

• *A spear gun propels a lock tip shaft at speed, v = 34 ft/sec. How long before the shaft impales a target grouper 9 ft away?*

$$v = \frac{ds}{dt}, \quad dt = \frac{ds}{v} = \frac{9}{34} \, sec = .26 \, sec$$

• *What is the average speed of a Zodiac covering distance, ds = 23 miles, in time dt = 30 min?*

$$v = \frac{ds}{dt} = \frac{23}{.5} \, mi/hr = 46 \, mi/hr$$

Docking, the Zodiac stops in time, dt = 5.6 sec. What is the magnitude of the deceleration, a?

$$a = \frac{dv}{dt} = \frac{-46}{5.6} \times \frac{5280}{3600} \, ft/sec^2 = -12 \, ft/sec$$

- *What is the change in speed, dv, of a hydroplane accelerating for time, dt = 6 sec, with acceleration, a = 24 ft/sec²?*

$$dv = adt = 24 \times 6 \; ft/sec = 144 \; ft/sec$$

- *A diver surfacing from 150 fsw covers the first 90 fsw in 90 sec, and the remaining 60 fsw in 30 sec. What is the average ascent rate, r?*

$$r = \frac{ds}{dt} = \frac{150}{90+30} \; fsw/sec = 1.25 \; fsw/sec$$

- *A submersible of mass, m, moves underwater with speed, v. If the speed is doubled, with is the increase in kinetic energy, ΔK, of the submersible?*

$$\Delta K = \frac{1}{2}m(2v)^2 - \frac{1}{2}mv^2 = \frac{3}{2}mv^2$$

If the speed is tripled, what is the change in momentum, Δp?

$$\Delta p = 3mv - mv = 2mv$$

- *What are the momentum, p, and kinetic energy, K, of a light diver propulsion vehicle (DPV), m = 32 kg, moving with velocity, v = 6 m/sec?*

$$p = mv = 32 \times 6 \; kg \, m/sec = 192 \; kg \, m/sec$$

$$K = \frac{1}{2}mv^2 = \frac{1}{2} \times 32 \times 36 \; kg \, m^2/sec^2 = 1.15 \; \times 10^3 \; j$$

What is the force, F, required to stop it in 8 sec?

$$dp = 192 \; kg \, m/sec, \;\; dt = 8 \; sec$$

$$F = \frac{dp}{dt} = \frac{192}{8} \; kg \, m/sec^2 = 24 \; newton$$

- *What is the increase in potential energy, U, for a diver of weight, mg = 150 lbs, who ascends from 60 fsw to the surface?*

$$U = mgh = 150 \times 60 \; ft \, lb = 9 \times 10^3 \; ft \, lb$$

- *A diver inflates his BC at depth, d = 10 msw, to approximately .015 m³. How much work, dW, does the diver do?*

$$dW = PdV$$

$$dW = 20.2 \times 10^4 \times .015 \; kg \, m^2/sec^2 = 3.03 \; \times 10^3 \; j$$

- *An 80 kg diver giant strides from the deck of a boat into the water 2.7 m below, taking .74 sec to hit the surface. What is the power, W, generated by the fall?*

$$W = \frac{dH}{dt}, \;\; dH = mgh, \;\; dt = .74 \; sec$$

$$dH = 80 \times 9.8 \times 2.7 \; kg \; m^2/sec^2 = 2.13 \times 10^3 \; j$$

$$W = \frac{2.13 \times 10^3}{.74} \; j/sec = 2.86 \times 10^3 \; watt$$

What is the kinetic energy, K, on impact, neglecting air resistance?

$$v = gt = 9.8 \times .74 \; m/sec = 7.3 \; m/sec$$

$$K = \frac{1}{2}mv^2 = \frac{1}{2} \times 80 \times 53.3 \; j = 2.13 \times 10^3 \; j$$

- *A UDT paradiver jumps (no chute) from a USN Seawolf helicopter with initial potential energy, $U_i = 12 \times 10^3 \; j$, and zero kinetic energy, $K_i = 0 \; j$ (all relative to the surface of the Earth). What is the kinetic energy, K_f, when the paradiver hits the water (neglecting air resistance) in the Gulf of Tonkin?*

$$E_i = K_i + U_i = E_f = K_f + U_f$$

$$U_i = 12 \times 10^3 \; j, \; U_f = 0 \; j, \; K_i = 0 \; j$$

$$K_f = K_i + U_i - U_f = 0 + 12 \times 10^3 - 0 \; j = 12 \times 10^3 \; j$$

At some point in the drop, the paradiver gains kinetic energy, $K = 9 \times 10^3 \; j$. What is the corresponding potential energy, U?

$$E = K + U = E_i = E_f = 12 \times 10^3 \; j$$

$$U = E - K = 12 \times 10^3 - 9 \times 10^3 \; j = 3 \times 10^3 \; j$$

- *What is the energy, ε, of a photon moving at the speed of light, c, and frequency, $f = 8.2 \times 10^{14} \; sec^{-1}$?*

$$h = 6.625 \times 10^{-34} \; j \; sec, \; f = 8.2 \times 10^{14} \; sec^{-1}$$

$$\varepsilon = hf = 6.625 \times 8.2 \times 10^{-20} \; j = 5.4 \times 10^{-19} \; j = 3.39 \times 10^{-3} \; keV$$

What is the corresponding photon wavelength, λ?

$$c = 2.99 \times 10^{10} \; cm/sec$$

$$\lambda = \frac{c}{f} = \frac{2.99 \times 10^{10}}{8.2 \times 10^{14}} \; cm = 3.6 \times 10^{-5} \; cm$$

- *What is the energy, E, of a lead weight, $m_0 = 1 \; kg$, moving at velocity, $v/c = .85$, aboard the Starship Enterprize initiating warp acceleration in the Sea Of Khan?*

$$c = 2.99 \times 10^8 \; m/sec, \; m_0 = 1 \; kg$$

$$E = \frac{m_0 c^2}{(1 - v^2/c^2)^{1/2}} = \frac{1 \times (2.99 \times 10^8)^2}{(1 - .85^2)^{1/2}} kg \; m^2/sec^2 = 1.72 \times 10^{17} \; j$$

What is the corresponding kinetic energy, K?

$$\gamma = (1 - v^2/c^2)^{-1/2} = .52^{-1/2} = 1.39$$

$$K = (\gamma - 1)m_0 c^2 = .39 \times 1 \times (2.99 \times 10^8)^2 \; kg \; m^2/sec^2 = 3.49 \times 10^{16} \; j$$

- What is the critical angle, ϕ_c, at the air-water interface, that is, in taking, $n_{air} = 1.0$, and, $n_{water} = 1.33$?

$$\sin \phi_c = \frac{n_{air}}{n_{water}} = \frac{1}{1.33} = .75$$

$$\phi_c = \sin^{-1}(.75) = 48.5^o$$

- What is the magnification, μ, and foreshortening, σ, across the quartz-air interface for an object in quartz, viewed in air?

$$\mu = \frac{n_{quartz}}{n_{air}}, \quad \sigma = \frac{n_{air}}{n_{quartz}}$$

$$\mu = \frac{1.456}{1.000} = 1.456, \quad \sigma = \frac{1.000}{1.456} = .687$$

- What is the magnification, μ, and foreshortening, σ, for an object in air, viewed in quartz?

$$\mu = \frac{n_{air}}{n_{quartz}}, \quad \sigma = \frac{n_{quartz}}{n_{air}}$$

$$\mu = .687, \quad \sigma = 1.456$$

- A coral head appears, $h_{wat} = 8$ ft, tall, and, $s_{wat} = 6$ ft, away in Truk Lagoon. What are the actual height, h, and distance, s?

$$\mu = 1.33, \quad \sigma = .75$$

$$h = \frac{h_{wat}}{\mu} = \frac{8}{\mu} \ ft = 6 \ ft$$

$$s = \frac{s_{wat}}{\sigma} = \frac{6}{.75} \ ft = 8 \ ft$$

- How long, dt, does it take a sound wave to propagate a distance, $d = 10,604$ m, in steel?

$$u = 5032 \ m/sec, \quad dt = \frac{ds}{u} = \frac{10604}{5302} \ sec = 2 \ sec$$

- A surface tender screams at a diver underwater with acoustical energy, $\varepsilon = 4.1$ btu. What is the energy, ε_R, reflected from the surface, and energy, ε_T, transmitted at the surface (absorbed in less than a cm)?

$$\varepsilon_R = R\varepsilon, \quad \varepsilon_T = T\varepsilon$$

$$\varepsilon_R = .9919 \times 4.1 \ btu = 4.066 \ btu, \quad \varepsilon_T = .0081 \times 4.1 \ btu = .034 \ btu$$

- What is the heat flux, ϕ, across a neoprene wetsuit of thickness, $dx = .64$ cm, for body temperature of $22.7 \ ^oC$ and water temperature of $4.1 \ ^oC$?

$$\phi = -K \frac{dT}{dx}$$

$$K = .0004 \ cal/cm \ ^oC \ sec, \quad dx = .64 \ cm, \quad dT = 22.7 - 4.1 \ ^oC = 18.6 \ ^oC$$

$$\phi = .0004 \times \frac{18.6}{.64} \ cal/cm^2 \ sec = 1.16 \times 10^{-2} \ cal/cm^2 \ sec$$

- *What heat flux, ϕ, does a light stick at 298 ^oK emit underwater, and what is the Centigrade temperature, (^oC), of the chemical candle?*

$$\phi = \sigma_0 T^4$$

$$T = 298\,^oK, \quad \sigma_0 = 5.67 \times 10^{-8}\ watts/m^2\ K^{o4}$$

$$\phi = 5.67 \times 10^{-8} \times 298^4 watts/m^2 = 447.1\ watts/m^2$$

$$^oC =^o K - 273 = 298 - 273 = 25^o$$

- *If an amount of heat, $dQ = 650$ cal, raises the temperature of a saline solution, $m = 50$ g, some, $dT = 14\,^oC$, at constant pressure, what is the specific heat, c_P?*

$$c_P = \frac{1}{m} \left[\frac{dQ}{dT} \right]_P = \frac{650}{50 \times 14}\ cal/g\,^oC = .928\ cal/g\,^oC$$

- *How many calories, Q, does it take to just melt 100 g ice?*

$$Q = lm, \quad l = 80\ cal/g, \quad m = 100\ g$$

$$Q = 80 \times 100\ cal = 8000\ cal$$

- *What additional amount of heat, dQ, does it take to raise the 100 g of water to its boiling point, $T = 100\,^oC$?*

$$dT = 100 - 0 = 100\,^oC, \quad c_P = 1.00\ cal/g^oC$$

$$dQ = mc_P dT = 1.00 \times 100 \times 100\ cal = 10^4\ cal$$

- *A welding thermometer is constructed using changes in resistance to calibrate temperature changes. If the thermometer is logarithmic in response, what is the temperature, T, at resistance, $X = 60$ ohms, for fixed points, $T_f = 500\,^oC$, $X_f = 80$ ohms, and $T_i = 100\,^oC$, $X_i = 20$ ohms?*

$$T - T_i = (T_f - T_i) \left[\frac{\ln X/X_i}{\ln X_f/X_i} \right]$$

$$T = 400 \times \left[\frac{\ln 60/20}{\ln 80/20} \right]\ ^oC = 417\,^oC$$

- *If an $i = .8$ amp current is passed over the $R = 60$ ohm resistor in the above welding thermometer, what is the corresponding potential drop, V?*

$$V = iR = .8 \times 60\ volts = 48\ volts$$

- *Sunlight striking the shallow azure water off the coast of Cozumel delivers, $\Gamma = 2\ cal/m^2$, to the surface. If, $\rho = .02$, is reflected, and, $\tau = .04$, is transmitted, what fraction, α, is absorbed?*

$$\rho = .02, \quad \tau = .04$$

$$\rho + \tau + \alpha = 1, \quad \alpha = 1 - \tau - \rho$$

$$\alpha = 1 - .04 - .02 = .94$$

What is the magnitude, Γ_r, of the reflected radiation?

$$\Gamma_r = \rho\Gamma, \quad \Gamma_r = .02 \times 2 \; cal/m^2 = .04 \; cal/m^2$$

• *What is the horizontal force, F, necessary to drag a 16.5 kg scuba tank across a flat iron plate at a fill station?*

$$\mu = .4, \quad N = mg$$

$$F = \mu N = .4 \times 16.5 \times 9.8 \; kg \; m/sec^2 = 64.7 \; newton$$

How much work, dH, is done in moving the tank a distance, ds = 12 m?

$$dH = Fds = 64.7 \times 12 \; j = 776.4 \; j$$

• *What is the change in internal energy, dU, of air in a compressor heated an amount, dQ = 100 cal, while doing piston expansion work, dW = 165 j?*

$$dQ = 100 \times 4.19 \; j = 419 \; j, \quad dW = 165 \; j$$

$$dU = dQ - dW = 419 - 165 \; j = 254 \; j$$

• *A steel anchor weighing, w, a massive 300 lbs in 200 fsw needs a lift bag of what volume, V, to just maintain it at the surface?*

$$w = 300 \; lbs, \quad \rho = 64.1 \; lbs/ft^3, \quad V = \frac{w}{\rho}$$

$$V = \frac{300}{64.1} \; ft^3 = 4.68^f t^3$$

If the bag is not vented on the way up, what will be the surfacing volume, Q?

$$P_{200} = 200 + 33 \; fsw = 233 \; fsw, \quad P_0 = 33 \; fsw, \quad V = 4.68 \; ft^3$$

$$P_{200}V = P_0 Q, \quad Q = \frac{P_{200}V}{P_0}$$

$$Q = \frac{233 \times 4.68}{33} \; ft^3 = 33.1 \; ft^3$$

If 10^{11} proton-antiproton pairs, n, annihilate in the BC of a diver making a stop at 60 fsw at temperature, T, of 20 °C and BC volume, V, of 3 ft^3, what would be the new temperature, T_f, at the same depth assuming all energy is deposited in the BC and nominal specific heat of air, c_P, is employed, that is, 0.24 $cal/g°C$, and air mass, m, of 1 g? Recall that proton-antiproton annihilation into two gamma rays is the most energetic reaction known in nature, with release of 1.88 GeV energy, R, for each reaction,

$$p + \bar{p} \rightarrow \gamma + \gamma \quad (1.88 \; GeV)$$

and that $1\ GeV = 3.82 \times 10^{-11}$ *cal. In the BC,*

$$c_P = 0.24\ cal/g\ ^oC,\ \ m = 1\ g,\ \ V = 3\ ft^3,\ \ T = 20\ ^oC$$

The energy released into the BC, dQ, is,

$$dQ = nR = 1.88 \times 10^{11}\ GeV = 3.82 \times 1.88\ cal = 7.18\ cal$$

with temperature change, dT,

$$c_P = \frac{1}{m}\frac{dQ}{dT},\ \ dT = \frac{1}{mc_P}dQ = \frac{7.18}{1 \times 0.24}\ ^oC = 29.9\ ^oC$$

The final BC temperature, T_f, is then,

$$dT = T_f - T,\ \ T_f = dT + T = 29.9 + 20\ ^oC = 49.9\ ^oC$$

What is the new BC volume, V_f?

$$T = 273 + 20\ ^oK = 293^oK,\ \ T_f = 273 + 49.9\ ^oK = 322.9\ ^oK$$

$$\frac{V}{T} = \frac{V_f}{T_f},\ \ V_f = V\frac{T_f}{T} = 3 \times \frac{322.9}{293}\ ft^3 = 3.30\ ft^3$$

- *All else the same, if the diver ascends to 30 fsw in the above problem, what is the new BC volume, V_f?*

$$P = 60 + 33\ fsw = 93\ fsw,\ \ P_f = 30 + 33\ fsw = 63\ fsw$$

$$\frac{PV}{T} = \frac{P_f V_f}{T_f},\ \ V_f = \frac{PVT_f}{P_f T} = \frac{93 \times 3 \times 322.9}{63 \times 293}\ ft^3 = 4.88\ ft^3$$

Appendix B

DIVEWARE AND PLANNING

Algorithms

Diveware is mainly focused on a few staging algorithms, namely the Buhlmann ZHL, Workman USN, full and modified RGBM, and VPM. While the ZHL, USN, and RGBM algorithms are validated by data, testing, and correlation analysis, the VPM is not, but boasts extensive usage in the technical diving community. The ZHL and USN algorithms are dissolved gas algorithms, while the RGBM and VPM are bubble algorithms. The former will yield shallow stop staging while the latter will result in deep stop staging. DCS spikes among users of all are not seen, suggesting rather safe staging protocols. User knobs allow conservative to liberal parameter settings depending on the vendor. In the dissolved gas algorithms, manipulation of critical tensions and gradients is the user knob. In the bubble algorithms, bubble size, permissible surfacing phase volume, and bubble gas diffusion lengths can be user manipulated.

For dissolved gas algorithms, the staging criteria is the usual $M - value$ approach, that is, for p the total tissue tension for all mixture gases (nitrogen and helium mainly) and M the critical tension for the particular tissue compartment, τ, we have,

$$p \leq M$$

always on ascent for all compartments. Stops are usually calculated for 10 fsw jumps upward with the longest wait across all compartments determining the stop time. Compartments range from $2 \leq \tau \leq 480$ min typically. Variations in M-values across software packages are small, usually in the so-called Spencer regime with M-values some $8 - -15\%$ below the classical USN (Workman) values and close to the Buhlmann ZHL M-values. Reduction factors, ξ, as published by Wienke in fitting bubble models within M-value frameworks, can be applied to reduce M-values and reproduce deep stops, according to,

$$M = \xi G + P$$

with P ambient pressure and G the critical gradient computed from fixed values of critical tensions and ambient pressures. The reduction factors, ξ, are also called gradient factors, GF, in the technical diving community and are free floated in value (not constrained to bubble model correlations) for dive planning, with, roughly,

$$0.45 \leq GF \leq 0.95$$

as some measure to give deep stops to an otherwise shallow stop algorithm. Unlike the classical M-values and bubble factors ξ, (pseudo) GFs are not correlated with data in any form today. A variant of the above is called ratio deco, whereby,

$$\frac{p}{P} \leq R$$

and is just another representation of the same approaches above with ξs and GFs. For,

$$R = \frac{M}{P}$$

standard Haldane staging obtains. For reduction factors, ξ, in the modified RGBM,

$$R = \frac{\xi G + P}{P}$$

and in the GF scheme, with ζ some other set of free floating constants,

$$R = \frac{\zeta M}{P}$$

and all previous comments remain the same concerning ξ and ζ.

In bubble models like RGBM and VPM, a critical gradient, G, is limited by bubble volume and growth rates according to the separated phase volume, Φ,

$$\int_0^\infty dt \int_{r_0}^\infty \frac{\partial}{\partial t}(p - P)B(r)dr \leq \Phi$$

at all points and time, t, in the dive and at the surface, with B a functional representation of the excited bubble distribution and r_0 some critical excitation radius for growth. The distribution, B, and anywhere between 3–5 model parameters have been correlated in the RGBM to dive profile data and outcomes. Risk functions are also obtained from the data.

Packages

A potpourri of software packages available on the market are described briefly in the following. They are chosen because of their widespread use, utility, historical perspectives, and diver popularity. New ones are coming online too. They might be broadly categorized as dissolved gas, dissolved gas with GFs, pseudo-bubble, and bubble models. Dissolved gas, dissolved gas with GFs, and pseudo-bubble models are collectively also termed neo-Haldane models. In neo-Haldane models, M-values are reduced compared to the original USN, RN or Swiss values. The RGBM and VPM are the only true, full bubble models of interest and commercially available in diveware and computers.

- ABYSS
ABYSS in the mid 90s first introduced the full Wienke RGBM into its diveware packages. The Buhlmann ZHL model was also included in the dissolved gas package. It has seen extensive use over the past 20 yrs or so in the technical diving area. A variety of user knobs on bubble parameters and M-values permit aggressive to conservative staging in both models. Both the ZHL and RGBM have been published and formally correlated with diving data. Later, the modified RGBM with ξs was incorporated into ABYSS. Modified RGBM with ξs was published and correlated with data in the late 90s and also served as the early basis for Suunto, Mares, Dacor, ConneXon, Cressi, UTC, HydroSpace, and other RGBM dive computers. The full RGBM was also incorporated into early HydroSpace computers. Output appears in Figure 67.

- VPlanner
VPlanner first introduced the VPM in the late 90s. Based on the original work of Yount and Hoffman, the software has seen extensive use by the technical diving community. No formal correlations of the VPM and VPlanner with data have been published. User knobs allow adjustment of bubble parameters for aggressive to conservative staging. VPlanner is also used in Liquivision and Advanced Diving Corporation computers for technical diving.

- ProPlanner
ProPlanner is a software package that uses modified M-values for diver staging. Buhlmann ZHL M-values with GFs are employed with user knobs for conservancy. The model is called the VGM by ProPlanner designers. Some GFs claim to mimic the VPM. Nothing has been formally published about the VGM and ProPlanner correlations.

- GAP
GAP is a software package similar to ABYSS offering the full RGBM, modified RGBM with ξs, and Buhlmann ZHL with GFs. Introduced in the mid 90s, it has seen extensive usage in the recreational and technical sectors. Apart from user GFs, the models and parameters in GAP have been published and correlated with diving data and profiles tested over years. Adjustable conservancy settings for all models can be selected. GAP has been keyed to the Atomic Aquatics and Liquivision dive computers. Figure 68 is sample GAP output.

- DecoPlanner
DecoPlanner is a diveware package offered by the GUE training agency. Both the VPM and Buhlmann ZHL with GFs are available in DecoPlanner. Evolving over the past 10 - 15 yrs, DecoPlanner also incorporates GUE *ratio deco*, p/P, approaches to modifying GFs. DecoPlanner correlations with data have not been published. It has seen extensive use in the technical diving community.

- RGBM Simulator

The RGBM Simulator is a software package marketed by HydroSpace Engineering and offers the full RGBM, modified RGBM with ξs, and Buhlmann ZHL algorithms. All of the algorithms have been correlated with data and published. As with all other diveware, conservancy settings allow adjustments of bubble parameters, ξs, and M-values. On the market since the late 90s, RGBM Simulator is also keyed to the HydroSpace dive computer. Sample output from RGBM Simulator is seen in Figure 69.

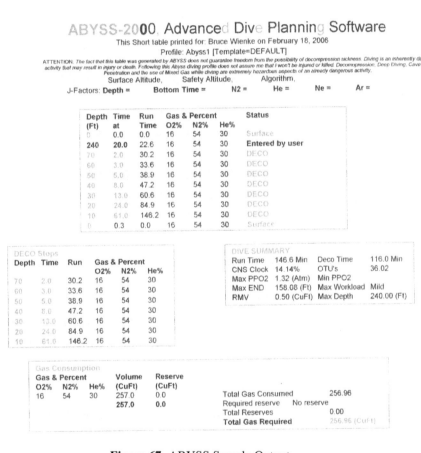

ABYSS-2000. Advanced Dive Planning Software

This Short table printed for: Bruce Wienke on February 18, 2006

Profile: Abyss1 [Template=DEFAULT]

ATTENTION. The fact that this table was generated by ABYSS does not guarantee freedom from the possibility of decompression sickness. Diving is an inherently dangerous activity that may result in injury or death. Following this Abyss diving profile does not assure me that I won't be injured or killed. Decompression, Deep Diving, Cave Penetration and the use of Mixed Gas while diving are extremely hazardous aspects of an already dangerous activity.

J-Factors: Depth =   Surface Altitude,   Safety Altitude,   Algorithm,
           Bottom Time =   N2 =   He =   Ne =   Ar =

Depth (Ft)	Time at	Run Time	O2%	N2%	He%	Status
0	0.0	0.0	16	54	30	Surface
240	20.0	22.6	16	54	30	Entered by user
70	2.0	30.2	16	54	30	DECO
60	3.0	33.6	16	54	30	DECO
50	5.0	38.9	16	54	30	DECO
40	8.0	47.2	16	54	30	DECO
30	13.0	60.6	16	54	30	DECO
20	24.0	84.9	16	54	30	DECO
10	61.0	146.2	16	54	30	DECO
0	0.3	0.0	16	54	30	Surface

DECO Stops

Depth	Time	Run	O2%	N2%	He%
70	2.0	30.2	16	54	30
60	3.0	33.6	16	54	30
50	5.0	38.9	16	54	30
40	8.0	47.2	16	54	30
30	13.0	60.6	16	54	30
20	24.0	84.9	16	54	30
10	61.0	146.2	16	54	30

DIVE SUMMARY

Run Time	146.6 Min	Deco Time	116.0 Min
CNS Clock	14.14%	OTU's	36.02
Max PPO2	1.32 (Atm)	Min PPO2	
Max END	158.08 (Ft)	Max Workload	Mild
RMV	0.50 (CuFt)	Max Depth	240.00 (Ft)

Gas Consumption

O2%	N2%	He%	Volume (CuFt)	Reserve (CuFt)
16	54	30	257.0	0.0
			257.0	0.0

Total Gas Consumed	256.96
Required reserve	No reserve
Total Reserves	0.00
Total Gas Required	256.96 (CuFt)

Figure 67. ABYSS Sample Output

Samples

Sample output from ABYSS, GAP, and RGBM Simulator are detailed in Figures 74-76. Output is typical of modern diveware. Platforms range from PCs to Droid devices as well as mainframes. Languages employed in codes include VIZ, BASIC, FORTRAN, C, and derivatives.

NAUI GAP - Dive Information

Created for: brwswe	Page 1/1	Creation Date 2/17/2006

The information presented here does in no way guarantee that you will not be injured or killed.
The authors accept no liability for your use of the information presented here.

deco schedule

NAUI-GAP (1530)
Model: RGBM   classic RGBM
mode: OC

Depth	Time (RT)	Gas	PO2
30 m	22.0 (29)	Tx32/40	1.28
6 m	2 (29)	Tx32/40	0.51
3 m	6 (35)	Tx32/40	0.42
0 m	– (35)	Tx32/40	0.00

Breathing gas	Volume
Tx32/40	2080.50 lit

Total CNS	Total OTU
13.5 %	35.8

Maximal Depth	Maximal Time
30.0 m	00:35 (= 35 min)

Maximal Po2 (B)	Maximal Po2 (D)
1.4 Bar	1.6 Bar

Maximal RMV (B)	Maximal RMV (D)
20.0 lit/min	10.0 lit/min

Maximal END
30.0 m

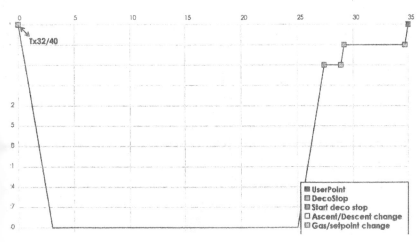

Figure 68. GAP Sample Output

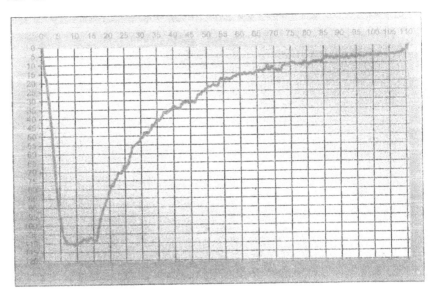

HS Explorer RGBM - Firmware 4.03.2   S/N: 0249

Dive Record Number - 406
Date - 09/27/05
  Lieu : Lac du Bourget
  Site : Le Focke-Wulf
Max Depth (m) - 0110.9
Avg Depth (m) - 0090.5
(before 1st stop)
Dive Time - 0110 min.
Time - 1152
Surface Interval - >1440 min.
Daily Dive Number - 01
Calculation Formula (CF) - 00
Alt - 00

Mix composition

No	%N	%He	%O2	Dir	Depth
0	79	0	21	-	-
1	79	0	21	-	-
2	26	63	11	-	-
3	44	36	20	Up	66
4	48	13	39	Up	30
5	0	0	100	Up	6
6	79	0	21	-	-
7	79	0	21	-	-
8	79	0	21	-	-
9	79	0	21	-	-

Capacité, pression et mélanges des blocs

Vol bloc	mélange	départ	arrivée	consommé (L)	l/mn
30	Tx11/63	230	85	4350	17.8
10	Tx20/36	220	40	1800	19.5
10	Tx39/13	220	20	2000	17.8
7	Oxygène	150	50	700	17.3

Figure 69. RGBM Simulator Sample Output

REFERENCES

References span a wide spectra of technical diving material and details, broaching historical to modern developments. Entries are alphabetically and chronologically listed.

Abramowitz M. and Stegun I.A. 1972. Handbook of Mathematical Functions, New York: Dover Publications.

Adamson A.W. 1976. The Physical Chemistry of Surfaces, New York: John Wiley and Sons.

Albano G., Griscuoli P.M. and Ciulla C. 1962. La Sindrome Neuropsichica Di Profundita, Lav. Um. 14: 351–358.

Allee W.C. 1992. Principals of Animal Ecology, Philadelphia: W.B. Saunders.

Atkins C.E., Lehner C.E., Beck K.A., Dubielzig R.R., Nordheim E.V. and Lanphier E.H. 1988. Experimental Respiratory Decompression Sickness in Sheep, J. Appl. Physiol. 65: 1163–1171.

Augenstein B.W., Bonner B.E., Mills F.E. and Nieto M.M. 1987. Antiproton Science and Technology, Singapore: World Scientific.

Bardach J. 1968. Harvest of the Sea, New York: Harper and Row.

Barnes H. 1969. Oceanography and Marine Biology, London: Allen and Unwin.

Bascom W. 1964. Waves and Beaches, New York: Doubleday Anchor.

Bassett B.E. 1979. And Yet Another Approach to the Problems of Altitude Diving and Flying after Diving, Decompression in Depth Proceedings, Professional Association of Diving Instructors, Santa Ana.

Batchelor G.K. 1953. Theory of Homogeneous Turbulence, New York: Cambridge University Press.

Bateman J.B. and Lang J. 1945. Formation and Growth of Bubbles in Aqueous Solutions, Canad. J. Res. E23: 22–31.

Beckwith B. 1969. Mechanical Measurement, Reading: Addison Wesley.

Bell G.I. and Glasstone S. 1970. Nuclear Reactor Theory, New York: Van Nostrand Reinhold.

Bell R.L. and Borgwardt R.E. 1976. The Theory of High Altitude Corrections to the US Navy Standard Decompression Tables, Undersea Biomed. Res. 3: 1–23.

Behnke A.R. 1971. Decompression Sickness: Advances and Interpretations, Aerospace Med. 42: 255–267.

Behnke A.R. 1967. The Isobaric (Oxygen Window) Principle of Decompression, Trans. Third Annual Conf. Marine Tech. Soc. 1: 213–228.

Behnke A.R. 1945. Decompression Sickness Incident to Deep Sea Diving and High Altitude, Medicine 24: 381–402.

Bennett P.B. and Elliot D.H. 1996. The Physiology and Medicine of Diving and Compressed Air Work, London: Bailliere Tindall and Cassell.

Bennett P.B. and Hayward A.J. 1968. Relative Decompression Sickness in Rats of Neon and Other Inert Gases, Aerospace Med. 39: 301–302.

Berghage T.E. and Durman D. 1980. US Navy Air Recompression Schedule Risk Analysis, Nav. Med. Res. Bull. 1: 1–22.

Bert P. 1878. La Pression Barometrique, Paris: Masson.

Boni M., Schibli R., Nussberger P. and Buhlmann A.A. 1976. Diving at Diminished Atmospheric Pressure: Air Decompression Tables for Different Altitudes, Undersea Biomed. Res. 3: 189–204.

Bookspan J. 1997. Diving Physiology in Plain English, Bethesda: Undersea and Hyperbaric Medical Society.

Bove A.A. and Davis J.C. 1990. Diving Medicine, Philadelphia: W.B. Saunders.

Bowker A.H. and Lieberman G.J. 1964. Engineering Statistics, Engelwood Cliffs: Prentice-Hall.

Boycott A.E., Damant G.C.C. and Haldane J.S. 1908. The Prevention of Compressed Air Illness, J. Hyg. 8: 342–443.

Brunt D. 1941. Physical and Dynamical Meteorology, London: Cambridge University Press.

Brereton R.G. 1974. US Navy SEAL Combat Manual, Memphis: Naval Technical Training.

Buckles R.G. 1968. The Physics of Bubble Formation and Growth, Aerospace Med. 39: 1062–1069.

Buhlmann A.A. 1984. Decompression/Decompression Sickness, Berlin: Springer Verlag.

Buhlmann A.A. 1966. Saturation and Desaturation With N_2 and He at 4 Atmospheres, J. Appl. Physiol. 23: 458–462.

Carslaw H.S. and Jaeger J.C. 1950. Conduction of Heat in Solids, Oxford: Clarendon Press.

Carter L.L. and Cashwell E.D. 1975. Particle Transport Simulations with The Monte Carlo Method, Oak Ridge: United States Energy and Research Development Administration.

Case K.M. and Zweifel P.F. 1977. Linear Transport Theory, Reading: Addison Wesley.

Chikazumi S. 1979. Physics of Magnetism, New York: John Wiley and Sons.

Commoner B., Corr M. and Stamler P.J. 1971. The Causes of Pollution, Environments 13: 2–19.

Conkin J. and Van Liew H.D. 1991. Failure of the Straight Line Boundary Between Safe and Unsafe Decompressions When Extrapolated to the Hypobaric Regime, Undersea Biomed. Res. 18: 16.

Crocker W.E. and Taylor H.J. 1952. A Method of Calculating Decompression Stages and the Formulation of New Diving Tables, Investigation into the Decompression Tables, Medical Research Council Report, UPS 131, London.

Cross E.R. 1970. High Altitude Decompression, Skin Diver Magazine 19: 17–18.

Darwin C.R. 1958. On the Origin of the Species by Means of Natural Selection, New York: New American Library.

Davidson W.M., Sutton B.M. and Taylor H.J. 1950. Decompression Ratio for Goats Following Long Exposure and Return to Atmospheric Pressure Without Stoppage, Medical Research Council Report, UPS 110, London.

Defant A. 1961. Physical Oceanography, New York: Doubleday.

Duffner G.J., Synder J.F. and Smith L.L. 1959. Adaptation of Helium-Oxygen to Mixed Gas Scuba, USN Navy Experimental Diving Unit Report, NEDU 3-59, Washington, DC.

Duxbury A.C. 1971. The Earth and its Oceans, Reading: Addison Wesley.

Eckenhoff R.G., Olstad C.E. and Carrod G.E. 1990. Human Dose Response Relationship for Decompression and Endogenous Bubble Formation, J. Appl. Physiol. 69: 914–918.

Eckenhoff R.G., Olstad C.E., Parker S.F. and Bondi K.R. 1986. Direct Ascent from Shallow Air Saturation Exposures, Undersea Biomed. Res. 13: 305–316.

Eckenhoff R.G. 1985. Doppler Bubble Detection, Undersea Biomed. Res. 12: 485–489.

Edmonds C., Lowry C. and Pennefather J. 1994. Diving and Subaquatic Medicine, Portland: Book News.

Edmonds C., McKenzie B. and Thomas R. 1997. Diving Medicine for Scuba Divers, Sydney: Aquaquest Publications.

Eisenberg P. 1953. Progress on the Mechanics of Cavitation, David Taylor Model Basin Rept. 842.

Epstein P.S. and Plesset M.S. 1950. On the Stability of Gas Bubbles in Liquid-Gas Solutions, J. Chm. Phys. 18: 1505–1509.

Ehrlich P. 1969. Ecocatastrophe, Ramparts 23–32.

Evans R.D. 1975. The Atomic Nucleus, New York: McGraw Hill.

Evans A. and Walder D.N. 1969. Significance of Gas Macronuclei in the Aetiology of Decompression Sickness, Nature London 222: 251–252.

Farm F.P., Hayashi E.M. and Beckman E.L. 1986. Diving and Decompression Sickness Treatment Practices Among Hawaii's Diving Fisherman, University of Hawaii Sea Grant Report, UNIHI-SEAGRANT-TP-86-01, Honolulu.

Feynman R.P., Leighton R.B. and Sands M. 1975. The Feynman Lectures on Physics I, II, III, Reading: Addison Wesley.

Fisher J.C. 1948. The Fracture of Liquids, J. Appl. Phys. 19: 1062–1067.

Fleagle R.G. and Businger J.A. 1963. Introduction to Atmospheric Physics, New York: Academic Press.

Frenkel J. 1946. Kinetic Theory of Liquids, New York: Oxford University Press.

Gasiorowicz S. 1967. Elementary Particle Physics, New York: John Wiley and Sons.

Geiger R. 1950. Climate Near The Ground, Cambridge: Harvard University Press.

Gernhardt M.L., Lambertsen C.J., Miller R.G. and Hopkins E. 1990. Evaluation of a Theoretical Model of Tissue Gas Phase Growth and Resolution During Decompression from Air Diving, Undersea Biomed. Res. 17: 95.

Gernhardt M.L. 1985. Tissue Gas Bubble Dynamics During Hypobaric Exposures, Society of Automotive Engineers Report, SAE-851337, Warrendale.

Gerth W.A. and Vann R.D. 1997. Probabilistic Gas and Bubble Dynamics Models of Decompression Sickness Occurrence in Air and Nitrogen-Oxygen Diving, Undersea Hyp. Med. 24: 275–292.

Gerth W.D. and Vann R.D. 1996. Development of Iso-DCS Risk Air and Nitrox Decompression Tables Using Statistical Bubble Dynamics Models, National Oceanographic and Atmospheric Administration Report, NOAA-46RU0505, Washington DC.

Gilliam B., Webb D. and von Maier R. 1995. Deep Diving, San Diego: Watersports.

Golding F.C., Griffiths P.D., Paton W.D.M., Walder D.N. and Hempleman H.V. 1960. Decompression Sickness During Construction of the Dartford Tunnel, Brit. J. Ind. Med. 17: 167–180.

Goldstein H. 1969. Mechanics, Reading: Addison Wesley.

Gradshteyn I.S. and Ryzhik I.M. 1965. Table of Integrals, Series, and Products, New York: Academic Press.

Gray J.S., Masland R.L. and Mahady S.C. 1945. The Effects of Breathing Carbon Dioxide on Altitude Decompression Sickness, US Air Force School of Aviation Medicine Report, Project 409, Randolph Field.

Groen P. 1967. The Waters of the Sea, University Park: Pennsylvania State University Press.

Guillen M. 1995. Five Equations that Changed the World, New York: Hyperion.

Hamilton R.W. 1975. Development of Decompression Procedures for Depths in Excess of 400 Feet, Undersea and Hyperbaric Medical Society Report, WS: 2-28-76, Bethesda.

Harvey E.N. 1945. Decompression Sickness and Bubble Formation in Blood and Tissue, Bull. N.Y. Acad. Med. 21: 505–536.

Harvey E.N., Barnes D.K., McElroy W.D., Whiteley A.H., Pease D.C. and Cooper K.W. 1944. Bubble Formation in Animals. I. Physical Factors, J. Cell. Comp. Physiol. 24: 1–22.

Harvey E.N., Whiteley A.H., McElroy W.D., Pease D.C. and Barnes D.K. 1944. Bubble Formation in Animals. II. Gas Nuclei and their Distribution in Blood And Tissues, J. Cell Comp. Physiol. 24: 23–24.

Harvey E.N., McElroy W.D., Whiteley A.H., Warren G.H. and Pease D.C. 1944. Bubble Formation in Animals. III. An Analysis of Gas Tension and Hydrostatic Pressure in Cats, J. Cell. Comp. Physiol. 24: 117–132.

Hempleman H.V. 1957. Further Basic Facts on Decompression Sickness, Investigation into the Decompression Tables, Medical Research Council Report, UPS 168, London.

Hempleman H.V. 1952. A New Theoretical Basis for the Calculation of Decompression Tables, Medical research Council Report, UPS 131, London.

Heine J. 1991. Cold Water Diving, Flagstaff: Best.

Hennessy T.R. and Hempleman H.V. 1977. An Examination of the Critical Released Gas Concept in Decompression Sickness, Proc. Royal Soc. London B197: 299–313.

Hennessy T.R. 1974. The Interaction of Diffusion and Perfusion in Homogeneous Tissue, Bull. Math. Biol. 36: 505–527.

Hills B.A. 1977. Decompression Sickness, New York: John Wiley and Sons.

Hills B.A. 1976. Supersaturation by Counterdiffusion and Diffusion of Gases, J. Appl. Physiol. 43: 56–69.

Hills B.A. 1969. Radial Bulk Diffusion into Heterogeneous Tissue, Bull. Math. Biophys. 31: 25–34.

Hills B.A. 1968. Linear Bulk Diffusion into Heterogeneous Tissue, Bull. Math. Biophys. 30: 47–59.

Hills B.A. 1968. Variation in Susceptibility to Decompression Sickness, Int. J. Biometeor. 12: 343–349.

Hills B.A. 1968. Relevant Phase Conditions for Predicting the Occurrence of Decompression Sickness, J. Appl. Physiol. 25: 310–315.

Hirschfelder J.O., Curtiss C.F. and Bird R.B. 1964. Molecular Theory of Gases and Liquids, New York: John Wiley and Sons.

Holmes A. 1965. Principles of Physical Geology, Ontario: Nelson and Sons.

Huang K. 1973. Statistical Mechanics, New York: John Wiley and Sons.

Huggins K.E. 1987. Multiprocessor Applications to Multilevel Air Decompression Problems, Michigan Sea Grant Publication, MICHU-SG-87-201, Ann Arbor.

Irving J. and Mullineux N. 1972. Mathematics in Physics and Engineering, London: Academic Press.

Isacks B. 1968. Seismology and the New Global Plate Tectonics, J. Geophys. Res. 73: 5855–5899.

Jackson J.D. 1962. Classical Electrodynamics, New York: John Wiley and Sons.

Jenkins F.A. and White H.E. 1977. Fundamentals of Optics, New York: McGraw Hill.

Jessop N.M. 1970. Biosphere: A Study of Life, Englewood Cliffs: Prentice Hall.

Johnson L.W. and Riess R.D. 1962. Numerical Analysis, Reading: Addison Wesley.

Kahaner D., Moler C. and Nash S. 1989. Numerical Methods and Software, Englewood Cliffs: Prentice Hall.

Keen M.J. 1968. Introduction to Marine Geology, New York: Pergamon Press.

Keller H. and Buhlmann A.A. 1965. Deep Diving and Short Decompression By Breathing Mixed Gases, J. Appl. Physiol. 20: 1267.

Kummell B. 1961. Introduction to Historical Geology, San Francisco: W.H. Freeman.

Kunkle T.D. and Beckman E.L. 1983. Bubble Dissolution Physics and the Treatment of Decompression Sickness, Med. Phys. 10: 184–190.

Lamb J.S. 1999. The Practice of Oxygen Measurement for Divers, Flagstaff: Best.

Lambertsen J.L. and Bornmann R.C. 1979. Isobaric Inert Gas Counterdiffusion, Undersea and Hyperbaric Medical Society Publication 54WS(IC)1-11-82, Bethesda.

Lambertsen C.J. and Bardin H. 1973. Decompression from Acute and Chronic Exposure to High Pressure Nitrogen, Aerospace Med. 44: 834–836.

Landau L.D. and Lifshitz E.M. 1985. Fluid Mechanics, Reading: Addison Wesley.

Landau L.D. and Lifshitz E.M. 1980. Mechanics, Reading: Addison Wesley.

Landau L.D. and Lifshitz E.M. 1979. Theory of Elasticity, Reading: Addison Wesley.

Lang M.A. and Vann R.D. 1992. Proceedings of the American Academy of Underwater Sciences Repetitive Diving Workshop, AAUS Safety Publication AAUSDSP-RDW-02-92, Costa Mesa.

Lang M.A. and Egstrom G.H. 1990. Proceedings of the American Academy of Underwater Sciences Biomechanics of Safe Ascents Workshop, American Academy of Underwater Sciences Diving Safety Publication, AAUSDSP-BSA-01-90, Costa Mesa.

Lang M.A. and Hamilton R.W. 1989. Proceedings of the American Academy of Underwater Sciences Dive Computer Workshop, University of Southern California Sea Grant Publication, USCSG-TR-01-89, Los Angeles.

Leebaert D. 1991. Technology 2001: The Future of Computing and Communications, Cambridge: Massachusetts Institute of Technology Press.

Lehner C.E., Hei D.J., Palta M., Lightfoot E.N. and Lanphier E.H. 1988. Accelerated Onset of Decompression Sickness in Sheep after Short Deep Dives, University of Wisconsin Sea Grant College Program Report, WIS-SG-88-843, Madison.

Leitch D.R. and Barnard E.E.P. 1982. Observations on No Stop and Repetitive Air and Oxynitrogen Diving, Undersea Biomed. Res. 9: 113–129.

Le Messurier D.H. and Hills B.A. 1965. Decompression Sickness: A Study of Diving Techniques in the Torres Strait, Hvaldradets Skrifter 48: 54–84.

Le Pichon X. 1968. Sea Floor Spreading and Continental Drift, J. Geophys. Res. 73: 3661–3697.

Levine S.N. 1968. Desalination and Ocean Technology, New York: Dover.

Loyst K., Huggins K.E. and Steidley M. 1991. Dive Computers, San Diego: Watersports.

Martin D.F. 1978. Marine Chemistry, New York: Marcel Dekker.

Mathews J. and Walker R.L. 1975. Mathematical Methods of Physics, New York: W.A. Benjamin.

Milliman J.D. and Emery K.O. 1968. Sea Levels During the Past 35,000 Years, Science 73: 1121–1123.

Morgan W.J. 1968. Rises, Trenches, Great Faults, and Crustal Blocks, Geophys. Res. 73: 1959–1982.

Mount T. and Gilliam B. 1991. Mixed Gas Diving, San Diego: Watersport.

Neal J.G., O'Leary T.R. and Wienke B.R. 1999. Trimix Diving, Fort Lauderdale: Underwater Dynamics Incorporated.

Neuman T.S., Hall D.A. and Linaweaver P.G. 1976. Gas Phase Separation During Decompression in Man, Undersea Biomed. Res. 7: 107–112.

Nishi R.Y., Eatock B.C., Buckingham I.P. and Ridgewell B.A. 1982. Assessment of Decompression Profiles by Ultrasonic Monitoring: No Decompression Dives, Defense and Civil Institute of Environmental Medicine Report, D.C.IEM 82-R-38, Toronto.

O'Leary T.R. and Wienke B.R. 2012. The Technical Diver, National Association of Underwater Instructors Technical Publication, Tampa.

Parzen E. 1970. Modern Probability Theory and its Applications, New York: John Wiley and Sons.

Paton W.D.M. and Walder D.N. 1954. Compressed Air Illness, Medical Research Council Report, HMSO 281, London.

Pease D.C. and Blinks L.R. 1947. Cavitation from Solid Surfaces in the Absence of Gas Nuclei, J. Phys. Coll. Chem. 51: 556–567.

Pilmanis A.A. 1976. Intravenous Gas Emboli In Man After Compressed Air Ocean Diving, Office Of Naval Research Contract Report, N00014-67-A-0269-0026, Washington, DC.

Powell M.P. and Rogers R.E. 1989. Doppler Ultrasound Monitoring of Gas Phase Formation and Resolution in Repetitive Diving, Undersea Biomed. Res. 16: 69.

Powell C.F. 1928. Condensation Phenomena at Different Temperatures, Proc. Royal Soc. London A119: 553–577.

Press W., Teukolsky S., Vettering W. and Flannery B. 1992. Numerical Recipes in FORTRAN, New York: Cambridge University Press.

Rashbass C. 1955. New Tables, Investigation into the Decompression Tables, 243 Medical Research Council Report, UPS 151, London.

Riley J.P. and Skirrow G. 1965. Chemical Oceanography, New York: Academic Press.

Rogers R.E. and Powell M.R. 1989. Controlled Hyperbaric Chamber Tests of Multiday Repetitive Dives, Undersea Biomed. Res. 16: 68.

Rossier R.N. 2000. Recreational Nitrox Diving, Flagstaff: Best.

Roughton F.J.W. 1952. Diffusion and Chemical Reaction Velocity in Cylindrical And Spherical Systems Of Physiological Interest, Proc. Royal Soc. B140: 203–221.

Rutkowski D. 1989. Nitrox Manual, San Diego: International Association of Nitrox Divers (IAND).

Sagan H. 1971. Boundary and Eigenvalue Problems in Mathematical Physics, New York: John Wiley and Sons.

Sawatzky K.D. and Nishi R.Y. 1990. Intravascular Doppler Detected Bubbles and Decompression Sickness, Undersea Biomed. Res. 17: 34–39.

Schreiner H.R. and Hamilton R.W. 1987. Validation of Decompression Tables, Undersea and Hyperbaric Medical Society Publication 74 (VAL), Bethesda.

Sears F.W. 1969. Thermodynamics, Reading: Addison Wesley.

Shapiro A.H. 1958. Dynamics and Thermodynamics of Compressible Fluid Flow, New York: Ronald.

Sheffield P.J. 1990. Flying after Diving, Undersea and Hyperbaric Medical Society Publication 77 (FLYDIV), Bethesda.

Shreider Y.A. 1966. The Monte Carlo Method, New York: Pergamon Press.

Smith K.H. and Stayton L. 1978. Hyperbaric Decompression By Means of Bubble Detection, Office of Naval Research Report, N0001-469-C-0402, Washington DC.

Smith C.L. 1975. Altitude Procedures for the Ocean Diver, National Association of Underwater Instructors Technical Publication 5, Colton.

Somers L.H. 1991. The University of Michigan Diving Manual, Ann Arbor: University of Michigan Press.

Spar J. 1965. Earth, Sea, And Air: Survey Of The Geophysical Sciences, Reading: Addison Wesley.

Spencer M.P. 1976. Decompression Limits for Compressed Air Determined by Ultrasonically Detected Blood Bubbles, J. Appl. Physiol. 40: 229–235.

Spencer M.P. and Campbell S.D. 1968. The Development of Bubbles in the Venous And Arterial Blood During Hyperbaric Decompression, Bull. Mason Cli. 22: 26–32.

Strauss R.H. 1974. Bubble Formation in Gelatin: Implications for Prevention of Decompression Sickness, Undersea Biomed. Res. 1: 169–174.

Strauss R.H. and Kunkle T.D. 1974. Isobaric Bubble Growth: Consequence of Altering Atmospheric Gas, Science 186: 443–444.

Streeter V. 1981. Handbook of Fluid Mechanics, New York: McGraw Hill.

Srinivasan R.S., Gerth W.D. and Powell M.R. 1999. Mathematical Models of Diffusion Limited Gas Bubble Dynamics in Tissue, J. Appl. Physiol. 86: 732–741.

Thalman E.D., Parker E.C., Survanshi S.S. and Weathersby P.K. 1997. Improved Probabilistic Decompression Model Risk Predictions Using Linear-Exponential Kinetics, Undersea Hyp. Med. 24: 255–274.

Thompson A.M., Cavert H.M. and Lifson N. 1958. Kinetics Of D_2O And Antipyrine In Isolated Perfused Rat Liver, Amer. J. Physiol. 192: 531–537.

Tikuisis P. 1986. Modeling the Observations of *In Vivo* Bubble Formation With Hydrophobic Crevices, Undersea Biomed. Res. 13: 165–180.

Tikuisis P., Ward C.A. and Venter R.D. 1983. Bubble Evolution in a Stirred Volume of Liquid Closed to Mass Transport, J. Appl. Phys. 54: 1–9.

Tricker R.A. 1964. Bores, Breakers, Waves, and Wakes, New York: American Elsevier.

Van Liew H.D. and Hlastala M.P. 1969. Influence of Bubble Size and Blood Perfusion on Absorption of Gas Bubbles In Tissues, Resp. Physiol. 24: 111–121.

Van Liew H.D., Bishop B., Walder P.D. and Rahn H. 1975. Bubble Growth and Mechanical Properties of Tissue In Decompression, Undersea Biomed. Res. 2: 185–194.

Vann R.D., Dovenbarger J., Wachholz C. and Bennett P.B. 1989. Decompression Sickness in Dive Computer and Table Use, DAN Newsletter 3–6.

Vann R.D., Grimstad J. and Nielsen C.H. 1980. Evidence for Gas Nuclei in Decompressed Rats, Undersea Biomed. Res. 7: 107–112.

Vann R.D. and Clark H.G. 1975. Bubble Growth and Mechanical Properties of Tissue in Decompression, Undersea Biomed. Res. 2: 185–194.

Von Arx W.S. 1964. Introduction to Physical Oceanography, Reading: Addison Wesley.

Walder D.N., Evans A. and Hempleman H.V. 1968. Ultrasonic Monitoring Of Decompression, Lancet. 1: 897–898.

Walder D.N. 1968. Adaptation to Decompression Sickness in Caisson Work, Biometeor. 11: 350–359.

Wallace D. 1975. NOAA Diving Manual, Washington DC: US Government Printing Office.

Weathersby P.K., Survanshi S. and Homer L.D. 1985. Statistically Based Decompression Tables: Analysis of Standard Air Dives, 1950–1970, Naval Medical Research Institute report, NMRI 85-16, Bethesda.

Weathersby P.K., Homer L.D. and Flynn E.T. 1984. On the Likelihood of Decompression Sickness, J. Appl. Physiol. 57: 815–825.

Weinberg S. 1972. Gravitation and Cosmology, New York: John Wiley and Sons.

Wienke B.R. 2010. Computer Validation and Statistical Correlations of a Modern Decompression Diving Algorithm, Comp. Biol. Med. 40: 252–260.

Wienke B.R. 2010. Diving Physics with Bubble Mechanics and Decompression Theory in Depth, Flagstaff: Best.

Wienke B.R. 2009. Diving Decompression Models and Bubble Metrics: Modern Computer Syntheses, Comp. Biol. Med. 39: 309–331.

Wienke B.R. 2008. Hyperbaric Physics and Phase Mechanics, Flagstaff: Best.

Wienke B.R. and O'Leary T.R. 2008. Statistical Correlations and Risk Analysis Techniques for a Diving Dual Phase Bubble Model and Data Bank Using Massively Parallel Supercomputers, Comp. Biol. Med. 38: 583–600.

Wienke B.R. 2003. Reduced Gradient Bubble Model in Depth, Flagstaff: Best.

Wienke B.R.. 2001. Technical Diving in Depth, Flagstaff: Best.

Wienke B.R. 1998. Physics, Physiology, and Decompression Theory for the Technical and Commercial Diver, National Association of Underwater Instructors Publication, Tampa.

Wienke B.R. 1993. Diving Above Sea Level, Flagstaff: Best.

Wienke B.R. 1993. Basic Diving Physics and Applications, Flagstaff: Best.

Wienke B.R. 1992. Numerical Phase Algorithm for Decompression Computers And Application, Comp. Biol. Med. 22: 389–406.

Wienke B.R. 1991. Basic Decompression Theory and Application, Flagstaff: Best.

Wienke B.R. 1991. Bubble Number Saturation Curve and Asymptotics of Hypobaric and Hyperbaric Exposures, Int. J. Biomed. Comp. 29: 215–225.

Wienke B.R. 1991. High Altitude Diving, National Association of Underwater Instructors Technical Publication, Montclair.

Wienke B.R. 1990. Reduced Gradient Bubble Model, Int. J. Biomed. Comp. 26: 237–256.

Wienke B.R. 1990. Modeling Dissolved and Free Phase Gas Dynamics Under Decompression, Int. J. BioMed. Comp. 25: 193–205.

Wienke B.R. 1989. Equivalent Multitissue and Thermodynamic Decompression Algorithms, Int. J. BioMed. Comp. 24: 227–245.

Wienke B.R. 1989. Tissue Gas Exchange Models and Decompression Computations: A Review, Undersea Biomed. Res. 16: 53–89.

Wienke B.R. 1989. N_2 Transfer and Critical Pressures in Tissue Compartments, Math. Comp. Model. 12: 1–15.

Wienke B.R. 1987. Computational Decompression Models. Int. J. BioMed. Comp. 21: 205–221.

Wienke B.R. 1986. DECOMP: Computational Package for Nitrogen Transport Modeling in Tissues, Comp. Phys. Comm. 40: 327–336.

Wienke B.R. 1986. Phenomenological Models for Nitrogen Transport in Tissues, Il Nuovo Cimento 8D: 417–435.

Wilkes M.V. 1959. Oscillations of the Earth's Atmosphere, London: Cambridge University Press.

Wittenborn A.F. 1963. An Analytic Development of a Decompression Computer, Proc. Second Symp. Underwater Physiol., Washington, DC: National Academy Of Science 1: 82–90.

Workman R.D. 1965. Calculation of Decompression Schedules for Nitrogen-Oxygen and Helium-Oxygen Dives, USN Experimental Diving Unit Report, NEDU 6-65, Washington DC.

Yang W.J. 1971. Dynamics of Gas Bubbles in Whole Blood and Plasma, J. Biomech. 4 119–125.

Yarborough O.D. 1937. Calculations Of Decompression Tables, USN Experimental Diving Unit Report, EDU 12–37, Washington DC.

Yount D.E. and Hoffman D.C. 1986. On The Use of A Bubble Formation Model to Calculate Diving Tables, Aviat. Space Environ. Med. 57: 149–156.

Yount D.E., Gillary E.W. and Hoffman D.C. 1984. A Microscopic Investigation of Bubble Formation Nuclei, J. Acoust. Soc. Am. 76: 1511–1521.

Yount D.E. 1982. On the Evolution, Generation, and Regeneration of Gas Cavitation Nuclei, J. Acoust. Soc. Am. 71: 1473–1481.

Yount D.E. 1979. Skins of Varying Permeability: A Stabilization Mechanism for Gas Cavitation Nuclei, J. Acoust. Soc. Am. 65: 1431–1439.

Yount D.E., Yeung C.M., and Ingle F.W. 1979. Determination of the Radii of Gas Cavitation Nuclei by Filtering Gelatin, J. Acoust. Soc. Am. 65: 1440–1450.

Yount D.E. and Strauss R.H. 1976. Bubble Formation in Gelatin: A Model for Decompression Sickness, J. Appl. Phys. 47: 5081–5089.

Zhang J., Fife C.E., Currie M.S., Moon R.E., Pintadosi C.A. and Vann R.D. 1991. Venous Gas Emboli and Complement Activation After Deep Air Diving, Undersea Biomed. Res. 18: 293–302.

INDEX

404

Asymptotics 156, 183, 188, 306, 310, 318
Atlantic Ocean 41, 47, 69
Atlantis III 195
Atmosphere 1, 10, 11, 15, 18–21, 23, 26–34,
 40–42, 44, 54, 55, 66, 68, 69, 73–75, 109,
 124, 133, 150, 177, 190, 226, 270, 369, 373
Atmospheric pressure 32, 43, 56, 71, 72, 75, 91,
 96, 97, 130, 131, 133, 175–181, 190, 281,
 344
Atmospheric temperatures 20, 22, 23
Atomic Aquatics 266, 278, 280, 322, 389
Attenuation 10, 92, 112
Audibility range 113
Australia 36, 73, 78, 263, 264, 341
Australian pearl divers 263
Autochthonous bubbles 341
Avalanche 68
Avogadro number 189, 190, 352

B

Baden 279
Balance 21, 47, 67, 74, 103, 106, 107, 121, 123,
 142, 143, 200, 236, 258, 271, 344, 346, 371
Baltic Sea 41
Bandwidth 220, 231
barometer equation 177, 178, 189
barotraumas 317, 345
Baryons 379
BASIC 277, 390
Bassett 183
Beattie-Bridgman equation 136
Beckman 264
Beer's law 10
Bell 74, 176, 183, 280, 328, 371
Bends 63, 117, 124, 125, 128, 154, 166, 262, 263,
 266–268, 272–275, 302, 304, 314, 340–342,
 353
Bends depths 302
Bends sites 266
Benjamin Franklin 42
Bennett 114, 115, 195, 197, 217, 279, 309, 313,
 324
Bernoulli 74, 79, 107, 108
Bernoulli's generalized law 107
Best diving mixtures 201, 202, 216
Binding energy 83, 93, 356
Binomial distribution 295, 297, 298
Binomial probability 298, 305, 316, 326, 328
Biochemical reactions 345
Biophysics 252
Black body 9, 365
Black body radiation 9
Black hole 378
Blood 90–92, 107, 113, 115, 117–120, 122, 125,
 128–132, 140, 142, 144, 149, 152, 162–164,
 166, 175, 176, 194, 195, 198, 207, 226, 228,
 232, 234, 236, 252, 255–259, 261, 262,
 266–270, 273, 314, 342, 344, 346, 348–351

Body morphology 100
Boiling 64, 76, 128, 138, 226, 364, 370, 373, 384
Boltzmann 126, 137–139, 177, 189, 190, 364, 378
Boltzmann's constant 137–139, 190
Bores 66, 67, 75–77
Borgwardt 176, 183
Bounce diving 161, 250, 264, 273, 274, 300
Boundary conditions 74, 108, 141, 234–236, 256,
 261, 269
Bourdon 96–98, 111
Boyle expansion and contraction 318
Boyle's law 86–89, 92, 96, 98, 124, 149, 165, 272
Brahe 35
Brain tomography 218, 222
Breathholding 345, 346
Breathing loop 104, 105, 216
Brubakk 279, 341
Bubble 42, 81, 87–91, 95, 112–117, 120, 121,
 123–132, 140, 142–145, 148–150, 156–167,
 174–176, 183–185, 187, 194, 196, 200, 203,
 216, 219, 222, 226, 228, 229, 231, 233,
 238–243, 246, 249–253, 255, 257–281,
 283–285, 287–289, 295, 300–303, 306, 307,
 312–314, 316–318, 320–326, 328–330,
 337–342, 346, 348, 387–390
Buhlmann 151, 173, 174, 176, 180, 182, 183, 185,
 195, 203, 237, 251, 276, 279, 281, 308, 322,
 323, 387, 389, 390
Bulk 112, 123, 136, 140, 166–168, 234, 235, 248,
 256, 268, 273, 282, 287, 289, 343, 363
Buoyancy 84, 86–89, 94, 95, 101, 102, 109, 177,
 325
Bureau of Mines 198

C

C5 hurricane 70
Cabeo 374
Caisson workers 274
California 37, 50, 51, 65, 73, 280
Camille 70
Capillary gauges 96–98, 111, 179, 186
Capillary waves 62, 63, 76
Carbon dioxide 18, 19, 21–23, 26–29, 33, 46, 55,
 56, 93, 117–120, 122, 133, 193, 198–201,
 207, 217, 269, 343–345, 347, 350, 371, 372
Carbon steel 101
Caribbean 47, 68, 69, 74
Catalysis 122
Cavitating flows 128, 129, 222
Cavitation 125, 128–130, 132, 226, 260
cavitation number 129
Cavity radius 127
CCR 104, 105, 324, 335, 337, 372
Centigrade 134, 138, 146, 370, 371, 384
Central limit theorem 298, 305
Central nervous system (CNS) 104, 128, 193, 20?
 207–210, 215–217, 267, 273, 314, 326, 33?
 340, 342–344, 349
Central processing units 220

410

For Product Safety Concerns and Information please contact our EU
representative GPSR@taylorandfrancis.com
Taylor & Francis Verlag GmbH, Kaufingerstraße 24, 80331 München, Germany

www.ingramcontent.com/pod-product-compliance
Ingram Content Group UK Ltd.
Pitfield, Milton Keynes, MK11 3LW, UK
UKHW020932180425

457613UK00012B/327

* 9 7 8 0 3 6 7 7 3 8 2 7 3 *